Textbook of Neonatal Resuscitation, *7th Edition*

Editor

Gary M. Weiner, MD, FAAP

Associate Editor

Jeanette Zaichkin, RN, MN, NNP-BC

Editor Emeritus

John Kattwinkel, MD, FAAP

Assistant Editors

Anne Ades, MD, FAAP

Christopher Colby, MD, FAAP

Eric C. Eichenwald, MD, FAAP

Kimberly D. Ernst, MD, MSMI, FAAP

Marilyn Escobedo, MD, FAAP

John Gallagher, MPH, RRT-NPS

Louis P. Halamek, MD, FAAP

Jessica Illuzzi, MD, MS, FACOG

Vishal Kapadia, MD, MSCS, FAAP

Henry C. Lee, MD, FAAP

Linda McCarney, MSN, APRN,
    NNP-BC

Patrick McNamara, MB, FRCPC

Jeffrey M. Perlman, MB, ChB, FAAP

Steven Ringer, MD, PhD, FAAP

Marya L. Strand, MD, MS, FAAP

Myra H. Wyckoff, MD, FAAP

Educational Design Editor

Jerry Short, PhD

Managing Editors

Rachel Poulin, MPH

Wendy Marie Simon, MA, CAE

Based on original text by
    Ronald S. Bloom, MD, FAAP
    Catherine Cropley, RN, MN

***Textbook of Neonatal
Resuscitation, 7th Edition,
eSim Cases:***

Anne Ades, MD, FAAP

Kimberly D. Ernst, MD, MSMI, FAAP

Jeanette Zaichkin, RN, MN, NNP-BC

Published by the American Academy of Pediatrics
141 Northwest Point Blvd
Elk Grove Village, IL 60007-1019
Telephone: 847/434-4000
Facsimile: 847/228-1350
www.aap.org

The recommendations in this publication and the accompanying materials do not indicate an exclusive course of treatment or serve as a standard of care. Variations, taking into account individual circumstances, nature of medical oversight, and local protocols, may be appropriate.

Every effort has been made to ensure that contributors to the Neonatal Resuscitation Program materials are knowledgeable authorities in their fields. Readers are nonetheless advised that the statements and opinions expressed are provided as guidelines and should not be construed as official policy of the American Academy of Pediatrics or the American Heart Association.

This material is made available as part of the professional education programs of the American Academy of Pediatrics and the American Heart Association. No endorsement of any product or service should be inferred or is intended.

The American Academy of Pediatrics and the American Heart Association disclaim any liability or responsibility for the consequences of any actions taken in reliance on these statements or opinions.

The American Academy of Pediatrics reserves the right to disclose personal information related to course completion of course participants/providers for administrative purposes such as to verify participation or classes taken or to validate the status of any Course Completion Card. In no event shall the American Academy of Pediatrics or American Heart Association have any liability for disclosure or use of information for such purposes or responsibility for the consequences of any actions taken in reliance on such information.

Printed in the United States of America

NRP323

ISBN: 978-1-61002-024-4

eBook: 978-1-61002-025-1

Library of Congress Control Number: 2015950716

5-276/0416   1 2 3 4 5 6 7 8 9 10

Acknowledgments

NRP Steering Committee Members

Myra H. Wyckoff, MD, FAAP, Co-chair 2011-2015

Steven Ringer, MD, PhD, FAAP, Co-chair 2013-2015

Marilyn Escobedo, MD, FAAP, Co-chair 2015-2017

Anne Ades, MD, FAAP

Christopher Colby, MD, FAAP

Erich C. Eichenwald, MD, FAAP

Kimberly D. Ernst, MD, MSMI, FAAP

Vishal Kapadia, MD, FAAP

Henry C. Lee, MD, FAAP

Marya L. Strand, MD, MS, FAAP

Liaison Representatives

Eric C. Eichenwald, MD, FAAP
 AAP Committee on Fetus and Newborn

John Gallagher, MPH, RRT-NPS
 American Association for Respiratory Care

Jessica Illuzzi, MD, MS, FACOG
 American College of Obstetricians
 and Gynecologists

Linda McCarney, MSN, APRN, NNP-BC
 National Association of Neonatal Nurses

Patrick McNamara, MB, FRCPC
 Canadian Paediatric Society

Associated Education Materials for the *Textbook of Neonatal Resuscitation, 7th Edition*

Instructor Toolkit, Jeanette Zaichkin, RN, MN, NNP-BC, Editor

Instructor Course, Jeanette Zaichkin, RN, MN, NNP-BC, Editor; Vishal Kapadia, MD, MSCS, FAAP; Henry C. Lee, MD, FAAP; Taylor Sawyer, DO, MEd, FAAP; and Nicole K. Yamada, MD, FAAP, Contributors

NRP Online Examination for Instructors, Jeanetet Zaichkin, RN, MN, NNP-BC

NRP Online Examination for Providers, Steven Ringer, MD, PhD, FAAP, and Jerry Short, PhD, Editors

NRP Reference Chart, Code Cart Cards, and Pocket Cards, Vishal Kapadia, MD, MSCS, FAAP, Editor

NRP Key Behavioral Skills Poster, Louis P. Halamek, MD, FAAP, Editor

NRP Equipment Poster, Jeanette Zaichkin, RN, MN, NNP-BC, Editor

NRP App, Steven Ringer, MD, PhD, FAAP and Marya L. Strand, MD, MS, FAAP, Editors

Neonatal Resuscitation Scenarios, Jeanette Zaichkin, RN, MN, NNP-BC, Editor; Myra H. Wyckoff, MD, FAAP; Vishal Kapadia, MD, MSCS, FAAP; Marya L. Strand, MD, MS, FAAP, Contributors

The committee would like to express thanks to the following reviewers and contributors to this textbook:

American Academy of Pediatrics Committee on Fetus and Newborn

American Academy of Pediatrics Section on Bioethics

International Liaison Committee on Resuscitation, Neonatal Delegation
 Jeffrey M. Perlman, MB, ChB, FAAP, Co-chair
 Jonathan Wylie, MD, Co-chair

Errol R. Alden, MD, FAAP, AAP Board-appointed Reviewer

Steven M. Schexnayder, MD, FAAP, AHA-appointed Reviewer

Aviva L. Katz, MD, FAAP, AAP Committee on Bioethics Reviewer

American Heart Association

Allan R. de Caen, MD, Chair, AHA Pediatric Forum

Farhan Bhanji, MD, MSc, Chair, AHA Educational
Science and Programs Committee

Photo Credits

Benjamin Weatherston

Gigi O'Dea, RN

Mayo Foundation for Medical Education and Research

Copy Editor

Jill Rubino

AAP Publications Staff

Theresa Wiener

Shannan Martin

AAP Life Support Staff

Kirsten Nadler, MS

Rachel Poulin, MPH

Wendy Marie Simon, MA, CAE

Robyn Wheatley, MPH

Thaddeus Anderson

Kristy Crilly

Gina Pantone

Olyvia Phillips

**The committee would like to express thanks to the following contributors
to the *NRP 7th Edition*:**

Pacific Lutheran University MediaLab, Tacoma, WA

MultiCare Tacoma General Hospital, Tacoma, WA

Taylor Sawyer, DO, MEd, FAAP

Nicole K. Yamada, MD, FAAP

Betty Choate, RNC-NIC

Ronna Crandall, RNC-NIC

Martine DeLisle, MSN, RNC

Maria Luisa Flores, BSN, RNC

Susan Greenleaf, BSN, RNC

Susan Hope, RN

Alta Kendall, ARNP, MSN, NNP-BC

Mary Kuhns, NNP

Gayle Livernash, RRT

Aimee Madding, RN

Cheryl Major, BSN, RNC-NIC

Tracey McKinney, RN, CNS, DNP, MS, NNP

Monica Scrudder, MSN, RNC-NIC

Kerry Watrin, MD

Raymond Weinrich, RN

Stephanie K. Kukora, MD, FAAP, University of
Michigan, Ann Arbor, MI

NRP Instructor Development Task Force

Anne Ades, MD, FAAP

Eric C. Eichenwald, MD, FAAP

Emer Finan, MB, DCH, Med, MRCPI

Louis P. Halamek, MD, FAAP

Steven Ringer, MD, PhD, FAAP

Gary M. Weiner, MD, FAAP

Myra H. Wyckoff, MD, FAAP

Karen Kennally, BSN, RN

Linda McCarney, MSN, RN, NNP-BC, EMT-P

Wade Rich, RCP

Kandi Zackery, BSN, RN, CEN, EMT-B

Jeanette Zaichkin, RN, MN, NNP-BC

Contents

Preface

Being entrusted by parents to provide care for their newly born baby is both a privilege and an extraordinary responsibility. Since the first edition of the *Textbook of Neonatal Resuscitation*, the Neonatal Resuscitation Program® (NRP®) has helped more than 3 million health care providers fulfill this responsibility by providing the opportunity to acquire the knowledge and skills required to save newborn lives. The history and evolution of the NRP is fascinating and provides important lessons for health educators. A brief description is available on the NRP Web site and is well worth reading. Although the 7th edition includes several new recommendations, it emphasizes the same guiding principles that have been the foundation of the NRP for nearly 30 years.

The original NRP textbook, published in 1987, was based on current practice, rational conjecture, and an informal consensus among experts. Beginning in 2000, the recommendations in the NRP textbook have been developed using a formal international consensus process. The American Academy of Pediatrics (AAP) and American Heart Association (AHA) partner in the evaluation of resuscitation science through the International Liaison Committee on Resuscitation (ILCOR). Researchers from the ILCOR Neonatal Task Force meet at regular intervals to review the science relevant to neonatal resuscitation. In a rigorous process, questions reflecting key knowledge gaps are identified, information scientists perform extensive literature searches, Neonatal Task Force members complete systematic reviews, the quality of scientific evidence is graded, and draft summary statements are prepared and published online for public comment. Finally, the members of the Task Force meet and discuss the summaries until a consensus on science is reached and treatment recommendations are formulated. The most recent statement, called the *2015 International Consensus on Cardiopulmonary Resuscitation and Emergency Cardiovascular Care Science With Treatment Recommendations (CoSTR)*, is based on a review of 27 neonatal resuscitation questions evaluated by 38 task force members representing 13 countries. After the meeting, each ILCOR member organization develops clinical guidelines based on the *CoSTR* document. Although ILCOR members are committed to minimizing international differences, each organization's guidelines may vary based on geographic, economic, and logistic differences. The most recent guidelines for the United States are called the *Neonatal*

Resuscitation 2015 American Heart Association Guidelines Update for Cardiopulmonary Resuscitation and Emergency Cardiovascular Care. The guidelines and links to the systematic reviews supporting each recommendation are available online (http://pediatrics. aappublications.org/content/136/Supplement_2/S196). The NRP Steering Committee develops the educational materials that help learners acquire the skills necessary to implement the current resuscitation guidelines.

This edition of the textbook includes 11 lessons. Two new lessons are dedicated to preparing for resuscitation (Lesson 2) and post-resuscitation care (Lesson 8). Similar to the 6th edition, the textbook emphasizes the importance of adequate preparation, effective ventilation, and teamwork. The details of how to implement ventilation corrective steps have been expanded and supplemented with additional illustrations. Nearly all drawings have been replaced with full-color photographs to enhance clarity. The order of lessons has been revised to reflect the increased emphasis on intubation before initiating chest compressions. Important changes in practice recommendations include new guidelines for the timing of umbilical cord clamping, the concentration of oxygen during resuscitation, the use of positive end-expiratory pressure (PEEP) and continuous positive airway pressure (CPAP) during and after resuscitation, the management of meconium-stained amniotic fluid, electronic cardiac (ECG) monitoring during resuscitation, the estimation of endotracheal tube insertion depth, and methods of thermoregulation for preterm (less than 32 weeks' gestation) newborns. Within each lesson, new sections devoted to teamwork and frequently asked questions allow additional consideration of these topics in the context of the lesson content.

The production of a textbook as complex as the *Textbook of Neonatal Resuscitation* cannot be accomplished without the effort of a team of dedicated and talented individuals. The ongoing partnership between the AAP, AHA, and ILCOR provides the infrastructure required to complete rigorous systematic reviews and develop evidence-based international guidelines. The members of the NRP Steering Committee, its liaison representatives, and volunteers spend countless hours preparing, reviewing, and debating each word and illustration in the textbook in an effort to provide learners with practical guidance even when the evidence is insufficient to make a definitive recommendation. Continued support from our strategic alliance partner, Laerdal Medical, has allowed the NRP to offer tools and learning technologies that challenge participants at every skill level. Working with Anne Ades (University of Pennsylvania), Kimberly Ernst (University of Oklahoma), and Jeanette Zaichkin

(AAP), this creative partnership has developed a virtual learning environment that allows every NRP provider to participate in electronic simulation. Bringing the photographs and printed words to paper requires tremendous patience and attention to detail. Members of the NICU staff at St Joseph Mercy Hospital-Ann Arbor (Chris Adams, Jennifer Boyle, Anne Boyd, Ann Caid) and the University of Michigan (Anthony Iannetta, Wendy Kenyon, Shaili Rajput, Kate Stanley, Suzy Vesey), along with Jeanette Zaichkin, patiently modeled resuscitation skills for our unflappable medical photographer Benjamin Weatherston. Most of the live delivery room photographs were provided by Christopher Colby and his talented staff at the Mayo Clinic-Rochester. Diligent copyediting by Jill Rubino ensured consistency and clarity, while every detail involved in coordinating the planning, writing, production, and editing was expertly managed by Rachel Poulin.

Every effective team requires strong leadership, and the NRP has been guided by a group of exceptional leaders. Jeffrey Perlman (Weill Medical College), Jonathan Wylie (James Cook University Hospital), and Myra Wyckoff (University of Texas Southwestern) provided steadfast leadership culminating in the international science and treatment consensus statements. Throughout the production cycle, NRP Steering Committee Cochairs Jane McGowan (Drexel University), Myra Wyckoff, Steven Ringer (Dartmouth-Hitchcock Medical Center), and Marilyn Escobedo (University of Oklahoma) patiently moderated spirited debate. Lou Halamek (Stanford University) challenged the committee to focus on competence rather than compliance and remain dedicated to innovation for the future. Jerry Short (University of Virginia) has been responsible for ensuring that the program's educational design and assessment components remain consistent with adult learning principles and meet the needs of a wide range of learners. John Kattwinkel (University of Virginia) was a founding member of the NRP, served as the Steering Committee Cochair, edited the previous 4 editions of the textbook, and provided the words that expressed the nuances and complexities inherent in an international consensus statement. His advice and counsel have been critically important during the production of the 7th edition of the textbook. He is truly a giant in the world of neonatal resuscitation and continues to guide every aspect of the program with his calm demeanor and softly spoken wisdom.

No acknowledgement would be complete without recognizing the tireless efforts of Jeanette Zaichkin and Wendy Simon. Jeanette's creativity and boundless energy has been at the center of every recent NRP educational activity. Among her contributions, Jeanette is an accomplished instructor mentor, edits the NRP instructor materials, created the online Instructor Course, coedits the *NRP Instructor Update,* edits the NRP simulation scenarios, and has starred in every recent NRP educational video. She has been a partner in every phase of the 7th edition beginning with the first draft that was outlined at her dining room table. Jeanette carefully considers every sentence and instinctively understands the practical implications for readers. Oftentimes behind the scenes, Wendy Simon is the person who quietly ensures that everything related to the NRP and the ILCOR Neonatal Task Force works. She intuitively understands how to advocate for important causes, connect people, and facilitate complex international projects. Wendy's conviction inspires the group to achieve more than anyone thought possible. Although she rarely accepts compliments, parents of children from Boston to Beijing can thank Wendy for their newborn's healthy start.

Gary M. Weiner, MD

Gary M. Weiner, MD, FAAP

Neonatal Resuscitation Program® Provider Course Overview

Neonatal Resuscitation Scientific Guidelines

The Neonatal Resuscitation Program® (NRP®) materials are based on the American Academy of Pediatrics (AAP) and American Heart Association (AHA) Guidelines for Cardiopulmonary Resuscitation and Emergency Cardiovascular Care of the Neonate (*Circulation.* 2015;132:S543-S560). A reprint of the Guidelines appears in the Appendix. Please refer to the Guidelines if you have any questions about the rationale for the current program recommendations. The Guidelines, originally published in October 2015, are based on the International Liaison Committee on Resuscitation (ILCOR) consensus on science statement. The evidence-based reviews prepared by members of ILCOR, which serve as the basis for both documents, can be viewed in the Web-based integrated guidelines site (https://eccguidelines.heart.org/index.php/circulation/cpr-ecc-guidelines-2/).

Level of Responsibility

The NRP Provider Course consists of 11 lessons, and participants are required to complete all 11 lessons to receive an NRP Course Completion Card. Even though not all newborn health care providers can perform all steps in resuscitation, they may be called to help a team and need to be familiar with each step.

Special Note: Neonatal resuscitation is most effective when performed by a designated and coordinated team. It is important for you to know the neonatal resuscitation responsibilities of team members who are working with you. Periodic practice among team members will facilitate coordinated and effective care of the newborn.

NRP eSim

NRP eSim is a new online neonatal resuscitation simulation exercise required for achieving NRP provider status with the 7th edition. The eSim methodology allows learners to integrate the NRP flow diagram steps in a virtual environment. For additional information on eSim, including Web browser requirements, visit www.aap.org/nrp.

Lesson Completion

Successful completion of the online examination and eSim cases is required *before* learners attend the skills/simulation portion of the NRP course. Learners must attend the skills/simulation portion of the course within 90 days of completing the online examination and eSim cases. To successfully complete the course, participants must pass the online examination, complete eSim cases, demonstrate mastery of resuscitation skills in the Integrated Skills Station, and participate in simulated resuscitation scenarios, as determined by the course instructor(s).

Upon successful completion of these requirements, participants are eligible to receive a Course Completion Card. Following the skills/simulation portion of the course, learners will receive an e-mail with a link to complete an online course evaluation. Once the online course evaluation is completed, an electronic Course Completion Card will be available in the learner's NRP Database profile.

Completion Does Not Imply Competence

The NRP is an educational program that introduces the concepts and basic skills of neonatal resuscitation. Completion of the program does not imply that an individual has the competence to perform neonatal resuscitation. Each hospital is responsible for determining the level of competence and qualifications required for someone to assume clinical responsibility for neonatal resuscitation.

Standard Precautions

The US Centers for Disease Control and Prevention has recommended that standard precautions be taken whenever risk of exposure to blood or bodily fluids is high and the potential infection status of the patient is unknown, as is certainly the case in neonatal resuscitation.

All fluid products from patients (blood, urine, stool, saliva, vomitus, etc) should be treated as potentially infectious. Gloves should be worn when resuscitating a newborn, and the rescuer should not use his or her mouth to apply suction via a suction device. Mouth-to-mouth resuscitation should be avoided by having a resuscitation bag and mask or T-piece resuscitator always available for use during resuscitation. Masks and protective eyewear or face shields should be worn during procedures that are likely to generate droplets of blood or other bodily fluids. Gowns or aprons should be worn during procedures that probably will generate splashes of blood or other bodily fluids. Delivery rooms must be equipped with resuscitation bags, masks, laryngoscopes, endotracheal tubes, mechanical suction devices, and the necessary protective shields.

Foundations of Neonatal Resuscitation

1

What you will learn

- Why neonatal resuscitation skills are important
- Physiologic changes that occur during and after birth
- The format of the Neonatal Resuscitation Program® Flow Diagram
- Communication and teamwork skills used by effective resuscitation teams

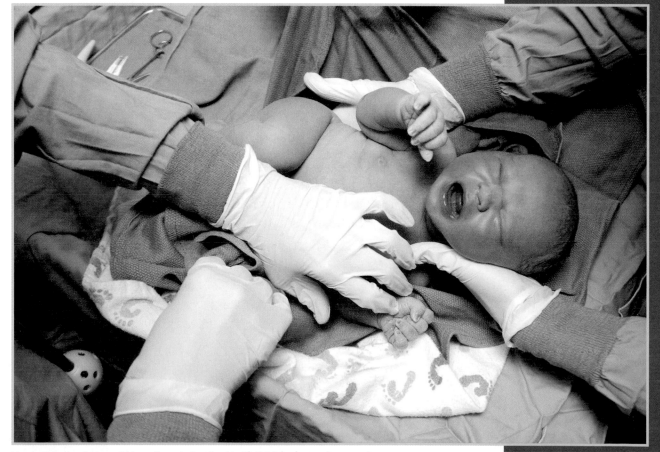

Used with permission of Mayo Foundation for Medical Education and Research.

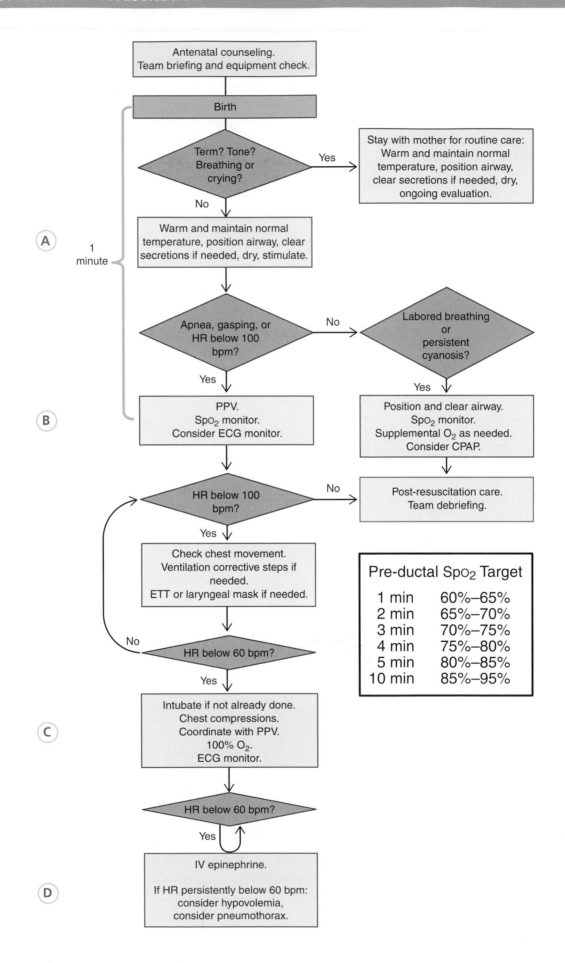

Antenatal counseling.
Team briefing and equipment check.

Birth

Term? Tone?
Breathing or
crying? — Yes → Stay with mother for routine care:
Warm and maintain normal
temperature, position airway,
clear secretions if needed, dry,
ongoing evaluation.

No

(A) 1 minute

Warm and maintain normal
temperature, position airway, clear
secretions if needed, dry, stimulate.

Apnea, gasping, or
HR below 100
bpm? — No → Labored breathing
or
persistent
cyanosis?

Yes

Yes

(B) PPV.
SpO₂ monitor.
Consider ECG monitor.

Position and clear airway.
SpO₂ monitor.
Supplemental O₂ as needed.
Consider CPAP.

HR below 100
bpm? — No → Post-resuscitation care.
Team debriefing.

Yes

Check chest movement.
Ventilation corrective steps if
needed.
ETT or laryngeal mask if needed.

No ← HR below 60 bpm?

Yes

(C) Intubate if not already done.
Chest compressions.
Coordinate with PPV.
100% O₂.
ECG monitor.

HR below 60 bpm?

Yes

(D) IV epinephrine.

If HR persistently below 60 bpm:
consider hypovolemia,
consider pneumothorax.

Pre-ductal SpO₂ Target

1 min	60%–65%
2 min	65%–70%
3 min	70%–75%
4 min	75%–80%
5 min	80%–85%
10 min	85%–95%

The Neonatal Resuscitation Program (NRP®) will help you learn the cognitive, technical, and teamwork skills that you need to resuscitate and stabilize newborns. Although most newborns make the cardiorespiratory transition to extrauterine life without intervention, many will require assistance to begin breathing and a small number will require extensive intervention. After birth, approximately 4% to 10% of term and late preterm newborns will receive positive-pressure ventilation (PPV), while only 1 to 3 per 1,000 will receive chest compressions or emergency medications. Because the need for assistance cannot always be predicted, teams need to be prepared to provide these lifesaving interventions quickly and efficiently at every birth. During your NRP course, your team will learn how to evaluate a newborn, make decisions about what actions to take, and practice the steps involved in resuscitation. As you practice together in simulated cases, your resuscitation team will gradually build proficiency and speed.

Why do newborns require a different approach to resuscitation than adults?

Most often, adult cardiac arrest is a complication of trauma or existing heart disease. It is caused by a sudden arrhythmia that prevents the heart from effectively circulating blood. As circulation to the brain decreases, the adult victim loses consciousness and stops breathing. At the time of arrest, the oxygen and carbon dioxide (CO_2) content of blood is usually normal. During adult cardiopulmonary resuscitation, chest compressions are used to maintain circulation until electrical defibrillation or medications restore cardiac function.

In contrast, most newborns requiring resuscitation have a healthy heart. When a newborn requires resuscitation, it is usually caused by a problem with respiration leading to inadequate gas exchange. Respiratory failure may occur either before or after birth. Before birth, fetal respiratory function is performed by the placenta. If the placenta is functioning normally, oxygen is transferred from the mother to the fetus and CO_2 is removed. When placental respiration fails, the fetus receives an insufficient supply of oxygen to support normal cellular functions and CO_2 cannot be removed. The blood level of acid increases as cells attempt to function without oxygen and CO_2 accumulates. Fetal monitoring may show a decrease in activity, loss of heart rate variability, and heart rate decelerations. If placental respiratory failure persists, the fetus will make a series of gasps followed by apnea and bradycardia. If the fetus is born in the early phase of respiratory failure, tactile stimulation may be sufficient to initiate spontaneous breathing and recovery. If the fetus is born in a later phase of respiratory failure, stimulation will not be sufficient and the newborn will require assisted ventilation for recovery. The most severely affected newborns may require chest compressions and epinephrine to allow the compromised heart muscle to restore circulation. At the time of birth, you may not know if the baby is in an early or a late phase of respiratory failure. After birth, respiratory failure occurs if the baby does not initiate or cannot maintain effective breathing effort. In either situation, the primary problem is a lack of gas exchange and *the focus of neonatal resuscitation is effective ventilation of the baby's lungs.*

Many concepts and skills are taught in this program. Establishing effective ventilation of the baby's lungs during neonatal resuscitation is the single most important concept emphasized throughout the program.

What happens during the transition from fetal to neonatal circulation?

Understanding the basic physiology of the cardiorespiratory transition from intrauterine to extrauterine life will help you understand the steps of neonatal resuscitation.

Fetal Respiration and Circulation

Before birth, the fetal lungs do not participate in gas exchange. All of the oxygen used by the fetus is supplied from the mother by diffusion across the placenta. CO_2 produced during fetal metabolism is transported across the placenta and removed by the mother's lungs. The fetal lungs are expanded in utero, but the potential air sacs (alveoli) are filled with fluid instead of air. The pulmonary vessels that will carry blood to the alveoli after birth are tightly constricted and very little blood flows into them.

In the placenta, oxygen diffuses from the mother's blood into adjacent fetal blood vessels. The oxygenated fetal blood leaves the placenta through the umbilical vein. The umbilical vein travels through the liver, joins the inferior vena cava, and enters the right side of the heart. Because the pulmonary vessels are constricted, only a small fraction of blood entering the right side of the heart travels to the fetal lungs. Instead, most of the blood bypasses the lungs, crossing to the left side of the heart through an opening in the atrial wall (patent foramen ovale) or flowing from the pulmonary artery directly into the aorta through the ductus arteriosus (Figures 1.1A and 1.1B). Blood in the aorta supplies oxygen and nutrients to the fetal organs. The most highly oxygenated blood flows to the fetal brain and heart. Some of the blood in the aorta returns to the placenta through the 2 umbilical arteries to deliver CO_2, receive more oxygen, and restart the circulation path. When blood follows this fetal circulation path and bypasses the lungs, it is called a *right-to-left shunt.*

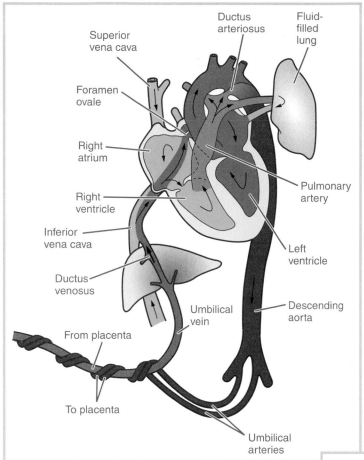

Figure 1.1A. Fetal Circulation Path: Only a small amount of blood travels to the lungs. There is no gas exchange in the lung. Blood returning to the right side of the heart from the umbilical vein has the highest oxygen saturation.

Figure 1.1B. Transitional Circulation Path: The baby breathes, pulmonary resistance decreases and blood travels to the lungs. Gas exchange occurs in the lungs. Blood returning to the left side of the heart from the lungs has the highest oxygen saturation.

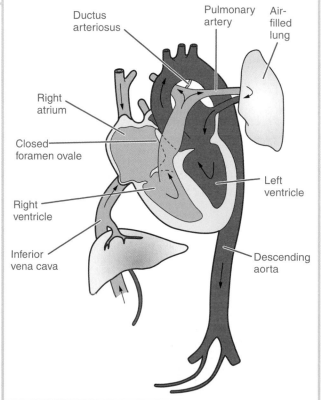

Transitional Circulation

A series of physiologic changes occur after birth that culminates in a successful transition from fetal to neonatal circulation. Table 1-1 summarizes 3 important physiologic changes that occur during this transition. When the baby breathes and the umbilical cord is clamped, the newborn uses the lungs for gas exchange. Fluid is absorbed quickly from the alveoli and the lungs fill with air. The previously constricted pulmonary blood vessels begin to dilate so that blood can reach the alveoli where oxygen will be absorbed and CO_2 will be removed (Figures 1.2A and 1.2B).

Table 1-1. Transition From Fetal to Neonatal Respiration

Change at Birth	Result
The baby breathes. The umbilical cord is clamped, separating the placenta from the baby.	The newborn uses the lungs, instead of the placenta, for gas exchange.
Fluid in the alveoli is absorbed.	Air replaces fluid in the alveoli. Oxygen moves from the alveoli into the pulmonary blood vessels and CO_2 moves into the alveoli to be exhaled.
Air in the alveoli causes blood vessels in the lung to dilate.	Pulmonary blood flow increases and the ductus arteriosus gradually constricts.

The baby's initial cries and deep breaths help to move fluid from the airways. In most circumstances, distention of the lungs with air provides sufficient oxygen (21%) to initiate relaxation of the pulmonary blood vessels. As blood levels of oxygen increase, the ductus arteriosus begins to constrict. Blood previously diverted through the foramen ovale and ductus arteriosus now flows from the right side of the heart into the lungs and the fetal "right-to-left shunt" gradually resolves. Oxygenated blood returning from the baby's lungs travels to the left side of the heart and is pumped through the aorta to tissues throughout the body.

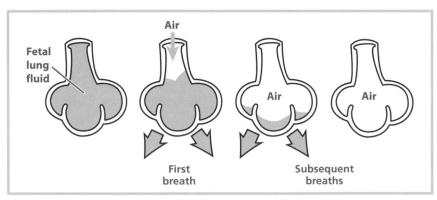

Figure 1.2A. Air replaces fluid in the alveoli.

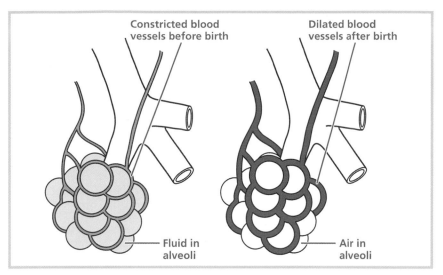

Constricted blood
vessels before birth

Dilated blood
vessels after birth

Fluid in
alveoli

Air in
alveoli

Figure 1.2B. Pulmonary blood vessels dilate.

Although the initial steps in a normal transition occur within a few
minutes of birth, the entire process may not be completed for hours or
even several days. For example, studies have shown it may take up to
10 minutes for a normal term newborn to achieve oxygen saturation
greater than 90%. It may take several hours for alveolar fluid to be
completely absorbed. Functional closure of the ductus arteriosus may
not occur for 24 to 48 hours after birth, and complete relaxation of the
pulmonary blood vessels does not occur for several months.

Review

1 Before birth, the alveoli in the fetal lungs are (collapsed)/
(expanded) and filled with (fluid)/(air).

2 Before birth, oxygen is supplied to the fetus by (the placenta)/(the
fetal lungs).

3 After birth, air in the alveoli causes vessels in the baby's lungs to
(constrict)/(relax).

Answers

1 Before birth, the alveoli in the fetal lungs are expanded and filled
with fluid.

2 Before birth, oxygen is supplied to the fetus by the placenta.

3 After birth, air in the alveoli causes vessels in the baby's lungs to
relax.

How does a newborn respond to an interruption in normal transition?

If there is an interruption in either placental function or neonatal respiration, gas exchange within tissues is decreased and the arterioles in the intestines, kidneys, muscles, and skin may constrict. A survival reflex maintains or increases blood flow to the heart and brain. This redistribution of blood flow helps to preserve function of these vital organs. If inadequate gas exchange continues, the heart begins to fail and blood flow to all organs decreases. The lack of adequate blood perfusion and tissue oxygenation interferes with cellular function and may lead to organ damage. Table 1-2 summarizes some of the clinical findings associated with an interruption in normal transition.

Table 1-2. Clinical Findings of Abnormal Transition

- Irregular or absent respiratory effort (apnea) or rapid breathing (tachypnea)
- Slow heart rate (bradycardia) or rapid heart rate (tachycardia)
- Decreased muscle tone
- Low oxygen saturation
- Low blood pressure

What is the Neonatal Resuscitation Program Flow Diagram?

The NRP Flow Diagram describes the steps that you will follow to evaluate and resuscitate a newborn. It is divided into 5 blocks beginning with birth and the initial assessment. Throughout the diagram, diamonds indicate assessments and rectangles show actions that may be required. Although it is important to work quickly and efficiently, *you must ensure that you have adequately performed the steps of each block before moving on to the next block.* Assessments are repeated at the end of each block and will determine if you need to proceed. The details of each block are described in subsequent lessons.

- *Initial Assessment:* Determine if the newborn can remain with the mother or should be moved to a radiant warmer for further evaluation.
- *Airway (A):* Perform the initial steps to establish an open *A*irway and support spontaneous respiration.
- *Breathing (B):* Positive-pressure ventilation is provided to assist *B*reathing for babies with apnea or bradycardia. Other interventions (continuous positive airway pressure [CPAP] or oxygen) may be appropriate if the baby has labored breathing or low oxygen saturation.

Take a moment to familiarize yourself with the layout of the NRP Flow Diagram.

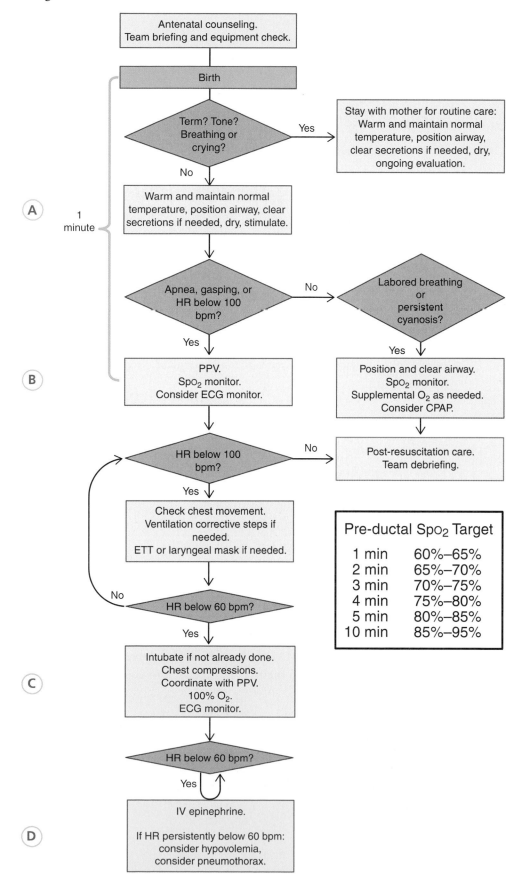

Pre-ductal SpO2 Target

1 min	60%–65%
2 min	65%–70%
3 min	70%–75%
4 min	75%–80%
5 min	80%–85%
10 min	85%–95%

9

- *Circulation (C):* If severe bradycardia persists despite assisted ventilation, *C*irculation is supported by performing chest compressions coordinated with PPV.
- *Drug (D):* If severe bradycardia persists despite assisted ventilation and coordinated compressions, the *D*rug epinephrine is administered as PPV and chest compressions continue.

Focus on Teamwork

Why are teamwork and communication emphasized throughout this program?

Effective teamwork and communication are essential skills during neonatal resuscitation. A Joint Commission investigation found that poor teamwork and communication were the most common root causes for potentially preventable infant deaths in the delivery room. During a complex resuscitation, providers will need to perform multiple procedures without delay. Confusion and inefficiency may occur because several teams of caregivers are working in a confined space at the same time. Even though each individual may have the knowledge and skills to perform a successful resuscitation, each person's skills will not be used optimally without effective coordination.

Pre-resuscitation team briefing

The first step in preparing for resuscitation is planning how your team will be contacted and who will respond. Once assembled, each team member needs to understand his or her role and the tasks he or she will be assigned. Perform a pre-resuscitation team briefing before every birth to review the clinical situation and the action plan. During the briefing, assess perinatal risk factors, identify a team leader, delegate tasks, identify who will document events as they occur, determine what supplies and equipment will be needed, and identify how to call for additional help (Figure 1.3). The pre-resuscitation team briefing is important even for well-established teams. A common analogy is to compare the medical team's pre-resuscitation briefing to an airline pilot's preflight check. Even pilots that have flown the same flight many times perform their preflight check to ensure their passengers' safety.

The team leader

Every resuscitation team needs to have an identified leader. Any team member who has mastery of the NRP Flow Diagram and effective leadership skills can be the team leader. Effective team leaders exemplify good communication skills by giving clear directions to

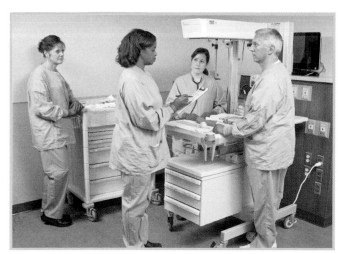

Pre-resuscitation Team Briefing
- Assess perinatal risk factors.
- Identify a team leader.
- Delegate tasks.
- Identify who will document events as they occur.
- Determine what supplies and equipment will be needed.
- Identify how to call for additional help.

Figure 1.3. Neonatal resuscitation team briefing

specific individuals, sharing information, delegating responsibilities to ensure coordinated care, and maintaining a professional environment. A skilled leader effectively utilizes her resources by allowing all team members to contribute their unique talents to the resuscitation process. It is important for the team leader to remain aware of the entire clinical situation, maintain a view of the "big picture" and not become distracted by a single activity. This is called *situational awareness*. If the leader is involved in a procedure that diverts her attention, the leader may need to appoint another qualified person to assume the leadership role. If the person in the leadership role changes during the resuscitation, a clear verbal statement should be made so that all team members know who is leading the team.

Effective communication

Although the team has a leader, every team member shares responsibility for ongoing assessment and ensuring that interventions are performed in the correct sequence with the correct technique. Successful coordination requires team members to share information and communicate with each other. Closed-loop communication is a technique that ensures instructions are heard and understood. When you give an instruction, direct the request to a specific individual, call your team member by name, make eye contact, and speak clearly. After giving an instruction, ask the receiver to report back as soon as the task is completed. After receiving an instruction, repeat the instruction back to the sender. For example,

> Sandy: *"Robert, I need a 3.5-mm endotracheal tube, with a stylet, and a laryngoscope with a size-1 blade. Tell me when they're ready."*
> Robert: *"You want a 3.5-mm endotracheal tube, with a stylet, and a laryngoscope with a size-1 blade."*
> Sandy: *"Correct."*

Once the equipment is ready,

> Robert: *"Sandy, a 3.5-mm endotracheal tube, with a stylet, and size-1 laryngoscope are ready now."*

Accurate documentation

Maintaining accurate documentation during an emergency is a skill demonstrated by highly effective teams. Complete records are important for clinical decision making and as a source for quality improvement data. The sense of urgency surrounding resuscitation can make accurate documentation challenging, but preparation can make this essential task easier. Events during resuscitation should be documented as they occur and supplemented with a retrospective narrative summary. Consider using a single time reference for accurately establishing the time that events occur. When team members use different watches or clocks during resuscitation, potential differences in the time readings can cause confusion and errors in documentation. Because multitasking can disrupt observation and communication, the recorder should not be responsible for other roles. Team members must announce interventions and assessments clearly and directly to the recorder. Consider using a paper form or electronic template designed specifically for neonatal resuscitation. Well-designed forms that follow the NRP Flow Diagram enable rapid data entry, allow the recorder to assist the team leader by providing prompts for the next intervention, and assist the leader in identifying delayed assessments. Ideally, the role of resuscitation recorder should be assigned to an experienced team member. Without experience, the recorder may have difficulty deciding what is important to record and providing decision support to the team leader. Practicing accurate documentation warrants the same preparation as any other resuscitation skill and should be included in mock codes and simulation.

Post-resuscitation team debriefing

Performing a post-resuscitation team debriefing reinforces good teamwork habits and helps your team identify areas for improvement. A quick debriefing can be performed immediately after the event while a more comprehensive debriefing may be scheduled a short time afterward. Your debriefings do not have to find major problems to be effective. Your team may identify a series of small changes that result in significant improvements in your team's performance.

The Neonatal Resuscitation Program Key Behavioral Skills

The 10 NRP Key Behavioral Skills, described in Table 1-3, are adapted from previously described models of effective teamwork (Center for Advanced Pediatric and Perinatal Education [CAPE], Lucile Packard Children's Hospital at Stanford University). In each of the lessons that

Table 1-3. Neonatal Resuscitation Program Key Behavioral Skills

Behavior	Examples
Know your environment.	• Perform an equipment check before the baby is delivered. • Know the location of resuscitation equipment and how to access it. • Know how to call for help and who is available.
Use available information.	• Know the prenatal and intrapartum history, including maternal complications, maternal medications, and other risk factors.
Anticipate and plan.	• Perform a pre-resuscitation team briefing to ensure all team members know the clinical situation. • Assign roles and responsibilities. • Discuss an action plan in the event of complications.

Clearly identify a team leader.	• Identify the team leader before the birth.
	• Effective leaders
	  – Clearly articulate goals.
	  – Delegate tasks as appropriate while monitoring the distribution of workload.
	  – Include other team members in assessment and planning.
	  – Think "out loud."
	  – Maintain situational awareness.
	  – Hand over leadership to another team member if he must become involved in a procedure.

Communicate effectively.	• Call team members by name. • Share information actively. • Inform your team if you identify a problem, error, or patient safety concern. • Order medications by name, dose, and route. • Use concise, clear language. • Use closed-loop communication. • Verify information. • Ensure that changes in information or assessments are shared with all team members. • Include family members in communication as appropriate.
Delegate workload optimally.	• Do not duplicate work or use more resources than necessary. • Change task assignments depending on skill sets and what is required at the moment. • Do not allow one person to become overloaded with tasks. • Do not allow the team to become fixated on a single task.
Allocate attention wisely.	• Maintain situational awareness by scanning and reassessing the clinical situation frequently. • Monitor each other's skill performance to ensure patient safety.
Use available resources.	• Know what personnel are available. • Know what additional or special supplies are available and how to access them.
Call for additional help when needed.	• Anticipate the need for additional team members based on risk factors and the progress of the resuscitation. • Call for additional help in a timely manner. • Know how you will call for additional help and the process for getting the right kind of assistance.
Maintain professional behavior.	• Use respectful verbal and nonverbal communication. • Actively seek and offer assistance. • Support and promote teamwork. • Respect and value your team.

follow, we will highlight how effective teams use these behavioral skills. Improving your teamwork and communication requires deliberate practice under conditions that are as realistic as possible. As you review each lesson and participate in simulation, think about how these behavioral skills can be used to improve your own team's performance.

Ethical Considerations

Neonatal resuscitation is a stressful event that frequently involves complicated ethical decision making for parents and health care providers. As you read the lessons in the textbook, ethical questions that are relevant to the material presented will be highlighted for your consideration. These concepts will be explored in detail in Lesson 11.

Questions to consider:

What is the difference between ethics and law?

What are the ethical principles that guide the care of newborns during resuscitation?

Key Points

1. Some newborns without any apparent risk factors will require resuscitation, including assisted ventilation.

2. Unlike adults, who experience cardiac arrest due to trauma or heart disease, newborn resuscitation is usually the result of respiratory failure, either before or after birth.

3. The most important and effective action in neonatal resuscitation is to ventilate the baby's lungs.

4. Very few newborns will require chest compressions or medication.

5. Prolonged lack of adequate perfusion and oxygenation can lead to organ damage.

6. Resuscitation should proceed quickly and efficiently; however, ensure that you have effectively completed the steps in each block of the Neonatal Resuscitation Program Flow Diagram before moving to the next.

7. Teamwork, leadership, and communication are critical to successful resuscitation of the newborn.

LESSON 1 REVIEW

1. Before birth, the alveoli in the fetal lungs are (collapsed)/ (expanded) and filled with (fluid)/(air).

2. Before birth, oxygen is supplied to the fetus by (the placenta)/ (the fetal lungs).

3. After birth, air in the alveoli causes vessels in the baby's lungs to (constrict)/(relax).

4. When resuscitating newborns, chest compressions and medication are (rarely)/(frequently) needed.

5. Members of an effective resuscitation team (share information)/ (work quietly and independently).

Answers

1. Before birth, the alveoli in the fetal lungs are expanded and filled with fluid.

2. Before birth, oxygen is supplied to the fetus by the placenta.

3. After birth, air in the alveoli causes vessels in the baby's lungs to relax.

4. When resuscitating newborns, chest compressions and medication are rarely needed.

5. Members of an effective resuscitation team share information.

Additional Reading

Dempsey E, Pammi M, Ryan AC, Barrington KJ. Standardised formal resuscitation training programmes for reducing mortality and morbidity in newborn infants. *Cochrane Database Syst Rev.* 2015 Sep 4;9

Sentinel Event Alert. Issue 30. Preventing infant death and injury during delivery. The Joint Commission for the Accreditation of Healthcare Organizations (JCAHO). 2004. http://www.jointcommission.org/ sentinel_event_alert_issue_30_preventing_infant death and injury_during_delivery/. Accessed March 23, 2015

Singhal N, McMillan DD, Yee WH, Akierman AR, Yee YJ. Evaluation of the effectiveness of the standardized neonatal resuscitation program. *J Perinatol.* 2001;21(6):388-392

Thomas EJ, Williams AL, Reichman EF, Lasky RE, Crandell S, Taggart WR. Team training in the neonatal resuscitation program for interns: teamwork and quality of resuscitations. *Pediatrics.* 2010;125(3):539-546

Preparing for Resuscitation

What you will learn

- Risk factors that can help predict which babies will require resuscitation
- How to assemble a resuscitation team
- Four key questions to ask the obstetric provider before birth
- How to perform a pre-resuscitation team briefing
- How to assemble and check resuscitation supplies and equipment

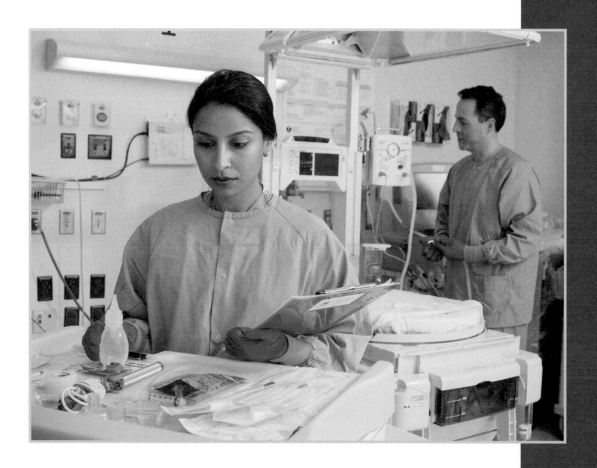

Case: Preparing for a birth with perinatal risk factors

A 30-year-old woman enters the hospital in labor at 36 weeks' gestation. She has insulin-requiring gestational diabetes and hypertension. She is found to have ruptured membranes with clear amniotic fluid. Fetal heart rate monitoring shows a Category II pattern (indeterminate pattern requiring evaluation, surveillance, and possibly other tests to ensure fetal well-being). Labor progresses rapidly and a vaginal birth is imminent. The obstetric provider calls your resuscitation team to attend the birth. As your team enters the room, you introduce yourselves, ask the obstetric provider 4 brief questions, and determine that there are several perinatal risk factors. The team proceeds to identify a team leader, performs a pre-resuscitation team briefing, discusses roles and responsibilities if interventions are required, and performs a complete equipment check.

Why is it important to anticipate the need for resuscitation before every birth?

You should be prepared to resuscitate the newborn at every birth. Table 2-1 describes risk factors that increase the likelihood that the newborn will require support with transition or resuscitation. Thoughtful consideration of these risk factors will help you identify the correct personnel to attend the birth. Although attention to these risk factors is helpful and will identify most newborns that require resuscitation after birth, some newborns without any apparent risk factors will require resuscitation.

Table 2-1. Perinatal Risk Factors Increasing the Likelihood of Neonatal Resuscitation

Antepartum Risk Factors	
Gestational age less than 36 0/7 weeks	Oligohydramnios
Gestational age greater than or equal to 41 0/7 weeks	Fetal hydrops
Preeclampsia or eclampsia	Fetal macrosomia
Maternal hypertension	Intrauterine growth restriction
Multiple gestation	Significant fetal malformations or anomalies
Fetal anemia	No prenatal care
Polyhydramnios	
Intrapartum Risk Factors	
Emergency cesarean delivery	Intrapartum bleeding
Forceps or vacuum-assisted delivery	Chorioamnionitis
Breech or other abnormal presentation	Narcotics administered to mother within 4 hours of delivery
Category II or III fetal heart rate pattern*	Shoulder dystocia
Maternal general anesthesia	Meconium-stained amniotic fluid
Maternal magnesium therapy	Prolapsed umbilical cord
Placental abruption	

*See Appendix 3 for description of fetal heart rate categories.

What questions should you ask before every birth?

It is important for the obstetric and newborn health care providers to coordinate care by establishing effective communication. Before every birth, review the antepartum and intrapartum risk factors described in Table 2-1. Ask the following 4 pre-birth questions:

① *What is the expected gestational age?*

② *Is the amniotic fluid clear?*

③ *How many babies are expected?*

④ *Are there any additional risk factors?*

Based on the responses to these questions, determine if you have assembled the necessary personnel and equipment.

What personnel should be present at delivery?

- Every birth should be attended by *at least 1 qualified individual*, skilled in the initial steps of newborn care and positive-pressure ventilation (PPV), whose only responsibility is management of the newly born baby.

- If risk factors are present (Table 2-1), *at least 2 qualified people should be present solely to manage the baby*. The number and qualifications of personnel will vary depending on the anticipated risk, the number of babies, and the hospital setting.

- A *qualified team with full resuscitation skills*, including endotracheal intubation, chest compressions, emergency vascular access and medication administration, should be identified and immediately available for every resuscitation.

  - The resuscitation team should be present at the time of birth if the need for extensive resuscitation measures is anticipated.

  - It is not sufficient to have the team with these advanced skills on call at home or in a remote area of the hospital. When resuscitation is needed, it must begin without delay.

For example, a nurse at an uncomplicated birth might evaluate gestational age, muscle tone, and respirations, and provide tactile stimulation. If the newborn does not respond appropriately, the nurse would position and clear the airway, start PPV, and initiate an emergency call for immediate assistance. Quickly, a second person comes to the warmer to assess the efficacy of PPV and places a pulse oximeter sensor. Another provider with full resuscitation skills, including intubation and umbilical vein catheter insertion, is in the immediate vicinity and arrives to assist the team.

In the case of an anticipated high-risk birth, such as an extremely premature baby or prolapsed umbilical cord, a team with sufficient personnel to provide PPV, intubate the trachea, perform chest compressions, obtain emergency vascular access, prepare medications, and document events should be assembled before the birth. Depending on the setting, this will likely require 4 or more qualified providers.

Each hospital must develop and practice a system for assembling a resuscitation team. Identify how the team will be alerted if risk factors are present, who will be called, and how additional help will be called if necessary. Practice a variety of scenarios to ensure that you have sufficient personnel immediately available to perform all of the necessary tasks.

Review

❶ What are the 4 pre-birth questions to ask the obstetric provider before every birth?

❷ Every delivery should be attended by at least 1 skilled person (whose only responsibility is the management of the newborn)/ (who shares responsibility for the mother and newborn's care).

Answers

❶ The 4 pre-birth questions are

    i. What is the expected gestational age?

    ii. Is the amniotic fluid clear?

    iii. How many babies are expected?

    iv. Are there any additional risk factors?

❷ Every delivery should be attended by at least 1 skilled person whose only responsibility is the management of the newborn.

Perform a pre-resuscitation team briefing.

Once your team is assembled, review the risk factors and any management plans developed during antenatal counseling. Identify the team leader, discuss the possible scenarios that your team may encounter, and assign roles and responsibilities. Use all of the available perinatal information to anticipate potential complications and plan your response. For example, if the obstetric provider tells you that the mother has just received narcotic analgesia, you will be prepared for a sedated baby that may require assisted ventilation. Discuss who will perform the initial assessment, who will stimulate the baby, who will start PPV if needed, and who will document the events. Sample scripts for performing pre-resuscitation team briefings are available on the Neonatal Resuscitation Program® (NRP®) Web site.

What supplies and equipment should be available?

All supplies and equipment necessary for a complete resuscitation must be readily available for every birth. When a high-risk newborn is expected, all appropriate supplies and equipment should have been checked and ready for immediate use. It is not sufficient to simply look at what is on the radiant warmer. It is much more effective to establish an organized routine, preferably with a standardized checklist, before every birth. In this way, you will confirm what is ready for immediate use and identify which pieces of equipment are missing.

The appendices of this lesson include 2 lists. The NRP Quick Equipment Checklist is a tool that you can use during your briefing to check the most essential supplies and equipment. The checklist follows the steps of the NRP Flow Diagram. Ask yourself, "Can I warm the baby, clear the airway, auscultate, ventilate, oxygenate, intubate, and medicate?" Consider keeping the NRP Quick Equipment Checklist near the radiant warmer so that it is accessible before every birth. The Neonatal Resuscitation Supplies and Equipment List is a comprehensive inventory of the supplies and equipment that should be available within the resuscitation area.

Focus on Teamwork

The preparation phase of neonatal resuscitation highlights several opportunities for effective teams to use the NRP Key Behavioral Skills.

Behavior	Example
Anticipate and plan.	Know which providers will be called to attend the birth based on the perinatal risk factors. Perform a standardized equipment check before every birth. Assign roles and responsibilities.
Use all available information. Use available resources.	Ask the obstetric provider the 4 pre-birth questions to identify risk factors. Prepare additional supplies and equipment, as necessary, based on these risk factors.
Know your environment.	Know how the resuscitation team is called and how additional personnel and resources can be summoned. Know how to access additional equipment and supplies for a complex resuscitation.
Clearly identify a leader.	If risk factors are present, identify a team leader before the birth and perform a pre-resuscitation team briefing to ensure that everyone is prepared and responsibilities are defined.

Frequently asked questions

What is the ideal number of people to have on the resuscitation team?

There is no single correct answer to this question. You must have sufficient personnel immediately available to perform all of the necessary tasks without delay. The personnel required at any particular birth will depend on the identified risk factors, the qualifications of the individuals on the team, and the setting. Simulate different scenarios to ensure that you have sufficient personnel on your team to perform all necessary procedures quickly and efficiently. For a complex resuscitation, this will require 4 or more people.

Who can be a team leader? Can the leadership role shift during resuscitation?

Any well-trained neonatal resuscitation care provider can be the team leader. A neonatal resuscitation team leader needs to fully understand the NRP Flow Diagram and have strong leadership skills. The leader does not have to be the most senior member of the team or the individual with the most advanced degree. That person may have technical skills that will be required during the resuscitation and may not be able to maintain her full attention on the baby's condition. The team leader needs to be in a position to observe and direct all of the team's activities. If the leader is performing a procedure that occupies her attention, it is appropriate to transfer the leadership role to another qualified team member. A clear verbal statement indicating the change in leadership helps to avoid confusion.

Ethical Considerations
Questions to consider
What laws apply to neonatal resuscitation?
What discussions should be held with parents prior to a very high-risk birth?
These questions are explored in detail in Lesson 11.

Key Points

1. Identify perinatal risk factors by asking the obstetric provider 4 questions prior to the birth.

    i. *What is the expected gestational age?*

    ii. *Is the amniotic fluid clear?*

    iii. *How many babies are expected?*

    iv. *Are there any additional risk factors?*

2 Many, but not all, babies who will require neonatal resuscitation can be identified by the presence of perinatal risk factors.

3 Every birth should be attended by at least 1 qualified individual, skilled in the initial steps of newborn care and PPV, whose only responsibility is management of the newly born baby.

4 If risk factors are present, *at least 2 qualified people should be present solely to manage the baby.* The number and qualifications of personnel will vary depending on the anticipated risk, the number of babies, and the hospital setting.

5 A qualified *team with full resuscitation skills*, including endotracheal intubation, chest compressions, emergency vascular access, and medication administration, should be identified and immediately available for every resuscitation. This team should be present at the birth if the need for extensive resuscitation measures is anticipated.

6 All supplies and equipment necessary for a complete resuscitation must be readily available and functional.

7 When a high-risk newborn is expected, all appropriate supplies and equipment should have been checked and ready for immediate use.

8 Use an organized equipment checklist that becomes a routine before every birth.

LESSON 2 REVIEW

1. What are the 4 pre-birth questions to ask the obstetric provider before every birth?

    i.

    ii.

    iii.

    iv.

2. Every delivery should be attended by at least 1 skilled person (whose only responsibility is the management of the newborn)/ (who shares responsibility for the mother and newborn's care).

3. If a high-risk birth is anticipated, (1 qualified person)/(a qualified team) should be present at the birth.

4. When a high-risk newborn is anticipated because of the presence of risk factors, resuscitation supplies and equipment (should)/(should not) be unpacked and ready for use.

5. During the pre-resuscitation team briefing, (prepare for a routine delivery because you do not know what will be needed)/(anticipate potential complications and discuss how responsibilities will be delegated).

6. A qualified nurse or respiratory care practitioner who has been trained in neonatal resuscitation and has strong leadership skills (can)/(cannot) be the team leader.

Answers

1. The 4 pre-birth questions are

   i. *What is the expected gestational age?*

   ii. *Is the amniotic fluid clear?*

   iii. *How many babies are expected?*

   iv. *Are there any additional risk factors?*

2. Every delivery should be attended by at least 1 skilled person whose only responsibility is the management of the newborn.

3. If a high-risk birth is anticipated, a qualified team should be present at the birth.

4. When a high-risk newborn is anticipated because of the presence of risk factors, resuscitation supplies and equipment should be unpacked and ready for use.

5. During the pre-resuscitation team briefing, anticipate potential complications and discuss how responsibilities will be delegated.

6. A qualified nurse or respiratory care practitioner who has been trained in neonatal resuscitation and has strong leadership skills can be the team leader.

Additional Reading

Aziz K, Chadwick M, Baker M, Andrews W. Ante- and intra-partum factors that predict increased need for neonatal resuscitation. *Resuscitation.* 2008;79(3):444-452

Katheria A, Rich W, Finer N. Development of a strategic process using checklists to facilitate team preparation and improve communication during neonatal resuscitation. *Resuscitation.* 2013;84(11):1552-1557

Appendix 1. Neonatal Resuscitation Program Quick Equipment Checklist

This checklist includes only the most essential supplies and equipment needed at the radiant warmer for most neonatal resuscitations. Tailor this list to meet your unit-specific needs. Ensure that an equipment check has been done prior to <u>every</u> birth.

Warm	• Preheated warmer
	• Warm towels or blankets
	• Temperature sensor and sensor cover for prolonged resuscitation
	• Hat
	• Plastic bag or plastic wrap (<32 weeks' gestation)
	• Thermal mattress (<32 weeks' gestation)
Clear airway	• Bulb syringe
	• 10F or 12F suction catheter attached to wall suction, set at 80 to 100 mm Hg
	• Meconium aspirator
Auscultate	• Stethoscope
Ventilate	• Flowmeter set to 10 L/min
	• Oxygen blender set to 21% *(21%-30% if <35 weeks' gestation)*
	• Positive-pressure ventilation (PPV) device
	• Term- and preterm-sized masks
	• 8F feeding tube and large syringe
Oxygenate	• Equipment to give free-flow oxygen
	• Pulse oximeter with sensor and cover
	• Target oxygen saturation table
Intubate	• Laryngoscope with size-0 and size-1 straight blades (size 00, optional)
	• Stylet (optional)
	• Endotracheal tubes (sizes 2.5, 3.0, 3.5)
	• Carbon dioxide (CO_2) detector
	• Measuring tape and/or endotracheal tube insertion depth table
	• Waterproof tape or tube-securing device
	• Scissors
	• Laryngeal mask (size 1) and 5-mL syringe
Medicate	Access to
	• 1:10,000 (0.1 mg/mL) epinephrine
	• Normal saline
	• Supplies for placing emergency umbilical venous catheter and administering medications
	• Electronic cardiac (ECG) monitor leads and ECG monitor

Appendix 2. Neonatal Resuscitation Supplies and Equipment List

Suction equipment

Bulb syringe
Mechanical suction and tubing
Suction catheters, 5F or 6F, 10F, 12F or 14F
8F feeding tube and large syringe
Meconium aspirator

Positive-pressure ventilation equipment

Device for delivering positive-pressure ventilation
Face masks, newborn and preterm sizes
Oxygen source
Compressed air source
Oxygen blender to mix oxygen and compressed air with flowmeter
    (flow rate set to 10 L/min) and tubing
Pulse oximeter with sensor and cover
Target oxygen saturation table

Intubation equipment

Laryngoscope with straight blades, No. 0 (preterm) and No. 1 (term)
Extra bulbs and batteries for laryngoscope
Endotracheal tubes, 2.5-, 3.0-, 3.5-mm internal diameter (ID)
Stylet (optional)
Measuring tape
Endotracheal tube insertion depth table
Scissors
Waterproof tape or tube-securing device
Alcohol pads
CO_2 detector or capnograph
Laryngeal mask (or similar supraglottic device) and 5-mL syringe
5F or 6F orogastric tube if insertion port present on laryngeal mask

Medications

Epinephrine 1:10,000 (0.1 mg/mL)—3-mL or 10-mL ampules
Normal saline for volume expansion—100 or 250 mL
Dextrose 10%, 250 mL (optional)
Normal saline for flushes
Syringes (1-mL, 3-mL or 5-mL, 20- to 60-mL)

Umbilical vessel catheterization supplies

Sterile gloves

Antiseptic prep solution

Umbilical tape

Small clamp (hemostat)

Forceps (optional)

Scalpel

Umbilical catheters (single lumen), 3.5F or 5F

Three-way stopcock

Syringes (3-5 mL)

Needle or puncture device for needleless system

Normal saline for flushes

Clear adhesive dressing to temporarily secure umbilical venous
catheter to abdomen (optional)

Miscellaneous

Gloves and appropriate personal protection

Radiant warmer or other heat source

Temperature sensor with sensor cover for radiant warmer (for use
during prolonged resuscitation)

Firm, padded resuscitation surface

Timer/clock with second hand

Warmed linens

Hat

Stethoscope (with neonatal head)

Tape, 1/2 or 3/4 inch

Electronic cardiac (ECG) monitor leads and ECG monitor

Intraosseous needle (optional)

For very preterm babies

Size-00 laryngoscope blade (optional)

Food-grade plastic bag (1-gallon size) or plastic wrap

Thermal mattress

Transport incubator to maintain baby's temperature during move to
the nursery

Appendix 3. Fetal Heart Rate Categories

Category I: This is a *normal* tracing and is predictive of normal fetal acid-base status at the time of the observation, and routine follow-up is indicated.

Category II: This is considered an *indeterminate* tracing. There is currently inadequate evidence to classify them as either normal or abnormal. Further evaluation, continued surveillance, and reevaluation are indicated.

Category III: This is an *abnormal* tracing and is predictive of abnormal fetal acid-base status at the time of the observation. A Category III tracing requires prompt evaluation and intervention.

Reference

Macones GA, Hankins GD, Spong CY, Hauth J, Moore T. The 2008 National Institute of Child Health and Human Development workshop report on electronic fetal monitoring: update on definitions, interpretation, and research guidelines. *Obstet Gynecol.* 2008;112(3): 661-666

Lesson 2: Performance Checklist

Preparing for Resuscitation

The Performance Checklist Is a Learning Tool

The learner uses the checklist as a reference during independent practice or as a guide for discussion and practice with a Neonatal Resuscitation Program (NRP) instructor. When the learner and instructor agree that the learner can perform the skills correctly and smoothly without coaching and within the context of a scenario, the learner may move on to the next lesson's Performance Checklist.

Note: If the institution policy is that a T-piece resuscitator normally is used in the delivery room, the learner should demonstrate proficiency with that device. However, he or she also should demonstrate ability to use a bag and mask.

Knowledge Check

1 What are the 4 pre-birth questions? What is the purpose of these questions?

2 Who can be the leader of a resuscitation? When might leadership shift?

3 What happens at a pre-resuscitation team briefing?

4 Where will you find the NRP Quick Equipment Checklist used in our birth setting?

Learning Objectives

1 Identify antepartum and intrapartum risk factors for neonatal resuscitation.

2 Demonstrate a pre-resuscitation team briefing.

3 Demonstrate an organized method for checking equipment and supplies.

Scenario

"You are notified that a woman has been admitted to the hospital in active labor. Check your supplies and equipment and prepare for the birth. As you work, say your thoughts and actions aloud so I will know what you are thinking and doing."

Instructor should check boxes as the learner responds correctly. The learner may refer to the NRP Quick Equipment Checklist or use a unit-specific checklist to ensure the availability and function of essential supplies and equipment.

✔	Critical Performance Steps
Ask the 4 pre-birth questions.	
	What is the expected gestational age? **"36 weeks' gestation" or "29 weeks' gestation"**
	Is the amniotic fluid clear? **"Yes" or "Blood stained"**
	How many babies are expected? **"1"**
	Are there any additional risk factors? **"Gestational hypertension" or "Preeclampsia"**
Assemble team.	
	Assembles team based on perinatal risk factors
Perform pre-resuscitation briefing.	
	Identifies team leader
	Discusses possible clinical scenarios and assign roles and responsibilities
Perform equipment check.	
	Demonstrates an organized routine to locate the most essential supplies needed for newborn resuscitation
Warm.	
	• Preheated warmer
	• Warm towels or blankets
	• Temperature sensor and sensor cover for prolonged resuscitation
	• Hat
	• Plastic bag or plastic wrap *(<32 weeks' gestation)*
	• Thermal mattress *(<32 weeks' gestation)*
Clear the airway.	
	• Bulb syringe
	• 10F or 12F suction catheter attached to wall suction, set at 80 to 100 mm Hg
	• Meconium aspirator
Auscultate.	
	• Stethoscope

✔	Critical Performance Steps
Ventilate.	
	• Flowmeter set to 10 L/min
	• Oxygen blender set to 21% *(21%-30% if <35 weeks' gestation)*
	• Positive-pressure ventilation (PPV) device
	• Term- and preterm-sized masks
	• 8F feeding tube and large syringe
Oxygenate.	
	• Equipment to give free-flow oxygen
	• Pulse oximeter with sensor and cover
	• Target oxygen saturation table
Intubate.	
	• Laryngoscope with size-0 and size-1 straight blades (size 00, optional)
	• Stylet (optional)
	• Endotracheal tubes (sizes 2.5, 3.0, 3.5)
	• Carbon dioxide (CO_2) detector
	• Measuring tape and/or endotracheal tube insertion depth table
	• Waterproof tape or tube-securing device
	• Scissors
	• Laryngeal mask (size 1) and 5-mL syringe
	• Electronic cardiac (ECG) monitor leads and ECG monitor
Medicate.	
	Access to
	• 1:10,000 (0.1 mg/mL) epinephrine
	• Normal saline
	• Supplies for placing emergency umbilical venous catheter and administering medications

Debrief

Instructor asks the learner debriefing questions to enable self-assessment, such as

1 Tell me how using this organized approach to checking resuscitation equipment works for you.

2 If all equipment and supplies are present, how long would it take you to confirm readiness for a birth?

3 Which of the NRP Key Behavioral Skills are demonstrated during preparation for resuscitation?

NRP Key Behavioral Skills

- Know your environment.
- Use available information.
- Anticipate and plan.
- Clearly identify a team leader.
- Communicate effectively.
- Delegate workload optimally.
- Allocate attention wisely.
- Use available resources.
- Call for additional help when needed.
- Maintain professional behavior.

Initial Steps of Newborn Care

What you will learn

- How to perform a rapid assessment of the newborn
- The initial steps of newborn care
- How to determine if additional steps are required
- What to do if a baby has persistent cyanosis or labored breathing
- How to use a pulse oximeter and interpret the results
- How to give supplemental oxygen
- When to consider using continuous positive airway pressure
- What to do when meconium-stained amniotic fluid is present

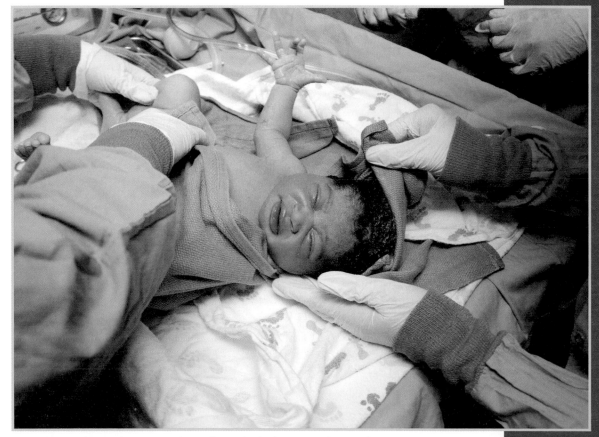

Used with permission of Mayo Foundation for Medical Education and Research.

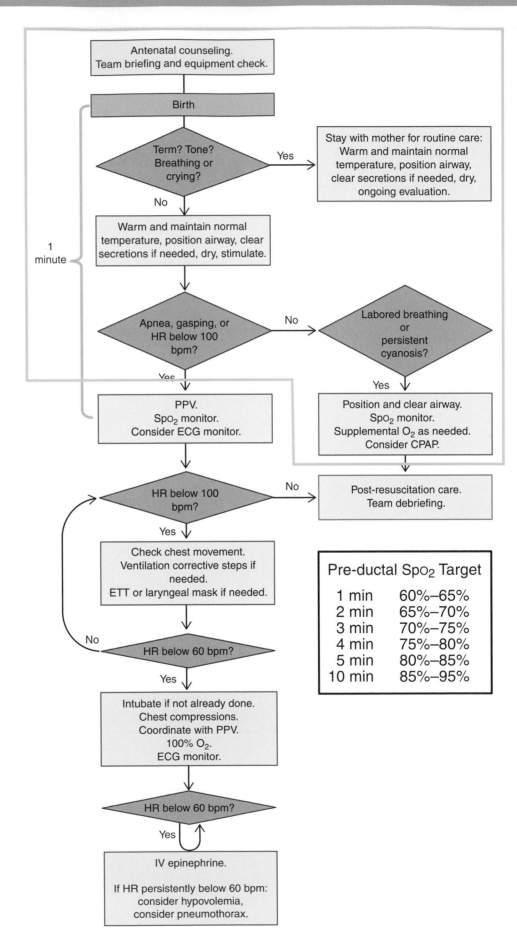

Antenatal counseling.
Team briefing and equipment check.

Birth

Term? Tone?
Breathing or
crying?

Yes → Stay with mother for routine care:
Warm and maintain normal
temperature, position airway,
clear secretions if needed, dry,
ongoing evaluation.

No

1 minute

Warm and maintain normal
temperature, position airway, clear
secretions if needed, dry, stimulate.

Apnea, gasping, or
HR below 100
bpm?

No → Labored breathing
or
persistent
cyanosis?

Yes

Yes

PPV.
SpO₂ monitor.
Consider ECG monitor.

Position and clear airway.
SpO₂ monitor.
Supplemental O₂ as needed.
Consider CPAP.

HR below 100
bpm?

No → Post-resuscitation care.
Team debriefing.

Yes

Check chest movement.
Ventilation corrective steps if
needed.
ETT or laryngeal mask if needed.

No

HR below 60 bpm?

Yes

Intubate if not already done.
Chest compressions.
Coordinate with PPV.
100% O₂.
ECG monitor.

HR below 60 bpm?

Yes

IV epinephrine.

If HR persistently below 60 bpm:
consider hypovolemia,
consider pneumothorax.

Pre-ductal SpO₂ Target

1 min	60%–65%
2 min	65%–70%
3 min	70%–75%
4 min	75%–80%
5 min	80%–85%
10 min	85%–95%

The following 2 cases are examples of how the initial steps of newborn care may be performed. As you read each case, imagine yourself as part of the resuscitation team.

Case 1: An uncomplicated birth

A healthy woman enters the hospital in active labor at 39 weeks' gestation. Her pregnancy has been uncomplicated. Her membranes rupture shortly after arrival and the amniotic fluid is clear. The nurse assigned to the baby's care completes a standardized equipment check to ensure that neonatal resuscitation equipment and supplies are ready for use if needed. Labor progresses without complications and a baby girl is born. She appears to be full-term, has good muscle tone, and cries vigorously. She is positioned skin-to-skin on her mother's chest and covered with a warm blanket. A nurse gently dries and stimulates her. One minute after birth, the cord is clamped and cut. Her color becomes increasingly pink as she continues to make the transition to newborn circulation. The nurse assigned to the baby's care continues to evaluate her respiratory effort, tone, color, and thermoregulation. Shortly after birth, her mother positions the newborn to initiate breastfeeding.

Case 2: Delayed transition

A multiparous woman presents at 39 weeks' gestation with active labor and ruptured membranes. Soon after admission, she develops a fever and receives intrapartum antibiotics for suspected chorioamnionitis. Fetal heart rate monitoring shows a Category II pattern (indeterminate pattern, requiring evaluation and surveillance and possibly other tests to ensure fetal well-being). Labor progresses and the obstetric providers call your resuscitation team to attend the vaginal birth. When you enter the room, you introduce the team to the laboring mother and ask the obstetric provider 4 pre-birth questions to assess perinatal risk factors. Your team completes a pre-resuscitation team briefing and equipment check.

Immediately after birth, the baby boy has poor tone and does not cry. The obstetric provider holds him in a warm blanket, gently suctions his mouth and nose with a bulb syringe, and stimulates him to breathe by gently rubbing his back. The baby still has poor tone and irregular respiratory effort. The cord is clamped and cut and he is brought to the radiant warmer. You position his head and neck to open his airway while an assistant continues to provide gentle stimulation. Another provider documents the events as they occur. His tone and respiratory effort quickly improve. Listening with a stethoscope, your assistant reports that the baby's heart rate is 120 beats per minute (bpm) and there are good breath sounds. Five minutes after birth, he still has central cyanosis and a pulse oximetry sensor is secured on his right hand. His oxygen saturation (SpO₂) is below the minute-specific value shown on the Flow Diagram, so he is given supplemental oxygen by holding oxygen tubing close to his face. The oxygen concentration is adjusted so that his oxygen saturation remains within the target range. By 10 minutes after birth, he is breathing regularly and supplemental oxygen has been discontinued. His oxygen saturation remains normal and he is placed skin-to-skin on his mother's chest to continue transition while vital signs and activity are closely monitored for possible deterioration. Shortly afterward, the care team conducts a short debriefing to evaluate its preparation, teamwork, and communication.

The time of birth and clamping the umbilical cord

At the time of birth, a large volume of blood remains in the placenta. If maternal blood is still flowing to the placenta and the umbilical cord is intact, placental gas exchange will continue while additional blood flows to the baby through the umbilical vein. The majority of this placental blood transfusion occurs during the first minute after birth and may play an important role in the transition from fetal to neonatal circulation.

Mark the *time of birth* by starting a timer when the last fetal part emerges from the mother's body. The ideal time for clamping the umbilical cord is the subject of ongoing research. Potential benefits of delayed cord clamping for preterm newborns include decreased mortality, higher blood pressure and blood volume, less need for blood transfusion after birth, fewer brain hemorrhages and a lower risk of necrotizing enterocolitis. In term newborns, delayed cord clamping may decrease the chance of developing iron-deficiency anemia and may improve neurodevelopmental outcomes. Potential adverse effects of delayed cord clamping include delaying resuscitation for compromised newborns and increased risks of polycythemia (high red blood cell concentration) and jaundice.

The current evidence suggests that clamping should be delayed for at least 30 to 60 seconds for most vigorous term and preterm newborns. If cord clamping is delayed, the baby should be placed skin-to-skin on the mother's chest or abdomen, or held securely in a warm, dry towel or blanket. Very preterm newborns may be wrapped in a warm blanket or polyethylene plastic to help maintain their temperature. During the interval between birth and umbilical cord clamping, the obstetric provider and neonatal team should evaluate the baby's tone and breathing effort and begin the initial steps of newborn care described in the remainder of this lesson.

If the placental circulation is not intact, such as after a placental abruption, bleeding placenta previa, bleeding vasa previa, or cord avulsion, the cord should be clamped immediately after birth. Most delayed cord clamping studies have excluded multiple gestations, so there is currently not enough evidence to evaluate the safety of delayed cord clamping in the setting of a multiple gestation birth. Similarly, other scenarios where safety data on delayed cord clamping are limited may benefit from a discussion between the neonatal and obstetric providers to plan whether cord clamping should be delayed. These scenarios may include fetal intrauterine growth restriction (IUGR), abnormal umbilical artery Doppler measurements, abnormal placentation, and other situations where utero-placental perfusion or umbilical cord blood flow are affected. There is not enough evidence to make a definitive recommendation whether umbilical cord clamping should be delayed in newborns who are not vigorous. If the placental circulation is intact, it may be reasonable to briefly delay cord clamping while the obstetric provider clears the airway and gently stimulates the baby to breathe. If the baby does not begin to breathe during this time, additional treatment may be required. The cord should be clamped and the baby brought to the radiant warmer.

Before birth, establish the plan for the timing of umbilical cord clamping with the obstetric providers.

How do you assess the newborn immediately after birth?

After birth, all newborns should have a rapid evaluation to determine if they can remain with their mother to continue transition or if they should be moved to a radiant warmer for further assessment. This initial evaluation may occur during the interval between birth and umbilical cord clamping. You will rapidly evaluate 3 questions.

1. **Does the baby appear to be term?**

   Determine if the baby's appearance is consistent with the expected gestational age. In some situations, the baby's gestational age is unknown before birth. If the baby appears to be term, proceed to the next evaluation question. If the baby appears preterm (less than 37 weeks' gestation), bring the baby to the radiant warmer for the initial steps.

A Rapid Evaluation for Every Newborn

- Term?
- Tone?
- Breathing or crying?

Preterm babies are more likely to require interventions during the transition to extrauterine life. For example, they have more difficulty expanding their lungs, establishing good respiratory effort, and maintaining their body temperature. Because of these risks, preterm babies should have the initial steps of newborn care performed under a radiant warmer. If the baby is born at a late-preterm gestation (34 to 36 weeks) and has stable vital signs with good respiratory effort, the baby can be brought to the mother within several minutes to continue transition.

2. **Does the baby have good muscle tone?**

   Quickly observe the baby's muscle tone. Healthy term babies should be active with flexed extremities (Figure 3.1). Newborns requiring intervention may have flaccid, extended extremities (Figure 3.2).

3. **Is the baby breathing or crying?**

   A vigorous cry is a clear indicator of strong respiratory effort (Figure 3.1). If the baby is not crying (Figure 3.2), observe the baby's chest for breathing effort. Be careful not to be misled by a baby who is gasping. Gasping is a series of deep, single or stacked inspirations that occurs in the setting of severely impaired gas exchange. A gasping baby requires intervention and must be brought to the radiant warmer.

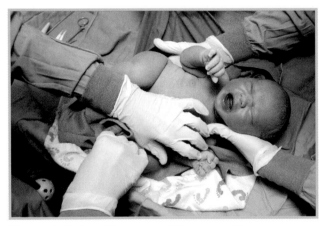

Figure 3.1. Low-risk newborn: full-term, good tone, crying. (Used with permission of Mayo Foundation for Medical Education and Research.)

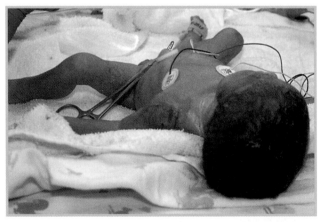

Figure 3.2. High-risk newborn: preterm, poor tone, not crying

What are the initial steps of newborn care?

The initial steps include providing warmth, positioning the head and neck so that the airway is open, clearing the airway of secretions if needed, drying, and providing gentle tactile stimulation. These steps may be initiated during the interval between birth and umbilical cord clamping and should be completed within approximately 30 seconds of birth.

Initial Steps of Newborn Care
• Provide warmth.
• Position the head and neck.
• Clear secretions if needed.
• Dry.
• Stimulate.

Vigorous, term newborn

If the answers to all 3 rapid evaluation questions are "*Yes*" (the baby has been born at term, has good muscle tone, and is breathing or crying), the baby can remain with the mother and have the initial steps performed on the mother's chest or abdomen. Warmth is maintained by direct skin-to-skin contact and covering the baby with a warm towel or blanket (Figure 3.3). If necessary, secretions in the upper airway can be cleared by wiping the baby's mouth and nose with a cloth. Gentle suction with a bulb syringe should be reserved for babies that have meconium-stained fluid, secretions that are obstructing the baby's breathing, and those that are having difficulty clearing their secretions. After the initial steps are completed, continue monitoring the newborn's breathing, tone, activity, color, and temperature to determine if additional interventions are required.

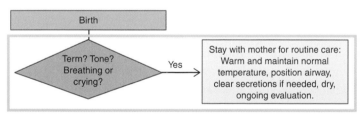

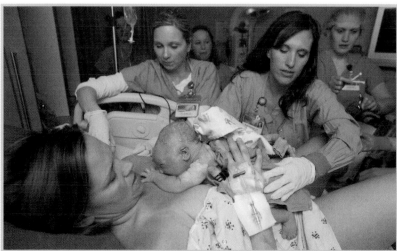

Figure 3.3. Vigorous, term newborn. Initial steps are performed skin-to-skin with mother. (Used with permission of Mayo Foundation for Medical Education and Research.)

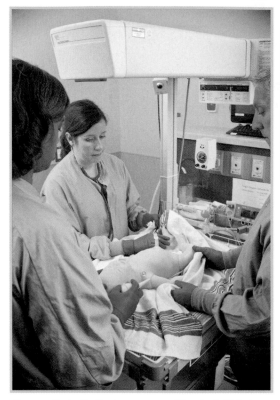

Figure 3.4. Radiant warmer used for the initial steps with high-risk newborns

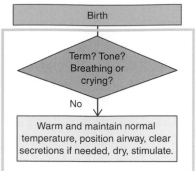

Birth

Term? Tone? Breathing or crying?

No

Warm and maintain normal temperature, position airway, clear secretions if needed, dry, stimulate.

Non-vigorous and preterm newborns

If the answer to any of the initial assessment questions is "*No*", the baby should be brought to a radiant warmer because additional interventions may be required.

- **Provide warmth.**

The baby should be placed under a radiant warmer so that the resuscitation team has easy access to the baby without causing excessive heat loss (Figure 3.4). Leave the baby uncovered to allow full visualization and to permit the radiant heat to reach the baby. If you anticipate that the baby will remain under the warmer for more than a few minutes, apply a servo-controlled temperature sensor to the baby's skin to monitor and control the baby's body temperature. Avoid both hypothermia* and overheating. During resuscitation and stabilization, the baby's body temperature should be maintained between 36.5°C and 37.5°C.

- **Position the head and neck to open the airway.**

The baby should be positioned on her back (supine), with the head and neck neutral or slightly extended in the "sniffing the morning air" position (Figure 3.5). This position opens the airway and allows unrestricted air entry. Avoid hyperextension (Figure 3.6) or flexion of the neck (Figure 3.7) because these positions may interfere with air

---

*After resuscitation, therapeutic hypothermia is indicated for certain high-risk newborns and is further described in Lesson 8.

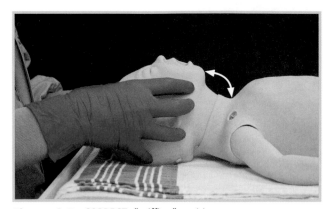

Figure 3.5. CORRECT: "sniffing" position

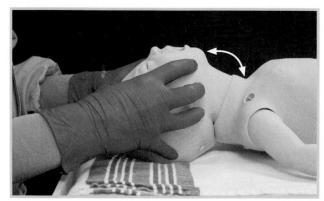

Figure 3.6. INCORRECT: Hyperextension

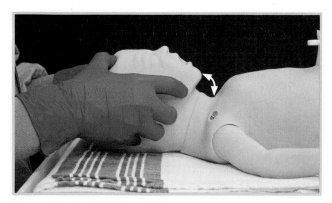

Figure 3.7. INCORRECT: Flexion

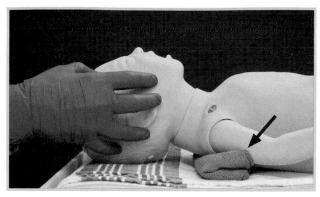

Figure 3.8. Optional shoulder roll for maintaining the "sniffing" position

entry. To help maintain the correct position, you may place a small, rolled towel under the baby's shoulders (Figure 3.8). A shoulder roll is particularly useful if the baby has a large occiput (back of head) from molding, edema, or prematurity.

- **If needed, clear secretions from the airway.**

Clear secretions from the airway if the baby is not breathing, is gasping, has poor tone, if secretions are obstructing the airway, if the baby is having difficulty clearing their secretions, if there is meconium-stained fluid, or if you anticipate starting positive-pressure ventilation (PPV). Secretions may be removed from the upper airway by suctioning gently with a bulb syringe. If the newborn has copious secretions coming from the mouth, turn the head to the side. This will allow secretions to collect in the cheek where they can be removed.

Brief, gentle suction usually is adequate to remove secretions. Suction the mouth before the nose to ensure that there is nothing for the newborn to aspirate if he should gasp when the nose is suctioned. You can remember "mouth before nose" by thinking "M" comes before "N" in the alphabet (Figure 3.9). *Be careful not to suction vigorously or*

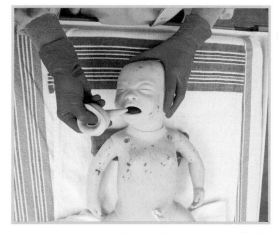
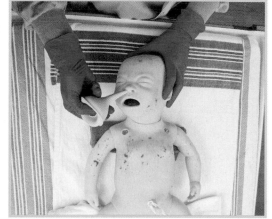

Figure 3.9. Suction the mouth then nose: "M" before "N".

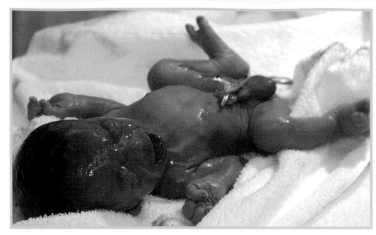

Figure 3.10. Wet skin promotes rapid body cooling.

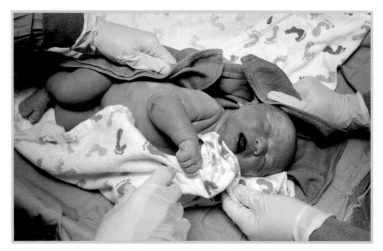

Figure 3.11. Dry the baby and remove wet linen to prevent heat loss and stimulate breathing. Gentle tactile stimulation may also initiate breathing. (Used with permission of Mayo Foundation for Medical Education and Research.)

deeply. Vigorous suction may injure tissues. Stimulation of the posterior pharynx during the first minutes after birth can produce a vagal response leading to bradycardia or apnea.

If using a suction catheter, the suction control should be set so that the negative pressure reads approximately 80 to 100 mm Hg when the tubing is occluded.

• **Dry.**

Wet skin increases evaporative heat loss (Figure 3.10). Place the baby on a warm towel or blanket and gently dry any fluid. If the first towel becomes wet, discard it and use fresh, warm towels or blankets for continued drying (Figure 3.11). If 2 people are present, the second person can be drying the baby while the first person is positioning and clearing the airway.

Drying is not necessary for very preterm babies less than 32 weeks' gestation because they should be covered immediately in polyethylene plastic. The interventions used to reduce heat loss in very preterm babies are described in Lesson 9.

• **Stimulate.**

Positioning, clearing secretions if needed, and drying the baby will frequently provide enough stimulation to initiate breathing. If the newborn does not have adequate respirations, *brief* additional tactile stimulation may stimulate breathing. Gently rub the newborn's back, trunk, or extremities. Overly vigorous stimulation is not helpful and can cause injury. **Never shake a baby.**

After a short period of impaired gas exchange, brief stimulation will initiate spontaneous breathing. However, after a prolonged period of impaired gas exchange, stimulation alone will not work and PPV will be required. If a newborn remains apneic despite rubbing the back or extremities for several seconds, begin PPV as described in the next lesson.

Review

1. Every newborn (does)/(does not) need an initial rapid evaluation of gestational age, muscle tone, and respiratory effort.

2. List the 3 rapid evaluation questions that determine which newborns should be brought to the radiant warmer for the initial steps.

3. List the 5 initial steps of newborn care.

4. When using suction to clear secretions, first suction the newborn's (mouth)/(nose).

5. Which image shows the correct way to position a newborn's head to open the airway (A, B, or C)? _____

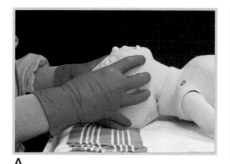
A

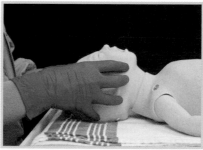
B

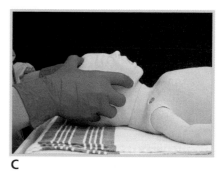
C

Answers

1. Every newborn does need an initial rapid evaluation of gestational age, muscle tone, and respiratory effort.

2. Is the baby term? Does the baby have good tone? Is the baby breathing or crying?

3. Provide warmth, position the head and neck to open the airway, clear secretions from the airway if necessary, dry, and stimulate.

4. When using suction to clear secretions, first suction the newborn's mouth.

5. Image B shows the correct way to position a newborn's head to open the airway.

How do you assess the newborn's response to the initial steps?

Evaluate the newborn's respirations and heart rate to determine if the baby is responding to the initial steps. This should take no more than an additional 30 seconds. If the baby does not have adequate spontaneous respirations and a heart rate of 100 bpm or higher within 1 minute of birth, you should begin PPV. **Remember:** *Ventilation of the baby's lungs is the most important and effective action during neonatal resuscitation.*

- **Respirations**

Assess if the baby is crying or breathing. If the baby is not breathing, or has gasping respirations, proceed directly to PPV. Remember, gasping respirations are ineffective and are treated the same as apnea. The baby's heart rate should be assessed while PPV begins.

- **Heart rate**

If the baby is breathing effectively, the heart rate should be at least 100 bpm. Your initial assessment of the heart rate will be made using a stethoscope. Auscultation along the left side of the chest is the most accurate physical examination method of determining a newborn's heart rate (Figure 3.12). Although pulsations may be felt at the umbilical cord base, palpation is less accurate and may underestimate the true heart rate. While listening, you may tap out the heartbeat on the bed so that your team will also know the heart rate. Estimate the heart rate by counting the number of beats in 6 seconds and multiplying by 10. For example, if you listen for 6 seconds and hear 12 beats, the heart rate is 120 bpm. Clearly report the heart rate to your team members ("*Heart rate is 120 per minute*").

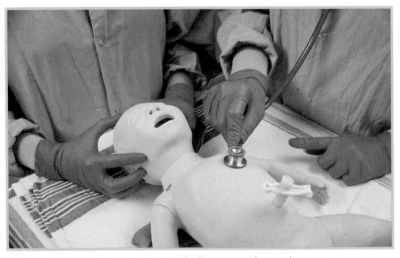

Figure 3.12. Assess the heart rate by listening with a stethoscope.

If you cannot determine the heart rate by physical examination and the baby is not vigorous, ask another team member to quickly connect a pulse oximetry sensor or electronic cardiac (ECG) monitor leads and evaluate the heart rate using a pulse oximeter or ECG monitor (Figure 3.13).

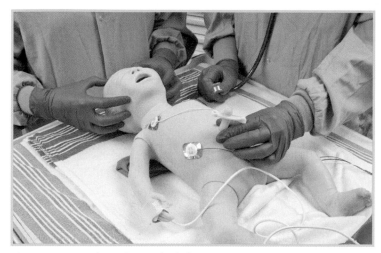

Figure 3.13. Alternative methods for assessing the heart rate: pulse oximetry and ECG monitor

Cautions: Pulse oximetry may not function if the baby's heart rate is low or if the baby has poor perfusion. In this case, monitoring the baby's heart rate with an ECG monitor is the preferred method. In unusual circumstances, an ECG monitor may show an electrical signal, although the heart is not actually pumping blood (pulseless electrical activity). In the newborn, pulseless electrical activity should be treated the same as an absent heart rate (asystole).

After the initial steps, what do you do if the baby is not breathing or the heart rate is low?

- Start PPV if the baby is not breathing (apnea) **OR** if the baby has gasping respirations.

- Start PPV if the baby appears to be breathing, but the heart rate is below 100 bpm.

- Call for immediate additional help if you are the only provider at the warmer.

If the baby has not responded to the initial steps within the first minute of life, *it is not appropriate to continue to provide only tactile stimulation.*

The details of providing PPV using a face mask are described in the next lesson.

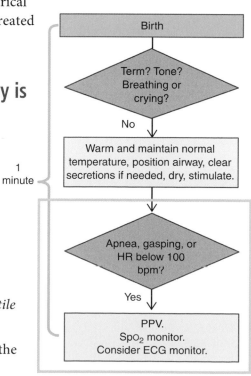

Birth

Term? Tone?
Breathing or
crying?

No

Warm and maintain normal
temperature, position airway, clear
secretions if needed, dry, stimulate.

1 minute

Apnea, gasping, or
HR below 100
bpm?

Yes

PPV.
SpO₂ monitor.
Consider ECG monitor.

What do you do if the baby is breathing and the heart rate is at least 100 bpm, but the baby appears persistently cyanotic?

Cyanosis

The term cyanosis describes skin or mucous membranes with a blue hue caused by poorly oxygenated blood. Cyanosis limited to the hands and feet (acrocyanosis) is a common finding in the newborn and does not indicate poor oxygenation (Figure 3.14). Low oxygen saturation causing the baby's lips, tongue, and torso to appear blue is called central cyanosis. Healthy babies may have central cyanosis for several minutes after birth. Studies have shown that visual assessment of cyanosis is not a reliable indicator of the baby's oxygen saturation and should not be used to guide oxygen therapy. If persistent central cyanosis is suspected, a pulse oximeter should be used to evaluate the baby's oxygenation.

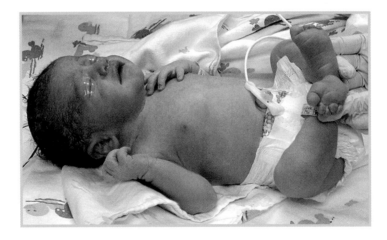

Figure 3.14. Acrocyanosis. This baby has cyanosis of the hands and feet, but the trunk and mucous membranes are pink. Acrocyanosis is normal. Supplemental oxygen is only needed if oxygen saturation is below the target range.

Pulse oximetry

Oxygen is carried by the hemoglobin inside red blood cells. Hemoglobin that is saturated with oxygen absorbs red light differently than hemoglobin that is not carrying oxygen. A pulse oximeter uses a light source and sensor to measure the absorption of red light passing through capillaries in the skin and estimates the portion of hemoglobin that is fully saturated with oxygen (Figure 3.15). The monitor displays the oxygen saturation, which ranges from 0% to 100%. This number is not the same as the partial pressure of oxygen (Po_2) measured by a blood gas machine. The oximeter also displays the baby's heart rate by sensing pulsatile blood flow in the capillaries.

Healthy newborns undergoing normal transition may take several minutes to increase their blood oxygen saturation from approximately 60%, which is the normal intrauterine state, to more than 90%, which

Indications for Pulse Oximetry

- When resuscitation is anticipated
- To confirm your perception of persistent central cyanosis
- When supplemental oxygen is administered
- When positive-pressure ventilation is required

is the eventual state of air-breathing healthy newborns. Figure 3.16 shows the time course of oxygen saturation changes after birth in healthy, full-term newborns breathing room air (21% oxygen). Oxygen saturation values following cesarean birth are slightly lower than those following vaginal birth.

Use pulse oximetry to guide your treatment when resuscitation is anticipated, to confirm your perception of persistent central cyanosis, if you give supplemental oxygen, or if PPV is required. Once the pulse oximeter sensor is attached to the baby, watch the monitor to ensure that it is detecting a pulse with each heartbeat. If you are monitoring the heart rate with an ECG monitor, the heart rate displayed on the pulse oximeter should be the same as the heart rate on the cardiac monitor. Most instruments will not display a saturation reading until a consistent pulse is detected. With good technique, a pulse oximeter will allow accurate assessment of the heart rate and oxygen saturation within approximately 1 to 2 minutes of birth. If the baby has a very low heart rate or poor perfusion, the oximeter may not be able to detect the pulse or oxygen saturation.

Tips for using a pulse oximeter

Proper placement of the pulse oximeter sensor is important.

- The sensor must be oriented correctly so that it can detect the transmitted red light. After placement, it may be helpful to cover the sensor to shield it from light in the room. If the oximeter is not detecting a consistent pulse, you may need to adjust the sensor to be sure that it is positioned opposite the light source.

- The heart and brain receive blood from an artery that attaches to the aorta before the ductus arteriosus. This is often referred to as pre-ductal blood. In most babies, the artery supplying the right arm also attaches to the aorta before the ductus arteriosus. The origin of blood flow to the left arm is less predictable. To measure the oxygen saturation of the pre-ductal blood that is perfusing the heart and brain, *place the pulse oximeter sensor on the right hand or wrist*. The left arm and both legs may have lower oxygen saturation because they may receive blood from the aorta after it has mixed with poorly oxygenated venous blood shunted from the right side of the heart through the ductus arteriosus (post-ductal).

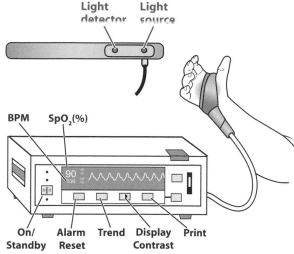

Figure 3.15. Oximeter with sensor attached to a baby's right hand on the hypothenar eminence

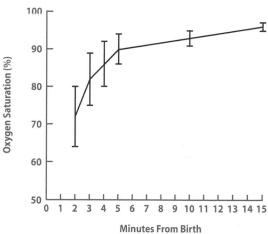

Figure 3.16. Pre-ductal oxygen saturation changes following birth (median and interquartile range). (From Mariani G, Dik PB, Ezquer A, et al. Pre-ductal and post-ductal O_2 saturation in healthy term neonates after birth. *J Pediatr.* 2007;150[4]:418-421.)

Table 3-1. Target Pre-ductal SpO$_2$ After Birth

1 min	60%-65%
2 min	65%-70%
3 min	70%-75%
4 min	75%-80%
5 min	80%-85%
10 min	85%-95%

Target pre-ductal oxygen saturations

When the oximeter has a reliable signal, compare the baby's pre-ductal oxygen saturation with the range of target values in Table 3-1. These values are based on oxygen saturations obtained from healthy, term babies breathing room air during the first 10 minutes of life. The ranges are approximations of the interquartile range and have been adjusted to provide values that are easier to remember. The ideal oxygen saturation after birth has not been established and there is ongoing controversy about which targets should be used. These targets have been selected to represent a consensus of acceptable values.

When is supplemental oxygen indicated and how is it administered?

Supplemental oxygen is used when the oximeter reading remains below the target range for the baby's age. Free-flow oxygen can be given to a spontaneously breathing baby by holding oxygen tubing close to the baby's mouth and nose (Figure 3.17). Free-flow oxygen is not effective if the baby is not breathing.

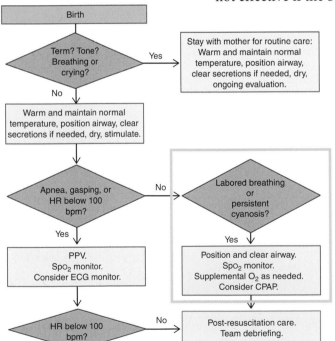

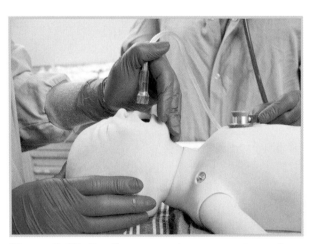

Figure 3.17. Free-flow oxygen given to a spontaneously breathing baby by holding oxygen tubing close to the baby's mouth and nose

You may also use one of the positive-pressure delivery devices described in Lesson 4 (Figure 3.18). If you are using a flow-inflating bag or T-piece resuscitator, hold the mask close to the face, but not so tight that pressure builds up within the mask. You **should not** attempt to administer free-flow oxygen through the mask of a self-inflating bag

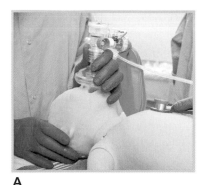
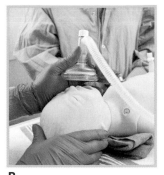
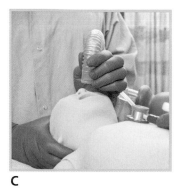

A   **B**   **C**

Figure 3.18. Free-flow oxygen given by a flow-inflating bag (A), a T-piece resuscitator (B), and the tail of a self-inflating bag with an open reservoir (C)
Note: For free-flow oxygen, the mask of a flow-inflating bag and T-piece resuscitator is NOT held tightly against the face.

because gas does not reliably flow through the mask unless the bag is being squeezed. Free-flow oxygen may be administered through the open reservoir ("tail") on some self-inflating bags. You will learn more about these devices in Lesson 4.

Adjusting the oxygen concentration

Guided by pulse oximetry, adjust the oxygen concentration to maintain the baby's minute-specific oxygen saturation within the target range described in Table 3-1. The goal is to prevent hypoxia without using excess oxygen and exposing the newborn to the potential risks of hyperoxia. Adjust the delivered oxygen concentration using compressed air and oxygen, an oxygen blender, and a flowmeter (Figure 3.19).

Compressed air and oxygen

Compressed gases may be built into the wall or obtained from portable tanks. Medical air (21% oxygen) is supplied from high-pressure hoses that are color-coded yellow, and 100% oxygen is supplied from high-pressure hoses that are color-coded green.

Oxygen blender and flowmeter

The compressed gases are connected to a blender, which has a dial that adjusts the gas mixture (21%-100%). The blended gas travels to an adjustable flowmeter. The flowmeter commonly has a floating ball that indicates the rate of gas flow leaving the device. Depending on the size

Free-flow Oxygen Delivery Devices
Oxygen tubing
Oxygen mask
Flow-inflating bag and mask
T-piece resuscitator and mask
Open reservoir ("tail") on a self-inflating bag

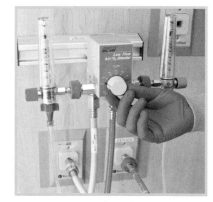

Figure 3.19. Adjust the oxygen concentration with compressed air (inflow from yellow hose), compressed oxygen (inflow from green hose), an oxygen blender, a flowmeter, and patient tubing (outflow from clear tubing). This image shows 2 flowmeters attached to the oxygen blender. Your system may only have 1 flowmeter.

of the flowmeter, you can adjust the dial to achieve gas flows between 0 L/min and 20 L/min. The blended gas, adjusted to the desired concentration and flow rate, is directed through tubing to the oxygen delivery device.

- For free-flow oxygen delivery, **adjust the flowmeter to 10 L/min.**

- Start free-flow oxygen supplementation with the blender set to 30% oxygen. Using the blender, adjust the oxygen concentration as needed to achieve the oxygen saturation target.

If the baby continues to require supplemental oxygen after the first few minutes, how should it be given?

Attempt to gradually decrease the oxygen concentration until the newborn can maintain saturation within the target range without supplemental oxygen. If respirations and heart rate are stable, but the newborn continues to require supplemental oxygen, use pulse oximetry to guide the appropriate oxygen concentration. Air and oxygen administered directly from a compressed source is cold and dry. To prevent heat loss, oxygen given to newborns for a prolonged period of time should be heated and humidified.

If the baby has labored breathing or oxygen saturation cannot be maintained within the target range despite 100% oxygen, you should consider a trial of continuous positive airway pressure (CPAP) or PPV.

What do you do if the baby has labored breathing or persistently low oxygen saturation?

CPAP

CPAP is a method of respiratory support that uses a continuous low gas pressure to keep a spontaneously breathing baby's lungs open. CPAP may be helpful if the airway is open, but the baby has signs of labored breathing or persistently low oxygen saturations. CPAP should only be considered in the delivery room if the baby is breathing and the baby's heart rate is at least 100 bpm.

A trial of CPAP in the delivery room can be given by using a flow-inflating bag or a T-piece resuscitator attached to a mask that is held tightly to the baby's face (Figure 3.20). CPAP **cannot** be given using a self-inflating bag. The equipment and method for administering CPAP are described in more detail in Lesson 4.

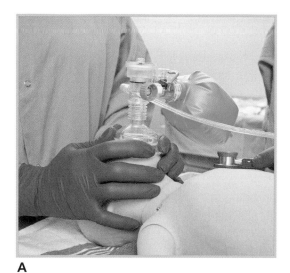 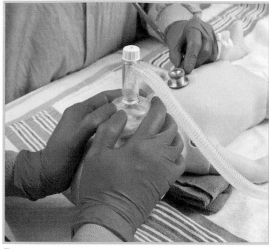

A **B**

Figure 3.20. Administering CPAP using a flow-inflating bag (A) or a T-piece resuscitator (B). Note: For CPAP, the mask is held tightly against the face to create a seal.

Does the presence of meconium-stained amniotic fluid change the approach to the initial steps?

The presence of meconium-stained amniotic fluid may indicate fetal distress and increases the risk that the baby will require resuscitation after birth.

- **Meconium-stained fluid and a vigorous newborn**

If the baby is vigorous with good respiratory effort and muscle tone, the baby may stay with the mother to receive the initial steps of newborn care. Simply use a bulb syringe to gently clear meconium-stained secretions from the mouth and nose.

- **Meconium-stained fluid and a non-vigorous newborn**

If a baby is born through meconium-stained amniotic fluid and has depressed respirations or poor muscle tone, bring the baby to the radiant warmer and perform the initial steps of newborn care as described in this lesson. You will use a bulb syringe to clear secretions from the mouth and nose. If the baby is not breathing or the heart rate is less than 100 bpm after the initial steps are completed, proceed with PPV.

Routine intubation for tracheal suction is not suggested. Previous editions of this textbook recommended routine endotracheal intubation and suction immediately after birth in an effort to reduce the chance of developing meconium aspiration syndrome; however, there is insufficient evidence to continue recommending this practice.

Focus on Teamwork

The initial steps of resuscitation highlight several opportunities for effective teams to use the Neonatal Resuscitation Program® (NRP®) Key Behavioral skills.

Behavior	Example
Anticipate and plan.	Ensure that you have enough personnel present at the time of delivery based on the identified risk factors.
Communicate effectively. Use available information.	Immediately after birth, the obstetric and neonatal care teams need to share their assessment of the newborn. Subsequent interventions will be based on this assessment. The care teams need to communicate their findings clearly and efficiently.
Know your environment.	Know how the pulse oximeter, compressed air and oxygen source, oxygen blender, and flowmeters work in your practice setting. Know what device is available to administer CPAP in your hospital. Know how to obtain an ECG monitor if needed.
Use available resources.	If you cannot auscultate or palpate a heart rate and the baby is not vigorous, quickly place a pulse oximeter sensor or ECG monitor leads and attach them to the appropriate monitor.
Call for additional help when needed.	After the initial steps, if you identify apnea, gasping, or a heart rate less than 100 bpm and you are alone, call for additional help. PPV is required and you will need additional personnel.

Frequently Asked Questions

After birth, do all babies need to have their mouth and nose suctioned with a bulb syringe?

No. Vigorous newborns that are breathing or crying and have good tone do not need to have their mouth and nose suctioned. If necessary, the upper airway can be cleared by wiping the baby's mouth and nose with a cloth. Gentle suction should be reserved for babies with meconium-stained fluid, difficulty clearing their secretions, and secretions obstructing their airway, and those who are not breathing or crying, have poor tone, or require PPV.

Does it matter if the pulse oximeter sensor is attached to the baby's hand or wrist?

For a small baby, some health care providers find it easier to secure the sensor to the baby's wrist; however, some manufacturers recommend placing the pulse oximeter sensor only on the baby's hand. There is evidence that an accurate reading can be obtained using a sensor placed on the baby's wrist. In the studies that established the normal progression of oxygen saturation in healthy newborns, the oximeter sensor was placed on the baby's wrist. Placement on either the hand or wrist is acceptable as long as the transmitted light is detected by the sensor and a reliable signal is obtained.

Previously, the Neonatal Resuscitation Program recommended routine endotracheal intubation and suction for non-vigorous babies born through meconium-stained amniotic fluid. Why is this no longer recommended?

Prior to each edition of the *Textbook of Neonatal Resuscitation,* questions are identified by the neonatology subgroup of the International Liaison Committee on Resuscitation (ILCOR). The scientific evidence is reviewed using a systematic approach and debated in a series of conferences. Treatment recommendations are developed using a method that evaluates the strength of supporting evidence (GRADE). The previous recommendation was largely based on small studies that did not use currently accepted methods to randomly assign babies to different treatment paths. As a result, the conclusions from these studies are subject to bias and the strength of evidence is considered very weak. The most recent ILCOR review determined that there was insufficient evidence to support routine endotracheal suction for non-vigorous babies born through meconium-stained fluid. The NRP Steering Committee's values include avoiding invasive procedures without good evidence of benefit for important outcomes. As a result, the NRP Steering Committee no longer suggests routine endotracheal suction for non-vigorous babies delivered through meconium-stained fluid until additional research demonstrates a benefit from this practice.

The presence of meconium-stained fluid is still considered a risk factor that increases the likelihood that the newborn will require resuscitation. At least 2 qualified people should be present at the time of birth solely to manage the baby. An individual with intubation skill should be identified and immediately available. If additional risk factors indicate that an extensive resuscitation is likely, a qualified team with full resuscitation skills should be present at the time of birth.

Ethical Considerations

Questions to consider

What is a surrogate decision maker?

What role should parents play in treatment decisions?

These questions are explored in detail in Lesson 11.

Key Points

1. Clamping the umbilical cord should be delayed for at least 30 to 60 seconds for most vigorous newborns not requiring resuscitation.

2. There is insufficient evidence to make a definitive recommendation on the timing of umbilical cord clamping for non-vigorous newborns.

3. All newborns require a rapid initial evaluation. Ask if the baby is term, has good muscle tone, and is breathing or crying. If the answer is "NO" to any of these, the newborn should be brought to the radiant warmer for the initial steps of newborn care.

4. A vigorous term newborn may have the initial steps of newborn care performed on the mother's chest or in her arms.

5. The 5 initial steps include the following: provide warmth, position the head and neck, clear secretions from the airway if needed, dry, and stimulate.

6. Avoid vigorous and deep suctioning of the posterior pharynx.

7. After the initial steps are completed, further decisions are based on assessment of breathing and heart rate.

8. Continued use of tactile stimulation in an apneic newborn wastes valuable time. Begin positive-pressure ventilation (PPV) if the baby has not responded to the initial steps within the first minute after birth.

9. To determine heart rate, listen with a stethoscope, count the number of beats in 6 seconds, and multiply the number of beats by 10 (add a zero to the beats counted).

10. If the heart rate cannot be determined by listening with a stethoscope and the baby is not vigorous, use an electronic monitor such as a pulse oximeter or an electronic cardiac (ECG) monitor.

11. Use pulse oximetry and the target oxygen saturation table to guide oxygen therapy when resuscitation is anticipated, to confirm your perception of persistent central cyanosis, if you give supplemental oxygen, or if PPV is required. Visual assessment of cyanosis is not reliable.

12. A healthy newborn breathing room air may take more than 10 minutes to achieve oxygen saturation greater than 90%.

⑬ Free-flow oxygen cannot be given reliably using a mask attached to a self-inflating bag; however, free-flow oxygen may be administered through the open reservoir ("tail") on some self-inflating bags.

⑭ Free-flow supplemental oxygen is not effective if the baby is not breathing.

⑮ CPAP may be helpful if the baby *is* breathing and the heart rate is *at least* 100 beats per minute (bpm), but respirations are labored or the oxygen saturation remains below the target.

⑯ If meconium-stained fluid is present and the baby is vigorous, suction the mouth and nose with a bulb syringe. The baby may remain with the mother for the initial steps. *If the baby is not vigorous*, bring the baby to the radiant warmer to perform the initial steps. Routine intubation for tracheal suction is not suggested.

LESSON 3 REVIEW

1. Every newborn (does)/(does not) need an initial rapid evaluation of gestational age, muscle tone, and respiratory effort.

2. List the 3 rapid evaluation questions that determine which newborns should be brought to the radiant warmer for the initial steps.

3. List the 5 initial steps of newborn care.

4. When using suction to clear secretions, first suction the newborn's (mouth)/(nose).

5. Which image shows the correct way to position a newborn's head to open the airway (A, B, or C)? _____

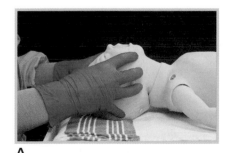

A

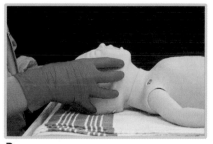

B

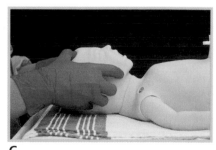

C

6. Which images show the correct way to give free-flow oxygen to a baby? Select all that are correct. (A, B, and/or C).

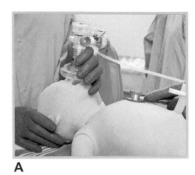 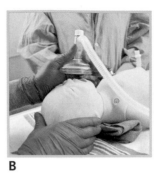 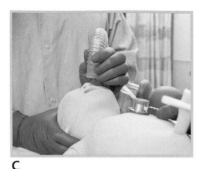

A   B   C

7. Oxygen saturation should be 85% to 95% by (2 minutes of age)/ (10 minutes of age).

8. A flow rate of (2 L/min)/(10 L/min) is used for free-flow oxygen administration.

9. You have provided warmth, positioned the head and neck, cleared the airway, dried, and stimulated a newborn. It is now 60 seconds after birth and she is still apneic and limp. Your next action is to

   A. Continue stimulation by vigorously rubbing her back and extremities.

   B. Give free-flow supplemental oxygen.

   C. Start positive-pressure ventilation.

10. You count a newborn's heartbeat for 6 seconds and count 6 beats. You report the heart rate as (36 beats per minute)/ (60 beats per minute).

11. If a baby *is* breathing, the heart rate is *above* 100 beats per minute, the airway is clear and correctly positioned, but the respirations are labored, you may consider (deep pharyngeal suction)/(CPAP).

Answers

1. Every newborn does need an initial rapid evaluation of gestational age, muscle tone, and respiratory effort.

2. Is the baby term? Does the baby have good tone? Is the baby breathing or crying?

3. Provide warmth, position the head and neck, clear secretions from the airway if necessary, dry, and stimulate.

4. When using suction to clear secretions, first suction the newborn's mouth.

5. Image B shows the correct way to position a newborn's head to open the airway.

6. All are correct.

7. Oxygen saturation should be 85% to 95% by 10 minutes of age.

8. A flow rate of 10 L/min is used for free-flow oxygen administration.

9. Your next action is to start positive-pressure ventilation (Answer C).

10. You report the heart rate as 60 beats per minute.

11. You may consider CPAP.

Additional Reading

Altuncu E, Ozek E, Bilgen H, Topuzoglu A, Kavuncuoglu S. Percentiles of oxygen saturations in healthy term newborns in the first minutes of life. *Eur J Pediatr.* 2008;167(6):687–688

Committee on Obstetric Practices, American College of Obstetricians and Gynecologists. Committee Opinion No. 543: Timing of umbilical cord clamping after birth. *Obstet Gynecol.* 2012;120(6):1522–1526

Katheria A, Rich W, Finer N. Electrocardiogram provides a continuous heart rate faster than oximetry during neonatal resuscitation. *Pediatrics.* 2012;130(5):e1177-e1181

Mariani, G, Dik PB, Ezquer A, et al. Pre-ductal and post-ductal O2 saturation in healthy term neonates after birth. *J Pediatr.* 2007;150(4):418-421

Owen CJ, Wyllie JP. Determination of heart rate in the baby at birth. *Resuscitation.* 2004;60(2):213–217

Phattraprayoon N, Sardesai S, Durand M, Ramanathan R. Accuracy of pulse oximeter readings from probe placement on newborn wrist and ankle. *J Perinatol.* 2012;32(4):276-280

Van Vonderen JJ, Hooper SB, Kroese JK, et al. Pulse oximetry measures a lower heart rate at birth compared with electrocardiography. *J Pediatr.* 2015;166(1):49-53

Lesson 3: Performance Checklist

Initial Steps of Newborn Care

The Performance Checklist Is a Learning Tool

The learner uses the checklist as a reference during independent practice or as a guide for discussion and practice with a Neonatal Resuscitation Program (NRP) instructor. When the learner and instructor agree that the learner can perform the skills correctly and smoothly without coaching and within the context of a scenario, the learner may move on to the next lesson's Performance Checklist.

Knowledge Check

1. What are the 3 rapid assessment questions that determine whether a newborn may stay with his mother or come to the radiant warmer?

2. Which newborns receive the initial steps? What are the 5 initial steps?

3. When do you start the Apgar timer?

4. How do you count a newborn's heart rate?

5. Why do you use pulse oximetry and when is it indicated?

6. What concentration of oxygen is used to initiate resuscitation for the term newborn? What concentration of oxygen is used when initiating free-flow oxygen supplementation?

Learning Objectives

1. Identify the newborn who requires initial steps of resuscitation at the radiant warmer.

2. Demonstrate correct technique for performing initial steps when the newborn stays with his mother, and when the newborn is received at the radiant warmer.

③ Demonstrate accuracy when counting an audible newborn heart rate.

④ Demonstrate correct placement of the oximeter sensor, interpretation of pulse oximetry, and administration of supplemental free-flow oxygen.

Scenario

"You are called to attend a vaginal birth. The mother is in active labor with ruptured membranes. How would you prepare for the birth of this baby? As you work, say your thoughts and actions aloud so I will know what you are thinking and doing."

Option 1: Clear fluid, vigorous term newborn

✔	Critical Performance Steps
Preparation for Resuscitation	
	Assesses perinatal risk (Learner asks 4 pre-birth questions.)
	Gestational age? **"39 weeks' gestation."**
	Clear fluid? **"Amniotic fluid is clear."**
	How many babies? **"One baby is expected."**
	Additional risk factors? **"There are no additional risk factors."**
	Assembles team
	• Identifies leader
	• Delegates tasks
	Performs equipment check
	<div align="center">**"The baby has been born."**</div>
Rapid Evaluation	
	Asks 3 rapid evaluation questions
	• Term? **"Yes."**
	• Muscle tone? **"Yes."**
	• Breathing or crying? **"Yes, the baby is crying."**
	Newborn stays with mother for initial steps
Initial Steps	
	Dries newborn, places skin-to-skin with mother, covers with warm blanket, continues ongoing evaluation of breathing, heart rate, tone, activity, color, and temperature

Option 2: Meconium-stained fluid, vigorous newborn, persistent cyanosis

✔	Critical Performance Steps
	Preparation for Resuscitation
	Assesses perinatal risk (Learner asks 4 pre-birth questions.)
	Gestational age? **"41 weeks' gestation."**
	Clear fluid? **"The fluid is meconium-stained."**
	How many babies? **"One baby is expected."**
	Additional risk factors? **"There are no additional risk factors."**
	Assembles team
	• Identifies leader
	• Delegates tasks
	Performs equipment check
	"The baby has been born."
	Rapid Evaluation
	Asks 3 rapid evaluation questions
	• Term? **"Yes."**
	• Muscle tone? **"Yes."**
	• Breathing or crying? **"Yes, the baby is crying."**
	Newborn stays with mother for initial steps
	Initial Steps
	Suctions mouth and nose with bulb syringe, dries newborn, places skin-to-skin with mother, covers with warm blanket, continues ongoing evaluation of breathing, heart rate, tone, activity, color, and temperature
	"The newborn is 5 minutes old and has central cyanosis that is not resolving."
	Checks breathing **"Breathing, no distress."**
	Checks heart rate **"Heart rate is 140 bpm."**
	Applies pulse oximeter sensor to right hand/wrist **"Pulse oximeter reads 68%."**
	Administers free-flow oxygen using correct technique **"Oxygen saturation is increasing."**
	Monitors oxygen saturation and adjusts blender appropriately per pulse oximetry. Continues to monitor saturation until within target range and stable without oxygen supplementation.

Option 3: Clear fluid, requires initial steps at warmer

✔	Critical Performance Steps
Preparation for Resuscitation	
	Assesses perinatal risk (Learner asks 4 pre-birth questions.) Gestational age? **"Term."** Clear fluid? **"Amniotic fluid is clear."** How many babies? **"One baby is expected."** Additional risk factors? **"Repeated fetal heart rate decelerations have been noted in the last 15 minutes."**
	Assembles team • Identifies leader • Delegates tasks
	Performs equipment check
"The baby has been born."	
Rapid Evaluation	
	Asks 3 rapid evaluation questions • Term? **"Yes."** • Muscle tone? **"No."** • Breathing or crying? **"No."**
Initial Steps	
	Receives baby at radiant warmer
	Positions airway
	Suctions mouth and nose
	Dries with towel or blanket, removes wet linen
	Stimulates by rubbing back or extremities
Checks Vital Signs	
	Checks breathing **"Yes, the baby is crying."**
	Checks heart rate **"The heart rate is 120 bpm."**

Option 4: Clear fluid, requires initial steps at warmer, remains apneic and bradycardic

✔	Critical Performance Steps
Preparation for Resuscitation	
	Assesses perinatal risk (Learner asks 4 pre-birth questions.)
	Gestational age? **"36 weeks' gestation."**
	Clear fluid? **"Amniotic fluid is clear."**
	How many babies? **"One baby is expected."**
	Additional risk factors? **"The mother has a fever."**
	Assembles team
	• Identifies leader
	• Delegates tasks
	Performs equipment check
"The baby has been born."	
Rapid Evaluation	
	Asks 3 rapid evaluation questions
	• Term? **"No, appears 36 weeks' gestation as expected."**
	• Muscle tone? **"No."**
	• Breathing or crying? **"No."**
Initial Steps	
	Receives baby at radiant warmer
	Positions airway
	Suctions mouth and nose
	Dries with towel or blanket, removes wet linen
	Stimulates by rubbing back or extremities
Vital Signs	
	Checks breathing **"Not breathing."**
	Indicates need for PPV (Scenario ends.)

Instructor asks the learner debriefing questions to enable self-assessment such as

1. What is going well so far as you prepare for a birth and make decisions about performing initial steps?

2. How did you know if the newborn required

   a. Initial steps at the radiant warmer?

   b. Supplemental oxygen?

3. How did you use pulse oximetry to guide your actions?

4. What would you do differently when preparing for resuscitation or performing initial steps in our next scenario?

5. Give me an example of how you used at least one of the NRP Key Behavioral Skills.

Neonatal Resuscitation Program Key Behavioral Skills

- Know your environment.
- Use available information.
- Anticipate and plan.
- Clearly identify a team leader.
- Communicate effectively.
- Delegate workload optimally.
- Allocate attention wisely.
- Use available resources.
- Call for additional help when needed.
- Maintain professional behavior.

Positive-Pressure Ventilation

What you will learn

- The characteristics of self-inflating bags, flow-inflating bags, and T-piece resuscitators
- When to give positive-pressure ventilation
- How to position the newborn's head for positive-pressure ventilation
- How to place a resuscitation mask on the newborn's face
- How to administer positive-pressure ventilation and assess effectiveness
- How to use ventilation corrective steps
- How to administer continuous positive airway pressure
- How to place an orogastric tube

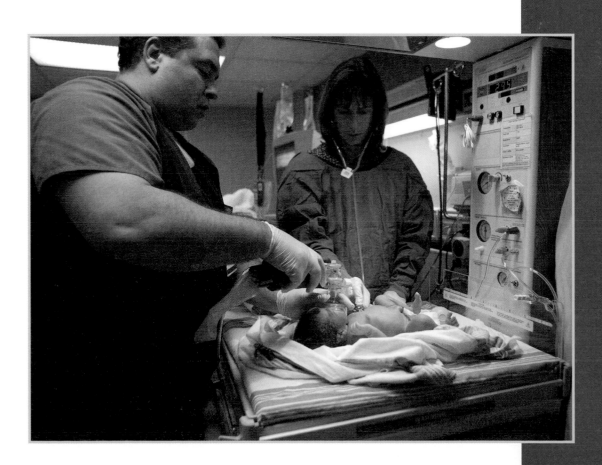

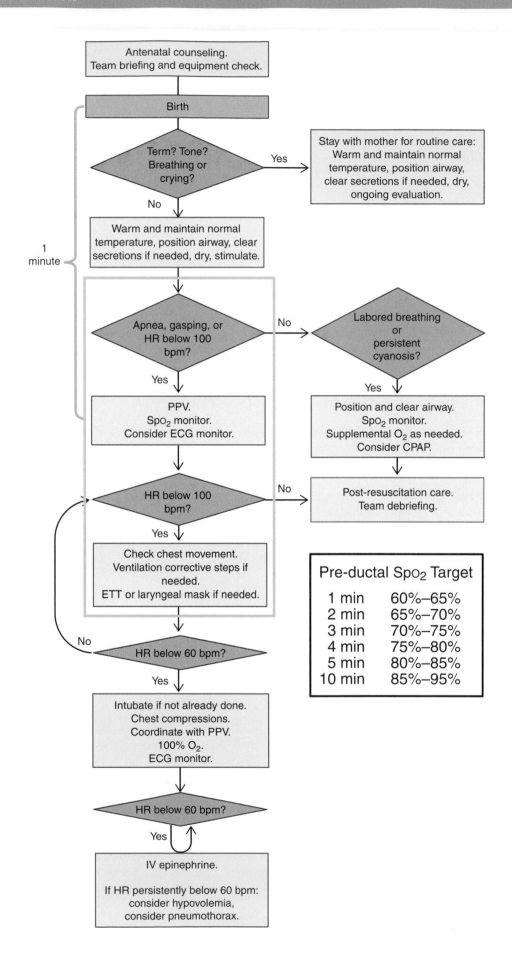

Antenatal counseling.
Team briefing and equipment check.

Birth

Term? Tone?
Breathing or
crying?

Yes → Stay with mother for routine care:
Warm and maintain normal
temperature, position airway,
clear secretions if needed, dry,
ongoing evaluation.

No

1 minute

Warm and maintain normal
temperature, position airway, clear
secretions if needed, dry, stimulate.

Apnea, gasping, or
HR below 100
bpm?

No → Labored breathing
or
persistent
cyanosis?

Yes

PPV.
SpO2 monitor.
Consider ECG monitor.

Yes → Position and clear airway.
SpO2 monitor.
Supplemental O2 as needed.
Consider CPAP.

HR below 100
bpm?

No → Post-resuscitation care.
Team debriefing.

Yes

Check chest movement.
Ventilation corrective steps if
needed.
ETT or laryngeal mask if needed.

HR below 60 bpm?

No

Yes

Intubate if not already done.
Chest compressions.
Coordinate with PPV.
100% O2.
ECG monitor.

HR below 60 bpm?

Yes

IV epinephrine.

If HR persistently below 60 bpm:
consider hypovolemia,
consider pneumothorax.

Pre-ductal SpO2 Target	
1 min	60%–65%
2 min	65%–70%
3 min	70%–75%
4 min	75%–80%
5 min	80%–85%
10 min	85%–95%

The following case is an example of how positive-pressure ventilation (PPV) is provided during resuscitation. As you read the case, imagine yourself as part of the resuscitation team.

Case: Resuscitation with positive-pressure ventilation using a resuscitation bag and mask

A woman with preeclampsia has labor induced at 36 weeks' gestation. During labor, several late fetal heart rate decelerations are noted and your resuscitation team is alerted. When your team arrives, you ask the obstetric provider about additional perinatal risk factors and are told that the baby has intrauterine growth restriction. You complete a pre-resuscitation team briefing and prepare your supplies and equipment. Shortly thereafter, a baby boy is born. The obstetrician gently stimulates him to breathe, but he remains limp and apneic. The umbilical cord is clamped and cut and he is moved to the radiant warmer.

After the initial steps are performed, he is still not breathing. You start PPV with 21% oxygen (room air) as an assistant listens to the baby's heart rate. The assistant reports that the baby's heart rate is 70 beats per minute (bpm), not increasing, and the chest is not moving with the assisted breaths. Another team member places a pulse oximeter sensor on the baby's right hand, attaches it to the oximeter, and begins documenting the events as they occur.

You initiate the ventilation corrective steps. First, you reapply the mask to the face and reposition the baby's head and neck. You restart PPV while your assistant watches the newborn's chest. The assistant reports that there is still no chest movement. You suction the mouth and nose with a bulb syringe and open the baby's mouth. Again, you start PPV, but there is still no chest movement. You gradually increase the inspiratory pressure and the assistant calls out, "*The chest is moving now.*" The assistant listens to the baby's heart rate and reports that it is increasing. Within 30 seconds of achieving ventilation that inflates the baby's lungs, the baby's heart rate is over 100 bpm and oxygen saturation is 64%. The assistant adjusts the oxygen concentration to maintain the baby's oxygen saturation within the minute-specific target range.

You continue PPV while monitoring the baby's respiratory effort. The baby begins to breathe and you gradually decrease the ventilation rate. When the baby is 4 minutes of age, he is breathing consistently, his heart rate is 140 bpm, and oxygen saturation is 80%. You discontinue PPV and use continuous positive airway pressure (CPAP) to maintain his oxygen saturation within the target range. While your team prepares to move the baby to the nursery for post-resuscitation care, you explain the next steps to his mother. Shortly afterward, you meet with your team and conduct a debriefing to evaluate your preparation, teamwork, and communication.

Why does the Neonatal Resuscitation Program® focus on positive-pressure ventilation?

Ventilation of the newborn's lungs is the single most important and effective step in neonatal resuscitation. Learning how to provide PPV is the foundation of neonatal resuscitation. This lesson focuses on assisted ventilation through a face mask. The next lesson describes how to provide ventilation through alternative airways.

Explain the common terminology used to describe positive-pressure ventilation.

Several terms and abbreviations are used to describe PPV (Figure 4.1).

- *Peak inspiratory pressure (PIP):* The highest pressure administered with each breath

- *Positive end-expiratory pressure (PEEP):* The gas pressure maintained in the lungs between breaths when the baby is receiving **assisted breaths**

- *Continuous positive airway pressure (CPAP):* The gas pressure maintained in the lungs between breaths when a baby is **breathing spontaneously**

- *Rate:* The number of assisted breaths administered per minute

- *Inspiratory time (IT):* The time duration (seconds) of the inspiratory phase of each positive-pressure breath

- *Manometer:* A gauge used to measure gas pressure

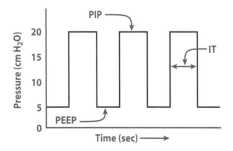

Figure 4.1. Pressure tracing during 3 positive-pressure breaths. PIP = Peak inspiratory pressure, PEEP = positive end-expiratory pressure, IT = inspiratory time.

What are the different types of resuscitation devices used to ventilate newborns?

Three types of devices are commonly used for ventilation.

❶ A *self-inflating bag* fills spontaneously with gas (air, oxygen, or a blend of both) after it has been squeezed and released (Figure 4.2).

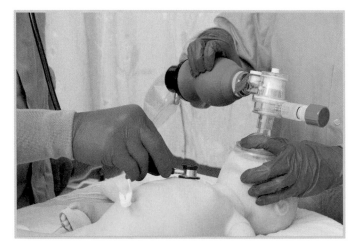

Figure 4.2. Self-inflating bag. Fills spontaneously. Does not need compressed gas or a tight seal to fill.

❷ A *flow-inflating bag* (also called an anesthesia bag) only fills when gas from a compressed source flows into it and the outlet is sealed (Figure 4.3).

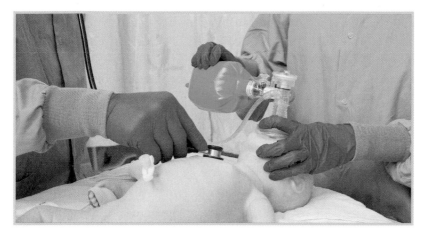

Figure 4.3. Flow-inflating bag. Requires compressed gas and a tight seal to fill.

❸ A *T-piece resuscitator* directs compressed gas toward the baby when an opening on the top of the T-shaped device is occluded (Figure 4.4).

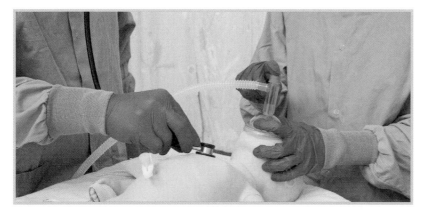

Figure 4.4. T-piece resuscitator. Requires compressed gas to function. Pressures are set by mechanical controls on the device.

Find out what kind of resuscitation device is used in your hospital. If your hospital uses flow-inflating bags or T-piece resuscitators, you should still learn how to use a self-inflating bag. A self-inflating bag should be readily available as a backup wherever resuscitation may be needed in case compressed gas is not available. The 3 devices are briefly described in the following text. Additional details are found in the Appendix to this lesson. You should read those sections of the Appendix that apply to the devices used in your hospital.

Self-inflating bags

A self-inflating bag remains fully inflated unless it is being squeezed (Figure 4.5). Once you release the bag, it recoils and draws fresh gas into the bag. If the bag is attached to an oxygen source, it fills with gas at the supplied oxygen concentration. If the bag is not attached to an oxygen source, it fills by drawing room air (21% oxygen) into the bag. Because the bag self-inflates, it does not require compressed gas or a tight seal at the outlet to remain inflated. The ventilation rate is determined by how often you squeeze the bag and the IT is determined by how quickly you squeeze the bag. Peak inspiratory pressure is controlled by how hard the bag is squeezed. PEEP may be administered if an additional valve is attached to the bag. Because gas does not flow out of the mask unless the bag is being squeezed, a self-inflating bag and mask cannot be used to administer CPAP or free-flow oxygen. Free-flow oxygen may be administered through the open reservoir ("tail") on some self-inflating bags.

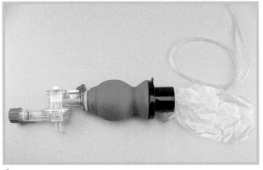 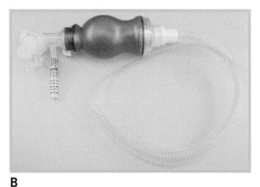

A   B

Figure 4.5. Self-inflating bags with a closed reservoir (A) and an open "tail" reservoir (B). Both bags reinflate automatically without compressed gas.

Most self-inflating bags have a pressure-release valve, also called a pop-off valve, which limits the peak pressure. These valves are usually set to release at 30 to 40 cm H_2O pressure, but they are not reliable and may not release until higher pressures are achieved. Some self-inflating bags have a device that allows the pressure-release valve to be temporarily occluded, allowing higher pressures to be administered. Occluding the pop-off valve should be an unusual occurrence and care must be taken not to use excessive pressure.

Flow-inflating bags

A flow-inflating bag inflates only when a compressed gas source is flowing into the bag and the outlet is sealed, such as when the mask is tightly applied to a baby's face (Figure 4.6A). If compressed gas is not flowing into the bag or the outlet is not sealed, the bag collapses and looks like a deflated balloon (Figure 4.6B). The ventilation rate is determined by how often you squeeze the bag and the IT is determined by how quickly you squeeze and release the bag. Peak inspiratory pressure is controlled by how hard the bag is squeezed and the balance between the amount of gas flowing into the bag and the gas escaping through an adjustable flow-control valve. PEEP, CPAP, and free-flow oxygen are also controlled by this balance in gas flow.

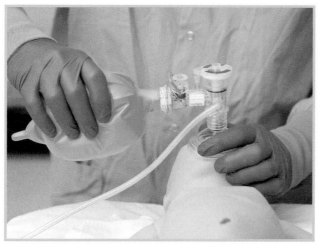
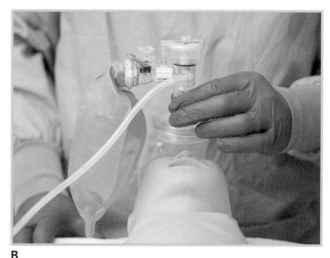

A **B**

Figure 4.6. Flow-inflating bag inflated with compressed gas and a tight seal against the baby's face (A). If compressed gas is not flowing into the bag or the outlet is not sealed, the bag collapses (B).

To ensure that the appropriate pressure is used, a manometer should always be used with a self-inflating or a flow-inflating bag. The manometer may be built into the bag or there may be an attachment site for an external manometer. If the attachment site is left open without a manometer attached, it will cause a large gas leak and prevent the baby from receiving the desired inspiratory pressure. A large leak may prevent a flow-inflating bag from filling.

T-piece resuscitator

A T-piece resuscitator is a mechanical device that uses valves to regulate the flow of compressed gas directed toward the patient (Figure 4.7). Similar to the flow-inflating bag, the device requires a compressed gas source. A breath is delivered by using a finger to alternately occlude and release a gas escape opening on the top of the T-piece cap. When the opening is occluded, gas is directed through the device and toward the baby. When the opening is released, some gas escapes through the cap. The rate is determined by how often you occlude the

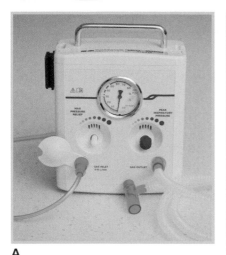
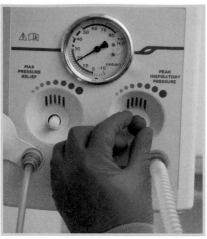
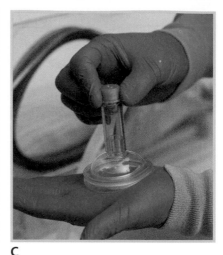

A   B   C

Figure 4.7. A T-piece resuscitator (A). The T-piece resuscitator's pressure is controlled by adjustable valves. Inspiratory pressure is adjusted by a dial on the machine (B) and PEEP is controlled by a dial on the T-piece cap (C).

opening on the cap and the IT is controlled by how long the opening is occluded. There are 2 control dials that are used to limit the inspiratory pressure. The *inspiratory pressure* control limits the PIP during each assisted breath. The *maximum pressure relief control* is a safety feature, similar to the pop-off valve on a self-inflating bag, which prevents the user from increasing the PIP beyond a preset value. This control dial may be covered by a removable shield. An adjustable dial on the T-piece cap controls how much gas is allowed to escape between breaths and, therefore, adjusts the PEEP and CPAP. A built-in manometer measures the inspiratory and expiratory pressure.

What are the indications for positive-pressure ventilation?

After completing the initial steps, PPV is indicated *if the baby is not breathing (apneic), OR if the baby is gasping, OR if the baby's heart rate is less than 100 bpm.* When indicated, PPV should be started within 1 minute of birth.

In addition, a trial of PPV may be considered if the baby is breathing and the heart rate is greater than or equal to 100 bpm, but the baby's oxygen saturation cannot be maintained within the target range despite free-flow oxygen or CPAP.

Immediately call for help if you are alone. Your assistant(s) will monitor the heart rate response to PPV, watch for chest movement, and attach a pulse oximeter to the right hand/wrist.

Indications for Positive-Pressure Ventilation

- Apnea (not breathing)
- Gasping
- Heart rate less than 100 bpm
- Oxygen saturation below the target range despite free-flow oxygen or CPAP

How do you prepare to begin positive-pressure ventilation?

1. Clear secretions from the airway.

If not done already, suction the mouth and nose to be certain that secretions will not obstruct PPV.

2. Position yourself at the baby's head.

The person responsible for positioning the airway and holding the mask on the baby's face is positioned at the baby's head (Figure 4.8). It is difficult to maintain the head, neck, and mask in the correct position when standing at the side or foot of the bed. Team members at the side of the bed are better positioned to assist with pulse oximeter placement and assess chest movement and breath sounds.

3. Position the baby's head and neck.

The baby's head and neck should be neutral or slightly extended in the sniffing position so that the baby's chin and nose are directed upward (Figure 4.9). Improper positioning is one of the most common reasons for ineffective mask ventilation. The airway will be obstructed if the neck is excessively flexed or extended. Because the back of a newborn's head (occiput) is prominent, it may be helpful to lift the shoulders

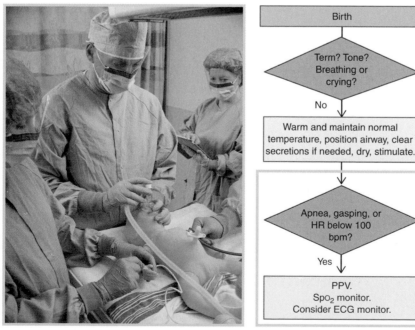

Birth

Term? Tone?
Breathing or
crying?

No

Warm and maintain normal
temperature, position airway, clear
secretions if needed, dry, stimulate.

Apnea, gasping, or
HR below 100
bpm?

Yes

PPV.
SpO$_2$ monitor.
Consider ECG monitor.

Figure 4.8. Position yourself at the baby's head to provide assisted ventilation.

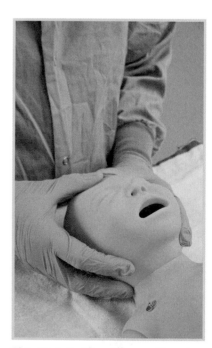

Figure 4.9. The sniffing position

slightly by placing a rolled towel or small blanket under the baby's shoulders (Figure 4.10).

How do you position the mask on the baby's face?

1. Select the correct mask.

A variety of mask sizes should be available at every delivery. Neonatal masks have a cushioned or soft pliable rim and come in 2 shapes—round and anatomically shaped (Figure 4.11). Anatomically shaped masks are made to be placed with the pointed part of the mask fitting over the nose. The mask should rest on the chin and cover the mouth and nose, but not the eyes. The correct mask will create a tight seal on the face (Figure 4.12).

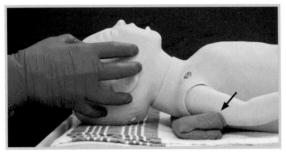

Figure 4.10. Shoulder roll used to position the head and neck

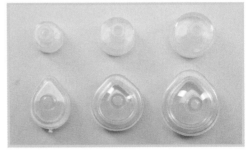

Figure 4.11. Round (top) and anatomic (bottom) face masks

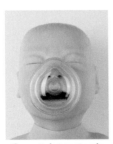 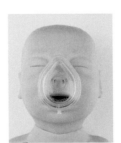 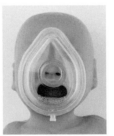 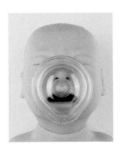

Correct size anatomic Incorrect (small) anatomic Incorrect (large) anatomic Incorrect (upside down) anatomic

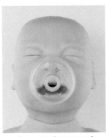 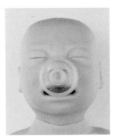 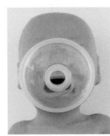

Correct size round Incorrect (small) round Incorrect (large) round

Figure 4.12. Correct and incorrect-sized anatomic and round face masks. The first mask in each row is correct. The remaining masks are incorrect. They are too small, too large, or upside down.

2. Place the mask on the baby's face.

An airtight seal between the rim of the mask and the face is necessary to achieve the pressure that will inflate the lungs *with any resuscitation device.* Ventilation will not be successful if there is a large air leak from an improperly placed mask.

One-Hand Technique:

Begin by cupping the chin in the bottom of an anatomic mask and then bring the mask over the mouth and nose (Figure 4.13). Hold the mask on the face with the thumb and index finger encircling the rim. Place the other 3 fingers under the bony angle of the jaw and gently lift the jaw upward toward the mask. Once the mask is positioned, an airtight seal can be formed by using even, downward pressure on the rim of the mask while holding the head in the sniffing position (Figure 4.14A).

Some round masks are designed to be held by the stem rather than the rim (Figure 4.14B). If you apply pressure to the rim of this type of mask, the mask shape is deformed and will leak.

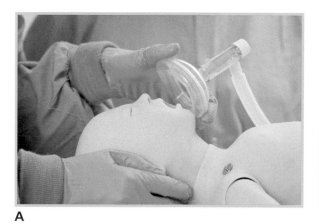 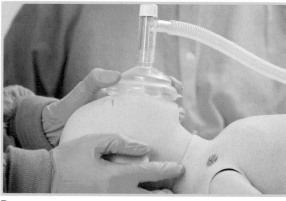

A   **B**

Figure 4.13. (A) Cup the chin in the mask. (B) Bring the mask over the mouth and nose.

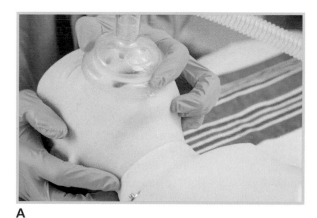 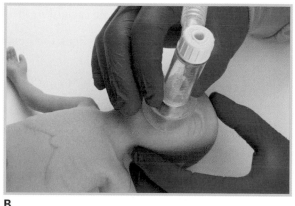

A   **B**

Figure 4.14. Maintaining a seal with the 1-hand technique using an anatomic mask (A) or a round mask (B).

Two-Hand Technique With Jaw Thrust:

It can be difficult to maintain a good seal and the correct head position with 1 hand. If you cannot achieve a good seal, use both hands to hold the mask with the jaw thrust technique. Use the thumb and first finger of both hands to hold the mask against the face. Place the other 3 fingers of each hand under the bony angle of the jaw and gently lift the jaw upward toward the mask (Figure 4.15). While you concentrate on making a good seal and maintaining the correct head position, another team member stands at the baby's side and squeezes the bag or occludes the T-piece cap. A third person monitors the baby's response.

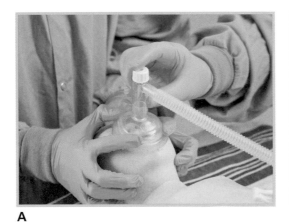
A

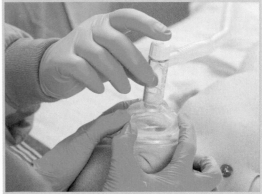
B

Figure 4.15. Two-hand technique with jaw thrust

Precautions

Care must be taken when holding the mask.

- Do not "jam" the mask down on the face. Too much pressure can obstruct the mask, cause air to leak around the side of the mask, inadvertently flex the baby's neck, or bruise the face.

- Be careful not to rest your hand on the baby's eyes.

- Be careful not to compress the soft tissue of the baby's neck.

- Recheck the position of the mask and the baby's head at intervals to make sure they are still correctly positioned.

What concentration of oxygen should be used to start positive-pressure ventilation?

Studies have shown that resuscitation started with 21% oxygen is just as effective as resuscitation started with 100% oxygen. In an attempt to balance the hazards possibly associated with extremes of oxygenation, this program recommends that your goal during and following resuscitation of a newborn should be to achieve an oxygen saturation, as measured by pulse oximetry, that closely mimics the saturation measured in healthy babies born at term. Before birth and throughout intrauterine development, the fetus has a blood oxygen saturation of approximately 60%. After birth, the oxygen saturation gradually increases above 90%. However, even healthy term newborns may take 10 minutes or longer to reach this saturation.

- For the initial resuscitation of newborns **greater than or equal to 35 weeks' gestation,** set the blender to **21% oxygen** (Figure 4.16).

- For the initial resuscitation of newborns **less than 35 weeks' gestation,** set the blender to **21% to 30% oxygen.**

- Set the flowmeter to **10 L/minute** (Figure 4.16).

- An assistant should place a pulse oximeter sensor on the right hand or wrist as soon as possible after PPV is started. Once the oximeter is reading reliably, compare the baby's pre-ductal oxygen saturation with the range of target values summarized in Table 4-1 and adjust the oxygen concentration as needed.

What ventilation rate should be used during positive-pressure ventilation?

Breaths should be given at a rate of *40 to 60 breaths per minute.*

Count out loud to help maintain the correct rate. Use the rhythm, "**Breathe**, *Two, Three*; **Breathe**, *Two, Three*; **Breathe**, *Two, Three*." Say "Breathe" as you squeeze the bag or occlude the T-piece cap and release while you say "Two, Three" (Figure 4.17).

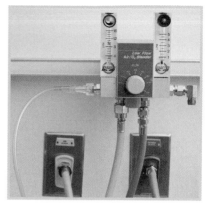

Figure 4.16. Flowmeter set to 10 L/min. Adjust blender to desired oxygen concentration.

Table 4-1. Oxygen saturation target range

Target Pre-ductal Spo$_2$ After Birth	
1 min	60%-65%
2 min	65%-70%
3 min	70%-75%
4 min	75%-80%
5 min	80%-85%
10 min	85%-95%

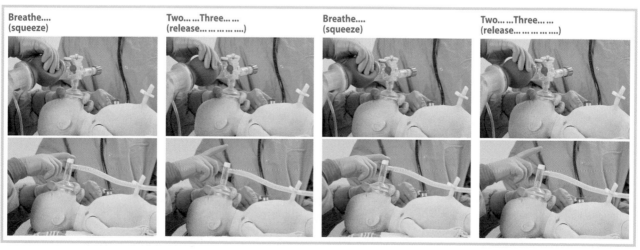

Breathe.... (squeeze)   Two......Three...... (release..............)   Breathe.... (squeeze)   Two......Three...... (release..............)

Figure 4.17. Count the rhythm out loud to maintain the correct rate.

How much pressure should be used to start positive-pressure ventilation?

After birth, fetal lung fluid within the alveoli must be replaced with air for gas exchange to occur. If the baby has not taken a spontaneous breath, the first few assisted breaths may require higher than usual pressure to move fluid out of the air spaces and inflate the alveoli. However, excessively high lung volumes and airway pressures can cause lung injury. The goal is to use just enough pressure to inflate and aerate the lungs so that the heart rate and oxygen saturation increase.

Start with a **PIP of 20 to 25 cm H_2O.** Full-term babies may require a higher inspiratory pressure for the first few breaths to inflate their lungs (30-40 cm H_2O). After the initial inflating breaths, you may be able to decrease the inspiratory pressure.

Administering PEEP with the initial inflating breaths helps to achieve stable lung inflation more quickly, remove fluid, and prevent the air spaces from collapsing during exhalation. **When PEEP is used, the suggested initial setting is 5 cm H_2O.**

Once you inflate the lungs, you should see a gentle rise and fall of the chest with each breath. If the baby appears to be taking very deep breaths during PPV, you are probably using too much pressure and the lungs may become overinflated. This increases the risk of producing an air leak within the lung (pneumothorax). Remember that the volume of a normal breath is much smaller than the amount of gas in your resuscitation bag.

If the baby is preterm, visual assessment of chest movement may be less reliable and the risk of injury from overinflation may be greater. It is possible to achieve successful ventilation without apparent chest movement. Additional details about providing assisted ventilation to preterm newborns are included in Lesson 9.

Review

1. The single most important and most effective step in neonatal resuscitation is (aggressive stimulation)/(ventilation of the lungs).

2. Positive-pressure ventilation is indicated if the baby is _____ or _____, or the heart rate is less than _____ beats per minute after the initial steps. *(Fill in the blanks.)*

3. A baby is born limp and apneic. You place her under a radiant warmer, position her airway, remove secretions, and dry and stimulate her. She does not improve. The next step is to (stimulate her more)/(begin positive-pressure ventilation).

④ If positive-pressure ventilation is given, at least (1)/(2) qualified providers will be needed at the radiant warmer to perform the necessary steps efficiently.

⑤ Which of these devices is a self-inflating bag, a flow-inflating bag, a T-piece resuscitator?

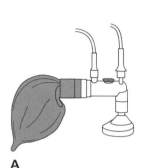 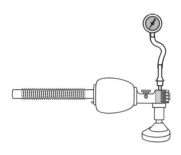 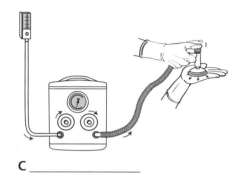

A _____   B _____   C _____

⑥ For positive-pressure ventilation, adjust the flowmeter to (5 L/min)/(10 L/min).

⑦ An anatomically shaped mask should be positioned with the (pointed)/(rounded) end over the newborn's nose.

⑧ Which mask is the correct size and correctly placed on the newborn's face? _____

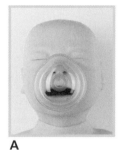 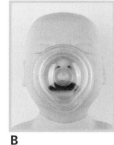 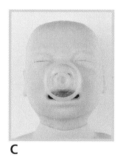

A   B   C

⑨ Administer positive-pressure ventilation at a rate of (20 to 25 breaths per minute)/(40 to 60 breaths per minute).

⑩ Begin positive-pressure ventilation with an inspiratory pressure of (20 to 25 cm H_2O)/(40 to 60 cm H_2O).

⑪ Ventilation of the term newborn begins with (21% oxygen)/(40% oxygen).

⑫ The oxygen concentration used during resuscitation is guided by the use of a (manometer)/(pulse oximeter) that measures the baby's oxygen saturation.

⑬ If you are using a device that administers positive end-expiratory pressure (PEEP), the recommended initial pressure is (5 cm H$_2$O)/ (10 cm H$_2$O).

Answers

① The single most important and most effective step in neonatal resuscitation is ventilation of the lungs.

② Positive-pressure ventilation is indicated if the baby is apneic or gasping, or the heart rate is less than 100 beats per minute after the initial steps.

③ The next step is to begin positive-pressure ventilation.

④ If positive-pressure ventilation is given, at least 2 qualified providers will be needed at the radiant warmer to perform the necessary steps efficiently.

⑤ Figure A= flow-inflating, Figure B= self-inflating, Figure C= T-piece resuscitator.

⑥ For positive-pressure ventilation, adjust the flowmeter to 10 L/min.

⑦ An anatomically shaped mask should be positioned with the pointed end over the newborn's nose.

⑧ Mask A is the correct size and is correctly placed on the newborn's face.

⑨ Administer positive-pressure ventilation at a rate of 40 to 60 breaths per minute.

⑩ Begin positive-pressure ventilation with an inspiratory pressure of 20 to 25 cm H$_2$O.

⑪ Ventilation of the term newborn begins with 21% oxygen.

⑫ The oxygen concentration used during resuscitation is guided by the use of a pulse oximeter that measures the baby's oxygen saturation.

⑬ If you are using a device that administers positive end-expiratory pressure (PEEP), the recommended initial pressure is 5 cm H$_2$O.

How do you evaluate the baby's response to positive-pressure ventilation?

The most important indicator of successful PPV is a rising heart rate. Initiate PPV at the recommended rate and pressure. An assistant will monitor the baby's heart rate response with a stethoscope, pulse oximeter, or an electronic cardiac (ECG) monitor. You will make 2 separate assessments of the baby's heart rate response to PPV. Your first assessment determines if the baby's heart rate is increasing with PPV.

First Heart Rate Assessment: Check the baby's heart rate after 15 seconds of positive-pressure ventilation.

If PPV was started because the baby had a low heart rate, **the baby's heart rate should begin to increase within the first 15 seconds of PPV.** If the heart rate does not increase, you must determine if you are inflating the baby's lungs and take corrective action if necessary.

Heart rate is increasing.

If the baby's heart rate is increasing, the assistant should announce *"Heart rate is increasing."* Continue PPV and do your *second assessment* of the baby's heart rate after another 15 seconds.

Heart rate is not increasing.

If the baby's heart rate is NOT increasing, the assistant should announce *"Heart rate is NOT increasing."* Check for chest movement with the assisted breaths, report the finding, and follow the steps below (Figure 4.19).

> ➤ **Heart rate not increasing - Chest IS moving.**

  - Announce *"Chest IS moving."*
  - Continue PPV that moves the chest.
  - Do your *second assessment* of the baby's heart rate after another 15 seconds of PPV that moves the chest.

> ➤ **Heart rate not increasing - Chest is NOT moving.**

  - Announce *"Chest is NOT moving."*
  - Ventilations are not inflating the lungs. Perform the ventilation corrective steps described in the following text until you achieve chest movement with ventilation.

- Alert the team when chest movement has been achieved.
- Continue PPV that moves the chest.
- Do your *second assessment* of the baby's heart rate after 30 seconds of PPV that moves the chest.

The ventilation corrective steps ("MR. SOPA steps")

The most likely reasons for ineffective mask ventilation are (1) leak around the mask, (2) airway obstruction, and (3) insufficient ventilating pressure. The 6 ventilation corrective steps address these common problems and are summarized in Table 4-2. You may use the mnemonic *"MR. SOPA"* to remember the 6 steps in order—**M**ask adjustment, **R**eposition head, **S**uction airway, **O**pen mouth, **P**ressure increase, and **A**lternative airway. You will perform the corrective steps until you achieve chest movement with assisted breaths. Once chest movement is achieved, the assistant will announce, "The *chest is moving NOW*." You will continue PPV for 30 seconds and assess the baby's heart rate response.

Table 4-2. The 6 Ventilation Corrective Steps: MR. SOPA

	Corrective Steps	Actions
M	Mask adjustment.	Reapply the mask. Consider the 2-hand technique.
R.	Reposition airway.	Place head neutral or slightly extended.
	Try PPV and reassess chest movement.	
S	Suction mouth and nose.	Use a bulb syringe or suction catheter.
O	Open mouth.	Open the mouth and lift the jaw forward.
	Try PPV and reassess chest movement.	
P	Pressure increase.	Increase pressure in 5 to 10 cm H_2O increments, maximum 40 cm H_2O.
	Try PPV and reassess chest movement.	
A	Alternative Airway	Place an endotracheal tube or laryngeal mask.
	Try PPV and assess chest movement and breath sounds.	

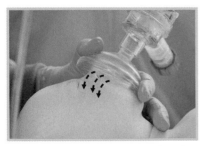

Figure 4.18. Inadequate mask seal on the face may result in ineffective ventilation. Air leak between the cheek and bridge of the nose is common.

M: Mask adjustment.

Reapply the **mask** to the face to form a better seal. Indicators of a good seal include achieving the desired PIP, maintaining the desired PEEP, and rapid reinflation of a flow-inflating bag between breaths. If a leak is present, use a little more pressure on the rim of the mask and lift the jaw upward. Do not press down hard on the baby's face. The most common place for a leak to occur is between the cheek and bridge of the nose (Figure 4.18). If you continue to have difficulty achieving a tight seal, use the **2-hand technique** described previously.

R: Reposition the baby's head.

The airway may be obstructed because the neck is flexed too far forward or is overextended. Reposition the baby's head and neck to ensure that it is neutral or slightly extended (the sniffing position).

After performing the M and R steps, try ventilating again while watching for chest movement. If the chest is not moving, proceed to the next 2 steps.

S: Suction the mouth and nose.

The airway may be blocked by thick secretions. Suction the mouth and nose with a bulb syringe. In unusual situations, thick secretions may be blocking the trachea, and endotracheal intubation for suction may be required.

O: Open the baby's mouth.

Use your finger to open the baby's mouth and reapply the mask.

After performing the S and O steps, try ventilating again while watching for chest movement. If the chest is still not moving, proceed to the next step.

P: Pressure increase.

Although you have an adequate seal and an open airway, inflating the baby's lungs may require a higher inspiratory pressure. Use the manometer to guide adjustments of the inspiratory pressure. Increase the pressure by 5 to 10 cm H_2O increments until you achieve chest movement. The maximum recommended pressure with face-mask ventilation for a term newborn is 40 cm H_2O.

If you are using a T-piece resuscitator, an assistant will need to adjust the PIP dial. If you are using a self-inflating bag, you may need to temporarily occlude the pop-off valve to achieve pressures greater than 30 cm H_2O. Use caution when occluding the pop-off valve.

Try ventilating with gradually increasing pressure while watching for chest movement. If the chest is still not moving with the maximum recommended pressure (40 cm H_2O for term newborn), proceed to the next step.

A: Alternative airway.

Mask ventilation techniques are not always sufficient to inflate the lungs. If you have completed the first 5 corrective steps and you still cannot achieve chest movement, you should insert an alternative airway such as an endotracheal tube or laryngeal mask (Lesson 5). Once an alternative airway is inserted, begin PPV and evaluate the baby's chest movement and breath sounds.

Alert the team when chest movement with ventilation is achieved.

Once you achieve chest movement with each assisted breath, announce, *"The chest is moving NOW."* Continue PPV for 30 seconds. This ensures that your whole team knows when to reevaluate the heart rate response.

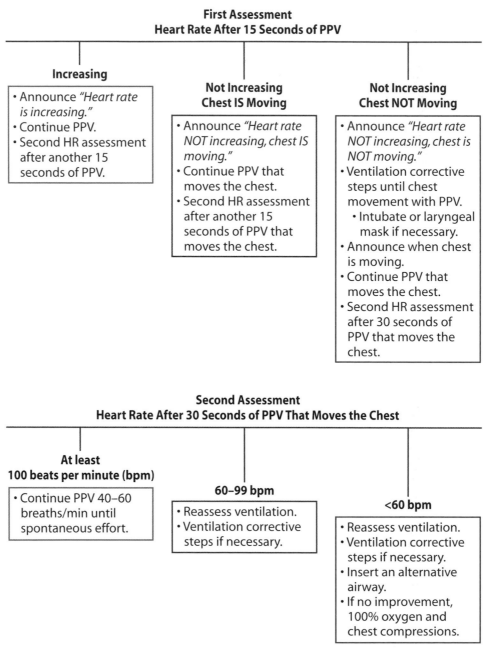

First Assessment
Heart Rate After 15 Seconds of PPV

Increasing
- Announce *"Heart rate is increasing."*
- Continue PPV.
- Second HR assessment after another 15 seconds of PPV.

Not Increasing
Chest IS Moving
- Announce *"Heart rate NOT increasing, chest IS moving."*
- Continue PPV that moves the chest.
- Second HR assessment after another 15 seconds of PPV that moves the chest.

Not Increasing
Chest NOT Moving
- Announce *"Heart rate NOT increasing, chest is NOT moving."*
- Ventilation corrective steps until chest movement with PPV.
  - Intubate or laryngeal mask if necessary.
- Announce when chest is moving.
- Continue PPV that moves the chest.
- Second HR assessment after 30 seconds of PPV that moves the chest.

Second Assessment
Heart Rate After 30 Seconds of PPV That Moves the Chest

At least
100 beats per minute (bpm)
- Continue PPV 40–60 breaths/min until spontaneous effort.

60–99 bpm
- Reassess ventilation.
- Ventilation corrective steps if necessary.

<60 bpm
- Reassess ventilation.
- Ventilation corrective steps if necessary.
- Insert an alternative airway.
- If no improvement, 100% oxygen and chest compressions.

Figure 4.19. Evaluating the baby's response to PPV determines your next steps. The first heart rate check is performed after 15 seconds of PPV. The second heart rate check is performed after 30 seconds of PPV that inflates the lungs.

You will do your *second assessment* of the baby's heart rate after 30 seconds of ventilation that inflates the lungs as indicated by chest movement.

If you have difficulty maintaining chest movement during this time, repeat the ventilation corrective steps as needed. Place an alternative airway if you have persistent difficulty maintaining effective ventilation with a face mask.

Second Heart Rate Assessment: Check the baby's heart rate after 30 seconds of ventilation that inflates the lungs.

> ➤ **The heart rate is greater than or equal to 100 bpm.**

Assisted ventilation has been successful. Continue ventilating at a rate of 40 to 60 breaths per minute (Figure 4.19). Monitor the baby's chest movement, heart rate, and respiratory effort. Adjust the oxygen concentration as needed based on pulse oximetry. When the heart rate is consistently more than 100 bpm, gradually reduce the rate and pressure of PPV, observe for effective spontaneous respirations, and stimulate the baby to breathe. Positive-pressure ventilation may be discontinued when the baby has a heart rate continuously over 100 bpm and sustained spontaneous breathing.

After PPV is stopped, continue to monitor the baby's oxygen saturation and breathing. Free-flow oxygen or CPAP may be required and can be weaned, as tolerated, based on pulse oximetry.

> ➤ **The heart rate is at least 60 bpm, but less than 100 bpm.**

Continue to administer PPV (40-60 breaths per minute) as long as the baby is showing steady improvement. Monitor the oxygen saturation and adjust the oxygen concentration to meet the target saturation range indicated on the table.

If the heart rate remains at least 60 bpm, but less than 100 bpm and **is not** improving, consider each of the following (Figure 4.19):

- Quickly reassess your ventilation technique.
  - Is the chest moving?
  - Does your assistant hear bilateral breath sounds?
  - Perform the ventilation corrective steps if necessary.

- Monitor heart rate, chest movement, respiratory effort, and oxygen saturation.

- Adjust the oxygen concentration to meet the target saturation.

- Consider inserting an alternative airway if one is not already in place.

- Call for additional expertise to help problem solve this situation.

> **The heart rate is less than 60 bpm.**

This uncommon situation occurs when the heart cannot respond to ventilation alone and requires additional support to bring oxygenated blood to the coronary arteries. Consider each of the following (Figure 4.19):

- Quickly reassess your ventilation technique.

  - Is the chest moving?

  - Does your assistant hear bilateral breath sounds?

  - Perform the ventilation corrective steps if necessary.

- Adjust the oxygen concentration to meet the target saturation.

- If not already done, inserting an alternative airway and providing 30 seconds of ventilation through the airway is strongly recommended.

- Call for additional help.

- If the baby's heart rate remains less than 60 bpm despite 30 seconds of PPV that inflates the lungs (chest movement), preferably through an alternative airway, increase the oxygen concentration (FiO_2) to 100% and begin chest compressions as described in Lesson 6.

What do you do if the baby is breathing spontaneously and has a heart rate at least 100 bpm, but has labored breathing or low oxygen saturation despite free-flow oxygen?

If the baby is breathing spontaneously and has a heart rate at least 100 bpm, but has labored respirations or low oxygen saturation, CPAP may be helpful. CPAP is **NOT** appropriate therapy for a baby who is not breathing spontaneously **or** whose heart rate is less than 100 bpm.

The distinction between PEEP and CPAP can be confusing. PEEP refers to pressure maintained between breaths when a baby is receiving assisted breaths. CPAP is a technique for maintaining pressure within the lungs of a *spontaneously breathing* baby. CPAP keeps the lungs slightly inflated at all times and may be helpful for preterm babies whose lungs are surfactant deficient causing the alveoli to collapse at the end of each exhalation. When CPAP is provided, the baby does not have to work as hard to reinflate the lungs with each breath. CPAP also may be beneficial for newborns with retained fetal lung fluid. Using early CPAP, you may be able to avoid the need for intubation and mechanical ventilation.

- ***Administering CPAP during the initial stabilization period***

CPAP is administered by making a tight seal between the baby's face and a mask attached to either a T-piece resuscitator or a flow-inflating bag. CPAP **cannot** be administered with a self-inflating bag even if a PEEP valve has been placed. The desired CPAP is achieved by adjusting the PEEP cap on the T-piece resuscitator or the flow-control valve on the flow-inflating bag (Figure 4.20). Test the amount of CPAP before applying the mask to the baby's face by holding the mask tightly against your hand and reading the pressure on the manometer (pressure gauge). Adjust the PEEP cap or the flow-control valve so that the manometer reads 5 cm H_2O pressure.

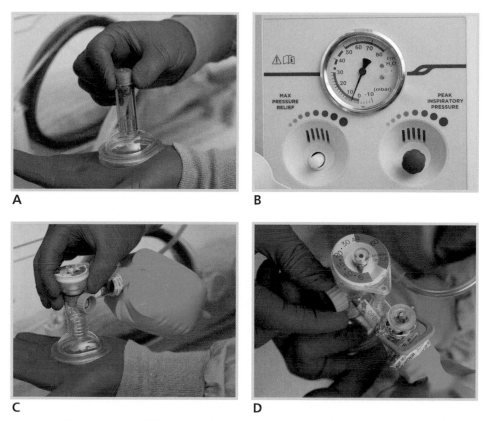

Figure 4.20. Adjust the CPAP pressure by turning the cap on the T-piece resuscitator (A, B) or the flow-control valve on the flow-inflating bag (C, D) before placing the mask on the baby's face.

After you have adjusted the CPAP to the desired pressure, place it firmly against the baby's face (Figure 4.21). Lift the baby's jaw into the mask instead of pushing the baby's head down into the mattress. Check that the pressure is still at the selected level. If it is lower, you may not have a tight seal of the mask on the baby's face. You may adjust the CPAP depending on how hard the baby is working to breathe. Do not use more than 8 cm H_2O. If the baby is not breathing effectively, you need to give PPV breaths instead of CPAP.

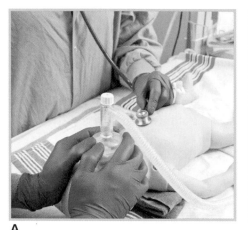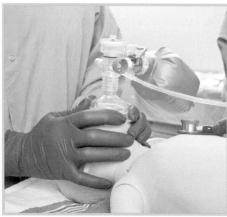

A **B**

Figure 4.21. Administering face-mask CPAP with a T-piece (A) and flow-inflating bag (B). The manometer shows the amount of CPAP administered. A tight seal must be maintained with the mask.

- *Administering CPAP after the initial stabilization period*

If CPAP will be administered for a prolonged period, you will use nasal prongs or a nasal mask (Figure 4.22). After the initial stabilization, CPAP can be administered with a bubbling water system, a dedicated CPAP device, or a mechanical ventilator.

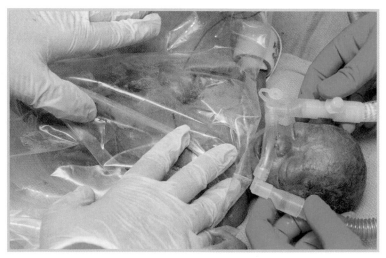

Figure 4.22. CPAP administered to a preterm newborn with nasal prongs.
(Used with permission of Mayo Foundation for Medical Education and Research.)

When should you insert an orogastric tube?

During CPAP or PPV with a mask, gas enters the esophagus and stomach (Figure 4.23). Gas in the stomach may interfere with ventilation. If a newborn requires CPAP or PPV with a mask for longer than several minutes, consider placing an orogastric tube and leaving it uncapped to act as a vent for the stomach.

Equipment needed:

- 8F feeding tube
- Large syringe
- Tape

Insertion steps:

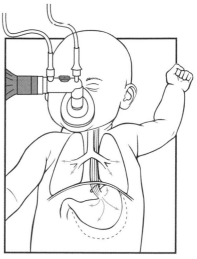

Figure 4.23. Excess gas in stomach from bag-mask ventilation

❶ Measure *the distance from the bridge of the nose to the earlobe and from the earlobe to a point halfway between the xiphoid process (the lower tip of the sternum) and the umbilicus.* Note the centimeter mark at this place on the tube (Figure 4.24). To minimize interruption of ventilation, measurement of the orogastric tube can be approximated with the mask in place.

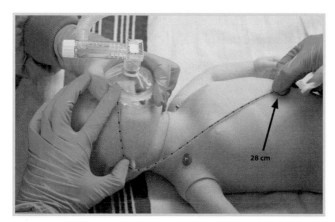

28 cm

Figure 4.24. Measuring the correct insertion depth for an orogastric tube. In this example, the tube should be inserted 28 cm.

❷ Insert the tube through the *mouth* (Figure 4.25A). Ventilation can be resumed as soon as the tube has been placed. Reassess the face-mask seal.

❸ Once the tube is inserted the desired distance, attach a syringe and remove the gastric contents (Figure 4.25B).

❹ Remove the syringe from the tube and leave the end of the tube *open* to provide a vent for air entering the stomach (Figure 4.25C).

❺ Tape the tube to the baby's cheek (Figure 4.25D).

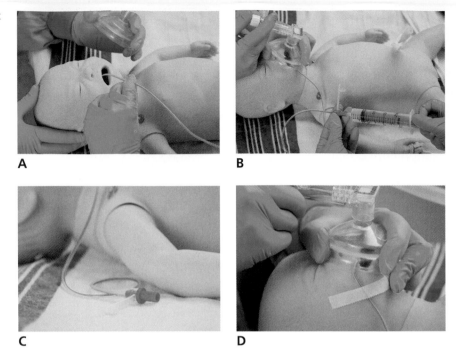

Figure 4.25. Insertion of an orogastric tube (A), aspirating the orogastric tube (B), opening the orogastric tube to vent (C), and securing the orogastric tube with tape (D)

Focus on Teamwork

Providing PPV highlights several opportunities for effective teams to use the Neonatal Resuscitation Program (NRP®) Key Behavioral skills.

Behavior	Example
Anticipate and plan.	Ensure that you have enough personnel present at the time of birth based on the risk factors you identified.
	During your pre-resuscitation team briefing, plan roles and divide responsibilities. Determine who performs PPV, auscultates the heart rate, assesses chest movement, places the pulse oximeter, and documents events as they occur.
Delegate workload optimally. Call for help when needed.	If PPV is required, at least 2 or 3 qualified providers are needed to perform all of the tasks quickly.
	If you have difficulty maintaining a good seal, the 2-hand technique may be required, which requires a second person to administer the assisted breath and a third person to evaluate the response.
	You may need to call for additional help if intubation is required.
Communicate effectively.	The individuals providing PPV and assessing the effectiveness of ventilation must share information and communicate with each other.
	If the ventilation corrective steps are required, frequent information sharing after each step is crucial. It is important to announce when chest movement has been achieved (*"Chest is moving NOW."*) so that the team knows when to evaluate the heart rate response.
Know your environment.	Know how to operate and troubleshoot your PPV device.
Use available resources.	Know how to obtain an electronic cardiac (ECG) monitor.

Frequently Asked Questions

Can a carbon dioxide (CO_2) detector be used to help assess the efficacy of ventilation during the corrective steps?

Yes, using a CO_2 detector during the ventilation corrective steps can provide a visual cue (Table 4-3) that helps you and your team identify when you have achieved ventilation that inflates the lungs. During effective mask ventilation, CO_2 from the baby's lungs will be exhaled through the mask. If you place a CO_2 detector between the mask and the PPV device (bag or T-piece) and you are providing effective ventilation, you should see the detector turn yellow during each exhalation (Figure 4.26). If the CO_2 detector does not turn yellow, your face-mask ventilation attempts may not be aerating the lungs. If the detector remains blue/purple after the first 5 corrective steps and the heart rate has not improved, it is another indication that you have not achieved effective ventilation and an alternative airway is needed.

Table 4-3. Interpreting the CO_2 detector with face-mask ventilation

CO_2 Detector Color	Interpretation
Blue/Purple	Not ventilating the lungs or low cardiac output.
Yellow	Ventilating the lungs.
Initially blue/purple then turns yellow after a ventilation corrective step	The ventilation corrective step was effective; heart rate will likely improve quickly.
Initially turns yellow then returns to blue/purple	Lung ventilation has been lost. Perform the ventilation corrective steps.

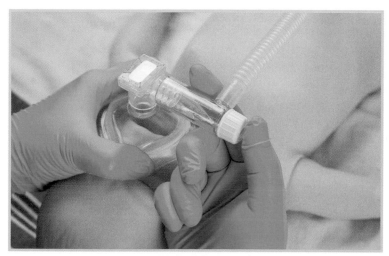

Figure 4.26. Colorimetric CO_2 detector used with face mask during ventilation corrective steps. Color change to yellow suggests ventilation of the lungs.

What are the advantages and disadvantages of each resuscitation device?

The *self-inflating bag* is often considered easier to use and requires little time to set up. Because it fully reinflates even without a seal, you will be less likely to know if you have a large leak between the mask and the baby's face. It is difficult to control the inspiratory time with a self-inflating bag. In addition, the mask cannot be used to administer CPAP to a spontaneously breathing baby.

The *flow-inflating bag* (also called an anesthesia bag) is more complicated to set up and takes more practice to use effectively. It requires a compressed gas source and adjustments to find the correct balance between gas inflow and outflow. The advantage is that you will know immediately if you lose gas pressure or have a leak between the bag and mask because the bag will deflate. Absent or partial inflation of the bag indicates that a tight seal has not been established. An effective face-mask seal is indicated by observing stable PEEP/CPAP on the manometer. The inspiratory time can be increased, if needed, by squeezing the bag for a longer period of time.

The *T-piece resuscitator* also requires some preparation time for setup prior to use. Similar to the flow-inflating bag, it requires a compressed gas source and adjustment to the dials controlling the PIP and PEEP. The primary advantage of the T-piece resuscitator is that it provides more consistent pressure with each breath than either the self-inflating or flow-inflating bag. An effective face-mask seal is indicated by observing stable PEEP/CPAP on the T-piece manometer. In addition, the users may not become fatigued because they are not repeatedly squeezing a bag. The inspiratory time can be increased, if needed, by occluding the hole on the T-piece cap for a longer period of time.

Can you give free-flow oxygen using a resuscitation device?

Free-flow oxygen cannot be given reliably via the mask of a self-inflating bag (Figures 4.27A and 4.27B). Free-flow oxygen may be given through the tail of an open reservoir. If your hospital has self-inflating bags with closed reservoirs, you will need separate tubing to administer free-flow oxygen.

Free-flow oxygen can be given via the mask of a flow-inflating bag or T-piece resuscitator (Figures 4.28A and 4.28B). The mask should be placed close to the face, allowing some gas to escape around the edges. If the mask is held tightly to the face, pressure will build up in the bag or in the T-piece device. If a flow-inflating bag is used, the bag *should not inflate* when used to provide free-flow oxygen. An inflated bag indicates that the mask is tight against the face and positive-pressure is

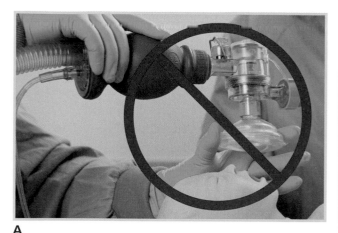

A

Figure 4.27A. INCORRECT. Free-flow oxygen CANNOT be given reliably through the mask of a self-inflating bag.

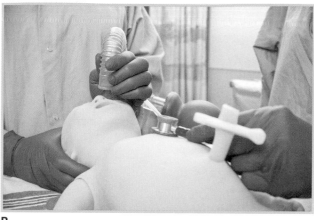

B

Figure 4.27B. CORRECT method for administering free-flow oxygen using the open tail reservoir of this self-inflating bag

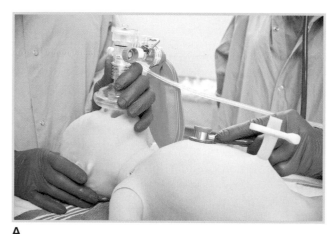

A

Figure 4.28A. Free-flow oxygen with a flow-inflating bag. The mask is held above the face without forming a seal.

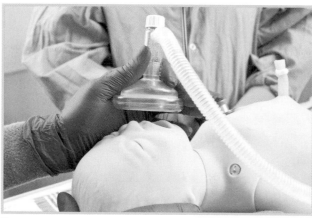

B

Figure 4.28B. Free-flow oxygen with a T-piece resuscitator. The opening on the cap is not occluded. The mask is held above the face without forming a seal.

being provided. If a T-piece is being used, the pressure manometer should read "zero" during free-flow oxygen administration.

Why not routinely use 100% oxygen during all neonatal resuscitations?

Multiple studies in both animals and humans have raised concerns about the safety of routinely using 100% oxygen during neonatal resuscitation. A series of human randomized and quasi-randomized studies over the last 2 decades have demonstrated that resuscitation with 21% oxygen is at least as effective as resuscitation with 100% oxygen. In meta-analyses of these studies, there was a statistically significant decrease in mortality among the babies resuscitated with

21% oxygen. Preterm babies exposed briefly to high oxygen concentration have been shown to have changes in cerebral blood flow and a higher risk of chronic lung disease. Because oxygen has been known to relax pulmonary blood vessels, some have expressed concern that babies resuscitated with lower oxygen concentrations will be more likely to develop pulmonary hypertension. Recent animal studies have shown that pulmonary vascular resistance decreases appropriately with 21% oxygen and that resuscitation with 21% oxygen may actually prevent rebound pulmonary hypertension and preserve the response to inhaled nitric oxide if pulmonary hypertension develops.

Key Points

1. Ventilation of the lungs is the single most important and most effective step in cardiopulmonary resuscitation of the compromised newborn.

2. After completing the initial steps, positive-pressure ventilation (PPV) is indicated if the baby is not breathing, <u>or</u> if the baby is gasping, <u>or</u> if the baby's heart rate is less than 100 beats per minute (bpm). When indicated, PPV should be started within 1 minute of birth. In addition, a trial of PPV may be considered if the baby is breathing and the heart rate is greater than or equal to 100 bpm, but the baby's oxygen saturation cannot be maintained within the target range despite free-flow oxygen or CPAP.

3. Once PPV starts, at least 2 qualified providers are needed to perform all of the necessary steps efficiently. If you are alone, call for immediate assistance.

4. During ventilation, the head should be neutral or slightly extended (sniffing position).

5. An airtight seal between the rim of the mask and the face is essential for providing PPV *with any resuscitation device.*

6. During PPV, the initial oxygen concentration for newborns greater than or equal to 35 weeks' gestation is 21%. The initial oxygen concentration for preterm newborns less than 35 weeks' gestation is 21% to 30%.

7. The ventilation rate is 40 to 60 breaths per minute.

8. The initial ventilation pressure is 20 to 25 cm H_2O.

⑨ The most important indicator of successful PPV is a rising heart rate.

⑩ Check the heart rate after the first 15 seconds of PPV.

⑪ If the heart rate is not increasing within the first 15 seconds of PPV, check for chest movement.

⑫ If the heart rate is not increasing within the first 15 seconds of PPV and you do not observe chest movement, start the ventilation corrective steps.

⑬ The 6 ventilation corrective steps *(MR. SOPA)* are

M: **M**ask adjustment

R: **R**eposition the head

_____

S: **S**uction mouth and nose

O: **O**pen the mouth

_____

P: **P**ressure increase (5-10 cm H_2O increments) to maximum 40 cm H_2O

_____

A: **A**lternative airway (endotracheal tube or laryngeal mask)

_____

⑭ Check the heart rate again after 30 seconds of PPV that inflates the lungs (moves the chest).

⑮ If the heart rate is at least 100 bpm, gradually reduce the rate and pressure of PPV while observing for effective spontaneous respirations and stimulating the baby. Positive-pressure ventilation may be discontinued when the heart rate is continuously greater than 100 bpm and the baby has sustained spontaneous breathing. After PPV is discontinued, use free-flow oxygen or CPAP as necessary to maintain the oxygen saturation within the target range.

⑯ If the heart rate is at least 60 bpm, but less than 100 bpm and not improving despite 30 seconds of PPV that inflates the lungs (chest movement), reassess your ventilation technique, perform the ventilation corrective steps if necessary, adjust the oxygen concentration as indicated by pulse oximetry, consider inserting an alternative airway if not already done, and call for additional expertise.

⑰ If the heart rate remains less than 60 bpm despite at least 30 seconds of PPV that inflates the lungs (chest movement), reassess your ventilation technique, perform the ventilation corrective steps if necessary, adjust the oxygen concentration as indicated by pulse oximetry, insertion of an alternative airway (endotracheal tube or laryngeal mask) is strongly recommended, and call for additional help. If no improvement, increase the oxygen concentration (FiO_2) to 100% and begin chest compressions.

⑱ If you must continue CPAP or PPV with a mask for more than several minutes, an orogastric tube should be inserted to act as a vent for the gas in the stomach during the remainder of the resuscitation.

⑲ To insert an orogastric tube, measure the distance from the bridge of the nose to the earlobe and from the earlobe to a point halfway between the xiphoid process (the lower tip of the sternum) and the umbilicus.

⑳ Self-inflating bags

- Do not require a compressed gas source

- Cannot be used to administer free-flow oxygen reliably through the mask

- Cannot be used to administer CPAP to a spontaneously breathing baby

㉑ Flow-inflating bags

- Require a compressed gas source

- Must have a tight seal to inflate

- Use a flow-control valve to regulate the peak inspiratory pressure (PIP) and positive-end expiratory pressure (PEEP)

- Can be used to administer free-flow oxygen through the mask

- Can be used to administer CPAP to a spontaneously breathing baby

㉒ T-piece resuscitators

- Require a compressed gas source

- Use adjustable dials to select the PIP and PEEP

- Can be used to administer free-flow oxygen through the mask

- Can be used to administer CPAP to a spontaneously breathing baby

LESSON 4 REVIEW

1. The single most important and most effective step in neonatal resuscitation is (aggressive stimulation)/(ventilation of the lungs).

2. Positive-pressure ventilation is indicated if the baby is _____ or _____, or the heart rate is less than _____ beats per minute after the initial steps. *(Fill in the blanks.)*

3. A baby is born limp and apneic. You place her under a radiant warmer, position her airway, remove secretions, and dry and stimulate her. She does not improve. The next step is to (stimulate her more)/(begin positive-pressure ventilation).

4. If positive-pressure ventilation is given, at least (1)/(2) qualified providers will be needed at the radiant warmer to perform the necessary steps efficiently.

5. Which of these devices is a self-inflating bag, a flow-inflating bag, a T-piece resuscitator?

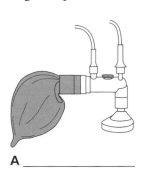 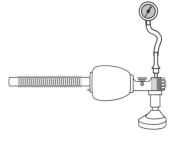 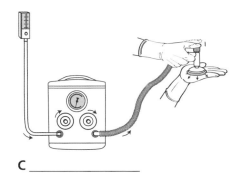

A _____ B _____ C _____

6. For positive-pressure ventilation, adjust the flowmeter to (5 L/min)/(10 L/min).

7. An anatomically shaped mask should be positioned with the (pointed)/(rounded) end over the newborn's nose.

8. Which mask is the correct size and correctly placed on the newborn's face? _____

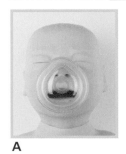 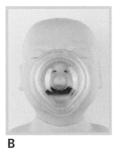 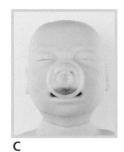

A   B   C

9. Administer positive-pressure ventilation at a rate of (20 to 25 breaths per minute)/(40 to 60 breaths per minute).

10. Begin positive-pressure ventilation with an inspiratory pressure of (20 to 25 cm H_2O)/(40 to 60 cm H_2O).

11. Ventilation of the term newborn begins with (21% oxygen)/(40% oxygen).

12. The oxygen concentration used during resuscitation is guided by the use of a (manometer)/(pulse oximeter) that measures the baby's oxygen saturation.

13. If you are using a device that administers positive end-expiratory pressure (PEEP), the recommended initial pressure is (5 cm H_2O)/(10 cm H_2O).

14. The mnemonic MR. SOPA can be used to remember the 6 ventilation corrective steps. What are each of the steps?
    M: _____ R: _____ then S: _____ O: _____ then P:_____ then A:_____

15. You have started positive-pressure ventilation for an apneic newborn. The heart rate is 40 beats per minute and is not improving with positive-pressure ventilation. Your assistant does not see chest movement. You should (start the ventilation corrective steps)/(proceed to chest compressions).

16. You have started positive-pressure ventilation for an apneic newborn. The heart rate has remained 40 beats per minute despite performing all of the ventilation corrective steps and ventilating through an endotracheal tube for 30 seconds. Your assistant sees chest movement with positive-pressure ventilation. You should (increase the ventilation rate to 100 breaths/minute)/(proceed to chest compressions).

17. You have administered positive-pressure ventilation for an apneic newborn. The baby's heart rate increased rapidly after the first few breaths. The heart rate is now 120 beats per minute, the oxygen saturation is 90%, and the baby is beginning to breathe spontaneously. You should (gradually discontinue positive-pressure ventilation)/(discontinue pulse oximetry).

18. When giving free-flow oxygen with a T-piece resuscitator or flow-inflating bag, you should (hold the mask above the baby's face, allowing some gas to escape around the edges of the mask)/(create a seal by holding the mask tightly to the baby's face).

19. To insert an orogastric tube, measure the distance from the bridge of the nose to the earlobe and from the earlobe (to the nipples)/(to a point halfway between the xiphoid process and the umbilicus).

Answers

1. The single most important and most effective step in neonatal resuscitation is ventilation of the lungs.

2. Positive-pressure ventilation is indicated if the baby is apneic or gasping, or the heart rate is less than 100 beats per minute after the initial steps.

3. The next step is to begin positive-pressure ventilation.

4. If positive-pressure ventilation is given, at least 2 qualified providers will be needed at the radiant warmer to perform the necessary steps efficiently.

5. Figure A= flow-inflating, Figure B= self-inflating, Figure C= T-piece resuscitator.

6. For positive-pressure ventilation, adjust the flowmeter to 10 L/min.

7. An anatomically shaped mask should be positioned with the pointed end over the newborn's nose.

8. Mask A is the correct size and is correctly placed on the newborn's face.

9. Administer positive-pressure ventilation at a rate of 40 to 60 breaths per minute.

10. Begin positive-pressure ventilation with an inspiratory pressure of 20 to 25 cm H_2O.

11. Ventilation of the term newborn begins with 21% oxygen.

12. The inspired oxygen concentration used during resuscitation is guided by the use of a pulse oximeter that measures the baby's oxygen saturation.

13. If you are using a device that administers positive end-expiratory pressure (PEEP), the recommended initial pressure is 5 cm H_2O.

14. **M**ask adjustment, **R**eposition the baby's head, then **S**uction the mouth and nose, **O**pen the baby's mouth, then **P**ressure increase, then **A**lternative airway.

15. You should start the ventilation corrective steps.

16. You should proceed to chest compressions.

17. You should gradually discontinue positive-pressure ventilation.

18. You should hold the mask above the baby's face, allowing some gas to escape around the edges of the mask.

19. Measure the distance from the bridge of the nose to the earlobe and from the earlobe to a point halfway between the xiphoid process and the umbilicus.

Additional Reading

Blank D, Rich W, Leone T, Garey D, Finer N. Pedi-cap color change precedes a significant increase in heart rate during neonatal resuscitation. *Resuscitation.* 2014;85(11):1568-1572

Boon AW, Milner AD, Hopkin IE. Lung expansion, tidal exchange, and formation of the functional residual capacity during resuscitation of asphyxiated neonates. *J Pediatr.* 1979;95(6):1031-1036

Hooper SB, Siew ML, Kitchen MJ, te Pas AB. Establishing functional residual capacity in the non-breathing infant. *Semin Fetal Neonatal Med.* 2013;18(6):336-343

Leone TA, Lange A, Rich W, Finer NN. Disposable colorimetric carbon dioxide detector use as an indicator of a patent airway during noninvasive mask ventilation. *Pediatrics.* 2006;118(1):e202-204

Milner AD, Sauders RA. Pressure and volume changes during the first breath of human neonates. *Arch Dis Child.* 1977;52(12):918-924

O'Donnell CP, Bruschettini M, Davis PG, et al. Sustained versus standard inflations during neonatal resuscitation to prevent mortality and improve respiratory outcomes. *Cochrane Database Syst Rev.* 2015;July 1;7:CD004953

Wood FE, Morley CJ. Face mask ventilation—the dos and don'ts. *Semin Fetal Neonatal Med.* 2013;18(6):344-351

Appendix

Read the section(s) that refers to the type of device used in your hospital.

A. Self-inflating resuscitation bag

What are the parts of a self-inflating bag?

There are 8 basic parts to a self-inflating bag (Figure 4A.1).

1 Gas outlet

2 PEEP valve (optional)

3 Manometer

4 Pressure-release valve

5 Gas inlet

6 Gas tubing

7 (A) Oxygen reservoir (closed type),
(B) Oxygen reservoir (open type)

8 Valve assembly

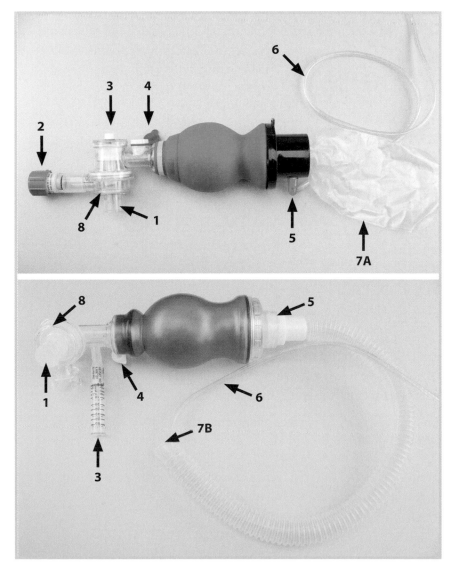

Figure 4A.1. Self-inflating bags with a closed (7A) and an open (7B) reservoir

The self-inflating bag reexpands after being squeezed and fills with gas from 3 locations. As the bag reinflates, air from the room is drawn in from openings in the back of the bag. Gas from the blender and flowmeter travels through *gas tubing* and enters the bag at the *gas inlet.* Gas from the blender collects in the *oxygen reservoir* and provides a third source for gas to fill the bag. Oxygen tubing does not need to be attached for the bag to provide positive-pressure with 21% oxygen. Oxygen tubing must be attached to a compressed gas source to deliver more than 21% oxygen.

The *gas outlet* is where gas exits from the bag to the baby and where a mask or alternative airway is attached.

A *manometer* (pressure gauge) measures the inflating pressure used during positive-pressure ventilation (PPV). Some bags will have a built-in manometer and others will need one attached. The attachment site is usually close to the patient outlet. If the manometer attachment site is left open, without a manometer attached, air will leak out and prevent you from achieving inspiratory pressure. Do not attach the oxygen inflow tubing to the manometer attachment site. This could generate undesired high pressure. Most self-inflating bags also have a *pressure-release (pop-off) valve*. These valves are usually set to release at 30 cm to 40 cm H$_2$O pressure, but they are not reliable and may not release until higher pressures are achieved.

Self-inflating bags have a *valve assembly* positioned between the bag and the patient outlet (Figure 4A.2). When the bag is squeezed during ventilation, the valve opens and directs gas to the patient. When the bag reinflates, the valve is closed. This prevents the patient's exhaled air from entering the bag and being rebreathed. Some self-inflating bags also have an adjustable *PEEP valve*.

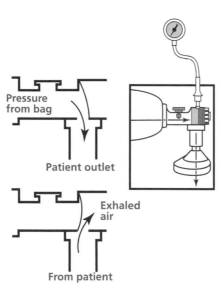

Figure 4A.2. Valve assembly within a self-inflating bag

Why is an oxygen reservoir used on a self-inflating bag?

An oxygen reservoir is an appliance that can be placed over the bag's air inlet. Gas from the blender collects in the reservoir. At very low flow rates, the reservoir prevents blended gas from being diluted with room air. Several different types of oxygen reservoirs are available, but they all perform the same function. Some have open ends ("tails") and others look like a bag covering the air inlet.

How do you test a self-inflating bag before use?

Block the mask or gas outlet with the palm of your hand and squeeze the bag (Figure 4A.3).

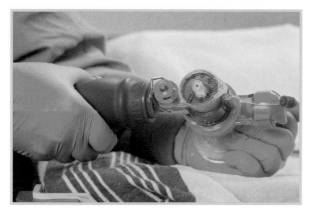

Figure 4A.3. Testing a self-inflating bag

Testing a self-inflating bag	
Block the mask or gas outlet.	If no,
• Do you feel pressure against your hand?	• Is there a crack or leak in the bag?
• Does the manometer register pressure when you squeeze the bag?	• Is the manometer missing, resulting in an open attachment site?
• Does the pressure-release valve open when the manometer registers 30 to 40 cm H_2O pressure?	• Is the pressure-release valve missing or blocked?
• Does the bag reinflate quickly when you release your grip?	

B. Flow-inflating resuscitation bag

What are the parts of a flow-inflating bag?

There are 6 parts to a flow-inflating bag (Figure 4A.4).

❶ Gas outlet

❷ Manometer

❸ Gas inlet

❹ Pressure-release valve (optional)

❺ Gas tubing

❻ Flow-control valve

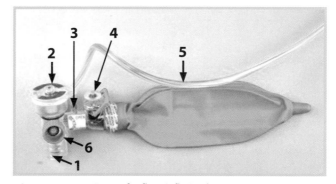

Figure 4A.4. Parts of a flow-inflating bag

Compressed gas from the blender and flowmeter enters the bag through oxygen tubing attached to the *gas inlet.*

The *gas outlet* is where gas exits from the bag to the baby and where a mask or alternative airway is attached. Even if you plan to use 21% oxygen for positive-pressure ventilation (PPV), you must have a compressed gas source to fill the flow-inflating bag.

The *flow-control* valve provides an adjustable leak that allows you to regulate the pressure in the bag when the bag is connected to an endotracheal tube or the mask is held tightly on the patient's face. The adjustable leak allows excess gas to escape rather than overinflate the bag or be forced into the patient.

Flow-inflating bags have a site for attaching a *manometer*. The attachment site usually is close to the patient outlet. A manometer must be attached or the site will be a source of leak and the bag will not inflate properly. A *pressure release (pop-off) valve* may also be present.

How does a flow-inflating bag work?

For a flow-inflating bag to work properly, there must be adequate gas flow from the source and a sealed system (Figure 4A.5). The bag inflation is controlled by the balance between gas entering the bag, gas exiting the adjustable flow-control valve, and gas exiting the gas outlet.

A flow-inflating bag will not inflate adequately if the mask is not properly sealed; flow from the gas source is insufficient, disconnected, or occluded; there is a hole in the bag; the flow-control valve is open too far; or the manometer attachment site has been left open.

Figure 4A.5. Reasons for insufficient inflation of a flow-inflating bag: (A) inadequate mask seal with leak, (B) insufficient gas inflow, (C) hole in bag, (D) flow-control valve open too far, (E) manometer attachment site open

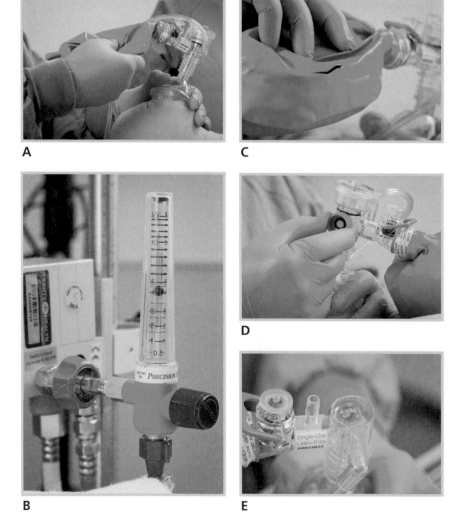

A

C

B

D

E

How do you test a flow-inflating bag before use?

To check a flow-inflating bag, attach it to a compressed gas source. Adjust the flowmeter to 10 L/min. Block the gas outlet to make sure the bag fills properly (Figure 4A.6). Do this by making a seal between the mask and the palm of your hand. Adjust the flow-control valve so that the bag is not over-distended. Watch the pressure gauge, and adjust the valve so that there is 5 cm H_2O pressure when the bag is not being squeezed (PEEP). Next, squeeze the bag at a rate of 40 to 60 times per minute. Check that the bag fills rapidly and you can achieve 30 to 40 cm H_2O pressure when the bag is squeezed firmly (inspiratory pressure). If the bag does not fill rapidly enough, decrease the leak at the flow-control valve or increase the gas flow from the flowmeter. Then, check to be sure that the pressure gauge still reads 5 cm H_2O pressure of PEEP when the bag is not being squeezed. You may need to make further adjustments in the flow-control valve to avoid excessive PEEP.

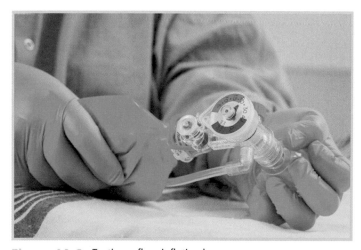

Figure 4A.6. Testing a flow-inflating bag

Testing a flow-inflating bag	
Block the mask or gas outlet. • Does the bag fill properly? • Adjust the flow-control valve to read 5 cm H_2O PEEP. Squeeze the bag 40 to 60 times per minute. • Does the bag reinflate quickly when you release your grip? • Adjust the flow-control valve to read 30 to 40 cm H_2O when squeezed firmly. • Check to be sure that the pressure still reads 5 cm H_2O when not being squeezed (PEEP).	If the bag does not fill correctly, • Is there a crack or hole in the bag? • Is the flow-control valve open too far? • Is the manometer attached? • Is the gas tubing connected securely? • Is the gas outlet sufficiently blocked?

How do you adjust the inflation of a flow-inflating bag?

There are 2 ways that you can adjust the pressure in the bag and thus the amount of inflation of the bag.

- By adjusting the incoming gas from the flowmeter, you regulate how much gas enters the bag.

- By adjusting the flow-control valve on the bag, you regulate how much gas escapes from the bag.

The flowmeter and flow-control valve should be set so that the bag is inflated to the point where it is comfortable to handle and does not completely deflate with each assisted breath (Figure 4A.7A). An overinflated bag (Figure 4A.7B) is difficult to manage and may deliver high pressure to the baby; a pneumothorax or other air leak may develop. An underinflated bag (Figure 4A.7C) makes it difficult to achieve the desired inflation pressure. With practice, you will be able to make the necessary adjustments to achieve a balance. If there is an adequate seal between the baby's face and the mask, you should be able to maintain the appropriate amount of inflation with the flowmeter set at 8 to 10 L/min.

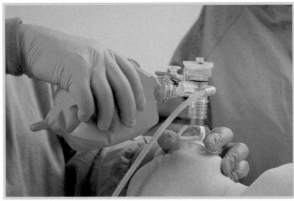

A

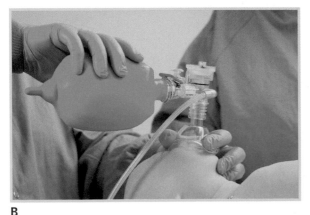

B

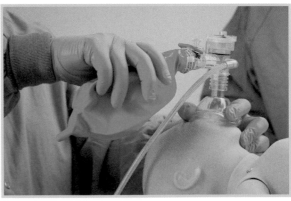

C

Figure 4A.7. Correct flow-inflating bag inflation (A), overinflation (B), and underinflation (C)

C. T-piece Resuscitator

What are the parts of a T-piece resuscitator?

There are 9 parts to a T-piece resuscitator (Figure 4A.8).

① Gas tubing

② Gas inlet

③ Maximum pressure-relief control

④ Manometer

⑤ Inspiratory pressure control

⑥ Gas outlet (proximal)

⑦ T-piece gas outlet (patient)

⑧ T-piece PEEP adjustment dial

⑨ Opening on T-piece cap

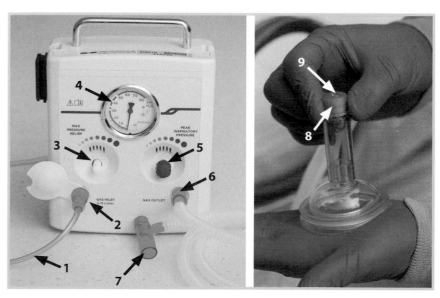

Figure 4A.8. Parts of a T-piece resuscitator

How does a T-piece resuscitator work?

Gas from a compressed source enters the T-piece resuscitator through *gas tubing* at the *gas inlet.* Gas exits the control box from the *gas outlet (proximal),* travels through corrugated tubing to the *T-piece gas outlet (patient),* where a mask or alternative airway attaches. When the *opening on the T-piece cap* is occluded by the operator, the preset inspiratory pressure is delivered to the patient for as long as the T-piece opening is occluded. The maximum pressure that can be used is regulated by the *maximum pressure relief control* valve. *PEEP* is adjusted using a dial on the T-piece cap.

How do you prepare the T-piece resuscitator for use?

Assemble the parts of the T-piece resuscitator as instructed by the manufacturer. Occlude the patient outlet (using a test lung, palm, or finger). Connect the device to the compressed gas source using gas tubing.

Adjust the pressure settings as follows:

- Adjust the blended gas flowmeter on the wall to regulate how much gas flows into the T-piece resuscitator. In most cases, **10 L/min is appropriate.**

- Set the *maximum pressure-relief control* by occluding the T-piece cap with your finger and adjusting the maximum pressure relief dial to a selected value (40 cm H_2O is the recommended maximum for term newborns, with a lower value for preterm newborns). Some manufacturers recommend that the maximum relief control be adjusted to an institution-defined limit when the device is put into original service and not be readjusted during regular use.

- Set the desired peak inspiratory pressure (PIP) by occluding the T-piece cap with your finger and adjusting the *inspiratory pressure control* to the selected pressure (Figure 4A.9).

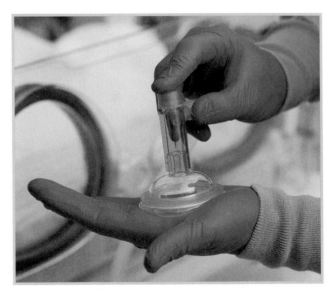
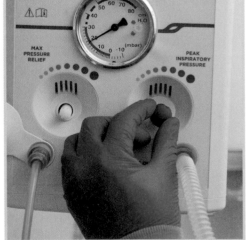

Figure 4A.9. Adjusting the peak inspiratory pressure

- Set the **PEEP** by removing your finger from the T-piece cap and adjusting the dial on the cap to the desired setting (5 cm H_2O is recommended) (Figure 4A.10).

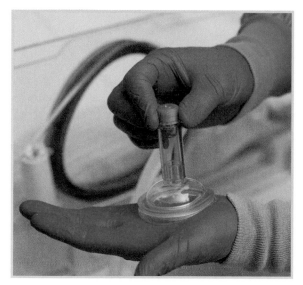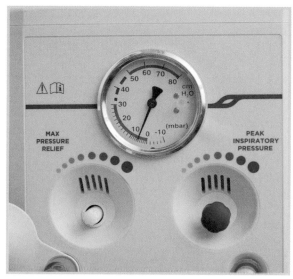

Figure 4A.10. Adjusting the PEEP

When the device is used to ventilate the baby, either by applying the mask to the baby's face or by connecting the device to an endotracheal tube, you administer a breath by alternately covering and releasing the opening on the T-piece cap. The inspiratory time is controlled by how long your finger covers the opening. Be careful not to become distracted and inadvertently cover the opening on the T-piece cap with your finger for a prolonged time.

How do you adjust the concentration of oxygen in a T-piece resuscitator?

The concentration of oxygen delivered by the T-piece resuscitator is controlled by the oxygen blender.

How do you test a T-piece resuscitator before use?

Testing a T-piece resuscitator	
Block the mask or T-piece gas outlet (patient) without occluding the opening on the T-piece cap. • Does the PEEP read 5 cm H_2O? Occlude the opening on the T-piece cap. • Does the peak pressure read 20 to 25 cm H_2O?	If the pressure is incorrect, • Is the T-piece gas outlet sealed? • Is the gas tubing connected to the gas inlet? • Is the gas flow sufficient? • Is the gas outlet (proximal) disconnected? • Is the maximum circuit pressure, peak inspiratory pressure, or PEEP incorrectly set?

Lesson 4: Performance Checklist

Positive-Pressure Ventilation

The Performance Checklist Is a Learning Tool

The learner uses the checklist as a reference during independent practice or as a guide for discussion and practice with a Neonatal Resuscitation Program (NRP) instructor. When the learner and instructor agree that the learner can perform the skills correctly and smoothly without coaching and within the context of a scenario, the learner may move on to the next lesson's Performance Checklist.

Note: If the learner's institution uses a T-piece resuscitator or flow-inflating bag, the learner should also demonstrate proficiency with a self-inflating bag to be used in case of emergency (loss of compressed gas).

Knowledge Check

1. What are the indications for positive-pressure ventilation (PPV)? When can you stop PPV?

2. What is peak inspiratory pressure (PIP)? What is positive end-expiratory pressure (PEEP)? How is continuous positive airway pressure (CPAP) different than PPV?

3. What is the recommended oxygen concentration for beginning PPV for a newborn greater than or equal to 35 weeks' gestation? For a newborn less than 35 weeks' gestation?

4. What is the recommended initial ventilation pressure and rate for a term newborn?

5. What is the most important indicator of ventilation that inflates the lungs?

6. What are the ventilation corrective steps (MR. SOPA)?

7. What is the purpose of an orogastric tube?

8. When can you proceed to chest compressions?

Learning Objectives

1 Identify the newborn that requires PPV.

2 Demonstrate correct technique for administering PPV.

3 Demonstrate the steps for assessing response to PPV.

4 Demonstrate the ventilation corrective steps (MR. SOPA).

5 Identify indications and method for discontinuing PPV.

6 Identify indications for CPAP in the delivery room and demonstrate correct technique for administering CPAP.

7 List pertinent NRP Key Behavioral Skills related to successful PPV.

Scenario

"You are called to attend a vaginal birth. Labor is progressing rapidly. Demonstrate how you would prepare for the birth of this baby. As you work, say your thoughts and actions aloud so I will know what you are thinking and doing."

✔	Critical Performance Steps
Preparation for Resuscitation	
	Assesses perinatal risk. (Learner asks 4 pre-birth questions.)
	Gestational age? **"38 weeks' gestation."**
	Clear fluid? **"Amniotic fluid is clear."**
	How many babies? **"One baby is expected."**
	Additional risk factors? **"Mom has pregnancy-induced hypertension and labor has been induced at 38 weeks' gestation. Several fetal heart rate decelerations have been noted."**
	Assembles team • Identifies leader • Delegates tasks
	Performs equipment check
	"The baby has been born."
Rapid Evaluation	
	Asks 3 rapid evaluation questions • Term? **"Yes."** • Muscle tone? **"No."** • Breathing or crying? **"No, not breathing or crying."**
Initial Steps at Radiant Warmer	
	Receives baby at radiant warmer, positions airway, suctions mouth and nose, dries, removes linen, stimulates

✔	Critical Performance Steps
Vital Signs	
	Checks breathing **"No."**
	Indicates need for PPV
Positive-Pressure Ventilation	
	Positions head in "sniffing" position
	Applies mask correctly
	Starts PPV in room air (21%) at 20-25 cm H_2O (PEEP of 5 cm H_2O if using T-piece or flow-inflating bag); rate 40-60 breaths per minute
	Calls for additional help if alone
	Requests pulse oximetry
	Requests ECG monitor (optional)
	Within 15 seconds of beginning PPV, requests heart rate check to assess if heart rate is increasing **"Heart rate about 40 bpm, not increasing."**
	Assesses chest movement **"No chest movement."**
Ventilation Corrective Steps (MR. SOPA)	
	Mask adjustment **R**epositions head Ventilates, assesses chest movement **"No chest movement."**
	Suctions mouth and nose **O**pens mouth Ventilates, assesses chest movement **"No chest movement, heart rate about 40 bpm."**
	Increases **P**ressure Ventilates, assesses chest movement **"Chest is moving with PPV."** Learner announces, "The chest is moving NOW. Continue PPV for 30 seconds."
Positive-Pressure Ventilation	
	Administers PPV with chest movement x 30 seconds Assesses heart rate **"Heart rate 120 bpm, oxygen saturation 64%, occasional respiratory effort."**
	Continues PPV Directs F_{IO_2} adjustment per oximetry Monitors respiratory effort **"Increasing spontaneous respiratory effort, muscle tone improving, heart rate 140 bpm, SpO_2 74%."**
	Gradually discontinues PPV **"Heart rate 140 bpm, strong and consistent spontaneous respiratory effort."**

✔	Critical Performance Steps
Free-flow Oxygen	
	Discontinues PPV
	Assesses need for free-flow oxygen after discontinuing PPV
	"Heart rate 140 bpm, SpO$_2$ 70%, good spontaneous respiratory effort."
	Administers free-flow oxygen correctly
	Assesses heart rate, oxygen saturation, respiratory status
	"Heart rate 140 bpm, SpO$_2$ 90%, good spontaneous effort."
	Weans and discontinues free-flow oxygen
Vital Signs	
	Monitors heart rate, breathing, oxygen saturation, temperature
	Plans post-resuscitation care
	Updates parents
Scenario Option: CPAP for labored respirations	
	"The newborn has labored breathing with grunting and retracting. Oxygen saturation is 80%, heart rate is 140 bpm."
	Applies CPAP at 5 cm H$_2$O pressure
	Adjust FIO$_2$ per pulse oximetry
	"Heart rate 140 bpm, SpO$_2$ 85%."
	Continues CPAP, adjusts FIO$_2$ per pulse oximetry
	"Baby is ___ minutes old, breathing effort has improved, heart rate 140 bpm, SpO$_2$ 90%."
	Measures placement depth for orogastric tube while CPAP is in progress
	Inserts orogastric tube and aspirates air and gastric contents; leaves orogastric tube open to air
Vital Signs	
	Monitors heart rate, breathing, oxygen saturation, temperature
	Prepares for transport to nursery
	Updates parents

Instructor asks the learner debriefing questions to enable self-assessment, such as

1 How did you know if the newborn required

    a. Positive-pressure ventilation?

    b. Supplemental oxygen after PPV was discontinued?

    c. CPAP in the delivery room?

2 What went well with this practice scenario? How is your team helping you make decisions?

3 What would you do differently when preparing for resuscitation or ventilating a newborn in our next scenario?

4 Give me an example of how you used at least one of the NRP Key Behavioral Skills.

Neonatal Resuscitation Program Key Behavioral Skills

- Know your environment.
- Use available information.
- Anticipate and plan.
- Clearly identify a team leader.
- Communicate effectively.
- Delegate workload optimally.
- Allocate attention wisely.
- Use available resources.
- Call for additional help when needed.
- Maintain professional behavior.

Alternative Airways: Endotracheal Tubes and Laryngeal Masks

What you will learn

- The indications for an alternative airway during resuscitation
- How to select and prepare the equipment for endotracheal intubation
- How to use a laryngoscope to insert an endotracheal tube
- How to determine if the endotracheal tube is in the trachea
- How to use an endotracheal tube to suction thick secretions from the trachea
- When to consider using a laryngeal mask for positive-pressure ventilation
- How to place a laryngeal mask

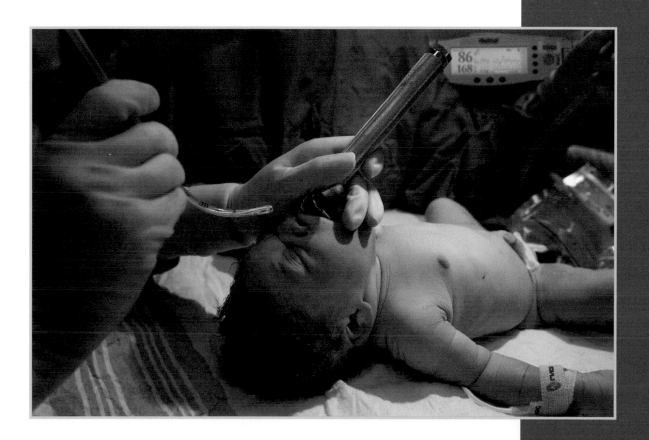

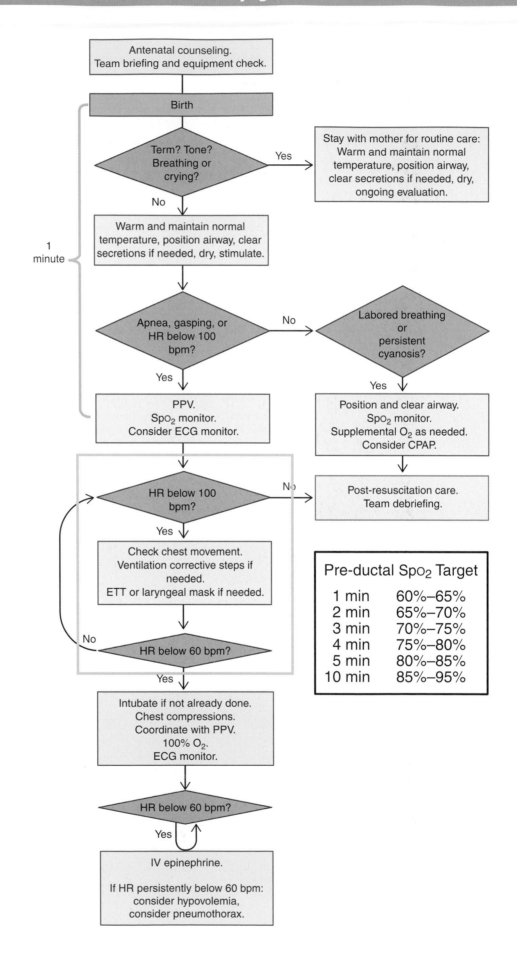

Antenatal counseling.
Team briefing and equipment check.

Birth

Term? Tone?
Breathing or
crying?

Yes → Stay with mother for routine care:
Warm and maintain normal
temperature, position airway,
clear secretions if needed, dry,
ongoing evaluation.

No

Warm and maintain normal
temperature, position airway, clear
secretions if needed, dry, stimulate.

1 minute

Apnea, gasping, or
HR below 100
bpm?

No → Labored breathing
or
persistent
cyanosis?

Yes

PPV.
SpO₂ monitor.
Consider ECG monitor.

Position and clear airway.
SpO₂ monitor.
Supplemental O₂ as needed.
Consider CPAP.

HR below 100
bpm?

No → Post-resuscitation care.
Team debriefing.

Yes

Check chest movement.
Ventilation corrective steps if
needed.
ETT or laryngeal mask if needed.

No

HR below 60 bpm?

Yes

Intubate if not already done.
Chest compressions.
Coordinate with PPV.
100% O₂.
ECG monitor.

HR below 60 bpm?

Yes

IV epinephrine.

If HR persistently below 60 bpm:
consider hypovolemia,
consider pneumothorax.

Pre-ductal SpO₂ Target	
1 min	60%–65%
2 min	65%–70%
3 min	70%–75%
4 min	75%–80%
5 min	80%–85%
10 min	85%–95%

Case 1: Resuscitation with positive-pressure ventilation using an endotracheal tube

A 25-year-old primiparous woman at 37 weeks' gestation is in active labor complicated by maternal fever and fetal tachycardia. Your resuscitation team is called to attend the anticipated vaginal birth. You ask the obstetric provider about perinatal risk factors and complete a pre-resuscitation team briefing. Shortly afterward, a baby girl is born. The obstetrician holds her in a dry blanket and gently stimulates her to breathe, but she remains limp and apneic. The umbilical cord is clamped and cut and she is moved to the radiant warmer where you complete the initial steps of newborn care. After completing the initial steps, she is still apneic and you start positive-pressure ventilation (PPV) while an assistant places a pulse oximeter on her right hand. Her heart rate is 50 beats per minute (bpm) and not increasing. You observe that the chest is not moving with PPV breaths and begin the ventilation corrective steps. After the first 5 corrective steps, the chest is still not moving consistently and your assistant reports that her heart rate is not improving. You decide that an alternative airway should be inserted to improve the effectiveness of PPV.

An assistant holds a 3.5-mm endotracheal tube, provides cricoid pressure, and monitors the procedure time while a qualified provider uses a laryngoscope with a size-1 blade to insert the endotracheal tube. A CO_2 detector is placed on the tube, ventilation is resumed, and the detector turns yellow, indicating that the tube is in the trachea. The baby's chest is moving and her heart rate rapidly increases. Based on the nasal-tragus length (NTL) measurement, the endotracheal tube is held with the 8-cm marking adjacent to the lip. Breath sounds are equal in both axillae, the tube is secured, and PPV continues. You adjust the oxygen concentration based on pulse oximetry. The baby still has poor tone and irregular respiratory effort. You quickly update her parents and transfer her to the nursery for a chest x-ray and additional care. Shortly afterward, your resuscitation team conducts a debriefing to discuss preparation, teamwork, and communication.

What alternative airways are available for neonatal resuscitation?

Endotracheal tubes

Endotracheal tubes (Figure 5.1) are thin tubes that are inserted through the glottis, between the vocal cords, and advanced into the trachea. Although digital intubation using only the operator's

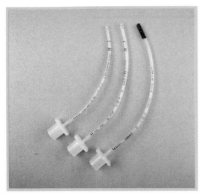

Figure 5.1. Endotracheal tubes (size 2.5, 3.0, 3.5)

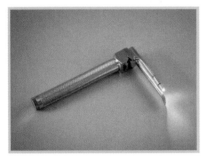

Figure 5.2. Laryngoscope

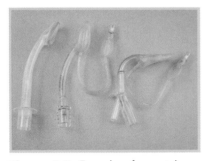

Figure 5.3. Examples of neonatal laryngeal masks (supraglottic devices)

finger has been described, endotracheal intubation typically requires the use of a lighted instrument (laryngoscope, [Figure 5.2]) to visualize the larynx and guide the placement of the tube between the vocal cords.

Laryngeal masks

A laryngeal mask is a small mask attached to an airway tube that is inserted into the mouth and advanced until the mask covers the glottis (Figure 5.3). An endotracheal tube is advanced through the glottis, but the laryngeal mask remains above the glottis, which is why the laryngeal mask is called a supraglottic airway device. The laryngeal mask is an effective alternative when attempts at face-mask ventilation and intubation are unsuccessful. Placement of a laryngeal mask does not require visualization of the larynx or the use of an instrument for insertion. Its use in preterm newborns is limited, in part because the smallest available size may be too large for smaller newborns.

When should an alternative airway be considered?

Insertion of an endotracheal tube or a laryngeal mask should be considered in the following circumstances:

- If PPV with a face mask does not result in clinical improvement, an endotracheal tube or laryngeal mask is strongly recommended to improve ventilation efficacy.

- If PPV lasts for more than a few minutes, an endotracheal tube or a laryngeal mask may improve the efficacy and ease of assisted ventilation.

Insertion of an endotracheal tube is strongly recommended in the following circumstances:

- If chest compressions are necessary, an endotracheal tube will maximize the efficacy of each positive-pressure breath and allow the compressor to give compressions from the head of the bed. If intubation is not successful or feasible, a laryngeal mask may be used.

- An endotracheal tube provides the most reliable airway access in special circumstances, such as (1) stabilization of a newborn with a suspected diaphragmatic hernia, (2) for surfactant administration, and (3) for direct tracheal suction if the airway is obstructed by thick secretions.

What are the important anatomic landmarks in the neonatal airway?

The anatomic landmarks are labeled in Figures 5.4 and 5.5.

❶ **Esophagus:** The passageway extending from the throat to the stomach

❷ **Epiglottis:** The lid-like structure overhanging the glottis

❸ **Vallecula:** The pouch formed by the base of the tongue and the epiglottis

❹ **Larynx:** Portion of the airway connecting the pharynx and trachea

❺ **Glottis:** The opening of the larynx leading to the trachea, flanked by the vocal cords

❻ **Vocal cords:** Mucous membrane-covered ligaments on both sides of the glottis

❼ **Thyroid and cricoid cartilage:** Lower portion of the cartilage protecting the larynx

❽ **Trachea:** Portion of the airway extending from the larynx to the carina

❾ **Carina:** Where the trachea branches into the 2 main bronchi

❿ **Main bronchi:** The 2 air passageways leading from the trachea to the lungs

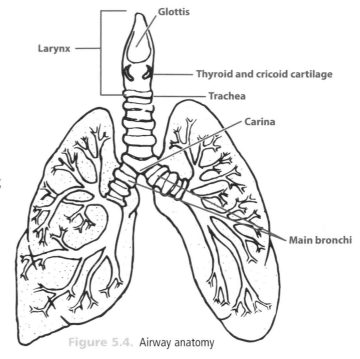

Figure 5.4. Airway anatomy

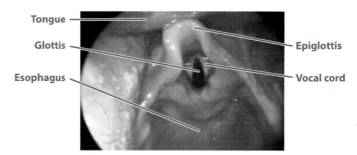

Figure 5.5. Laryngoscopic view of vocal cords and surrounding structures

What equipment should be available for airway insertion?

The equipment necessary to place an alternative airway should be kept together and readily accessible. It is important to anticipate the need for airway insertion and prepare the equipment before a high-risk delivery.

Each delivery room, nursery, and emergency department should have at least one complete set of the following items (Figure 5.6):

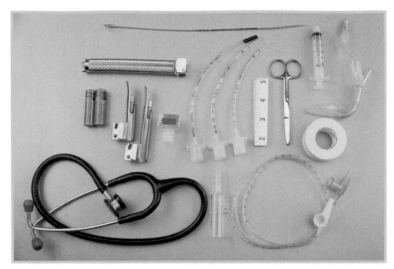

Figure 5.6. Neonatal airway equipment and supplies (supplies removed from sterile packaging for demonstration purposes)

1 Laryngoscope handle with an extra set of batteries and extra bulbs

2 Laryngoscope blades: No. 1 (term newborn), No. 0 (preterm newborn), No. 00 *(optional for very preterm newborn)*. Straight blades (Miller), rather than curved blades (Macintosh), are preferred

3 Endotracheal tubes with internal diameters of 2.5, 3.0, and 3.5 mm

4 Stylet *(optional)* that fits into the tracheal tube

5 CO_2 monitor or detector

6 Suction setup with suction catheters: size 10F or 12F (for suctioning the pharynx), size 8F, and either size 5F or 6F (for suctioning endotracheal tubes of various sizes)

7 Waterproof adhesive tape (1/2 or 3/4 inch), or other tube-securing device

8 Measuring tape and/or endotracheal tube insertion depth table

9 Scissors

10 Meconium aspirator

11 Stethoscope (with neonatal head)

⑫ Positive pressure ventilation device (bag or T-piece resuscitator) and tubing for blended air and oxygen

⑬ Pulse oximeter, sensor and cover

⑭ Laryngeal mask (size 1) or other supraglottic device and 5-mL syringe.

Airway placement should be performed as a clean procedure. All supplies should be protected from contamination by being opened, assembled, and placed back in their packaging until just before use. The laryngoscope blades and handle should be cleaned, following your hospital's procedures, after each use.

Endotracheal Intubation

What type of endotracheal tube should be used?

The endotracheal tube should have a uniform diameter throughout the length of the tube (Figure 5.7A). Tapered and cuffed tubes are not recommended for neonatal resuscitation. Endotracheal tubes have centimeter markings along the side measuring the distance to the tip of the tube. Many tubes will also have lines or markings (Figure 5.7B) near the tip that are intended to be a vocal cord guide. When the tube is inserted so that vocal cords are positioned between the 2 sets of lines, the tip of the tube is expected to be above the carina; however, the location and design of the lines varies considerably between manufacturers. *The vocal cord guide is only an approximation and may not reliably indicate the correct insertion depth.*

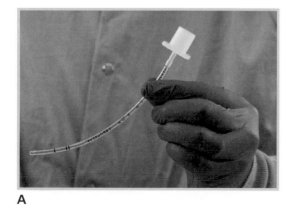
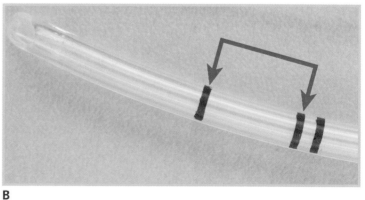

A   B

Figure 5.7. Neonatal endotracheal tube with a uniform diameter (A). This tube has a vocal cord guide that is used to approximate the insertion depth (B). The tube is inserted so that the vocal cords are positioned in the space between the double line and single line (indicated by the arrows). The vocal cord guide is only an approximation and may not reliably predict the correct insertion depth.

How do you prepare the endotracheal tube?

<u>Select the correct size.</u>

Endotracheal tubes are described by the size of their internal diameter (mm ID). The appropriate endotracheal tube diameter is estimated from the baby's weight or gestational age. Table 5-1 gives the recommended endotracheal tube size for various weight and gestational-age categories. Using a tube that is too small increases the resistance to air flow and the chance that it will become obstructed by secretions. Using a tube that is too large may traumatize the airway.

Table 5-1. Endotracheal tube size for babies of various weights and gestational ages

Weight (g)	Gestational Age (wks)	Endotracheal Tube Size (mm ID)
Below 1,000	Below 28	2.5
1,000-2,000	28-34	3.0
Greater than 2,000	Greater than 34	3.5

<u>Consider using a stylet.</u>

Many operators find it helpful to use a stylet with the endotracheal tube to provide additional rigidity and curvature (Figure 5.8). Use of a stylet is optional and depends on the operator's preference. When inserting a stylet, it is important to ensure that the tip is not protruding from either the end or side hole of the endotracheal tube. If the tip is protruding, it may cause trauma to the tissues. The stylet should be secured with a plug, or bent at the top, so that it cannot advance farther into the tube during the insertion procedure.

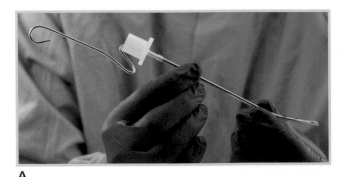

A

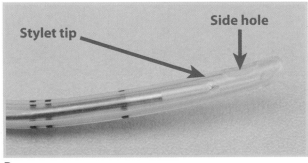

B

Figure 5.8. Optional stylet for increasing endotracheal tube stiffness and maintaining curvature during intubation

How do you prepare the laryngoscope and other equipment you will need?

The following steps describe how to prepare the equipment used for intubation:

1. Select the appropriate laryngoscope blade and attach it to the handle.

   a. Use a No. 1 blade for term newborns.

   b. Use a No. 0 blade for preterm newborns. Some operators may prefer to use a No. 00 blade for extremely preterm newborns.

2. Turn on the light by clicking the blade into the open position to verify that the batteries and light are working. If the light is dim or flickers, tighten or replace the bulb, insert a new battery, or replace the laryngoscope.

3. Prepare the suction equipment. Occlude the end of the suction tubing to ensure that the suction is set to 80 to 100 mm Hg. Connect a size 10F (or larger) suction catheter to remove secretions from the mouth and pharynx. Smaller suction catheters (size 8F and size 5F or 6F) should be available for removing secretions from the endotracheal tube, if necessary, after placement. Appropriate catheter sizes are listed in Table 5-2.

   A meconium aspirator can be attached to the endotracheal tube to directly suction meconium or thick secretions that obstruct the trachea. Some endotracheal tubes have an integrated suction port.

4. Prepare a PPV device with a mask to ventilate the baby, if necessary, between intubation attempts. Check the operation of the device as described in Lesson 4.

5. Place a CO_2 detector, stethoscope, measuring tape or insertion depth table, waterproof adhesive tape, and scissors (or a tube stabilizer) within reach.

Table 5-2. Suction catheter size for endotracheal tubes of various inner diameters

Endotracheal Tube Size (mm ID)	Catheter Size
2.5	5F or 6F
3.0	6F or 8F
3.5	8F

How should you position the newborn for intubation?

Place the baby's head in the midline, the neck slightly extended, and the body straight. It may be helpful to place a small roll under the baby's shoulders to maintain slight neck extension. This "sniffing" position aligns the trachea for optimal viewing by allowing a straight line of sight into the glottis once the laryngoscope has been properly placed. Your assistant should help to maintain good positioning throughout the procedure.

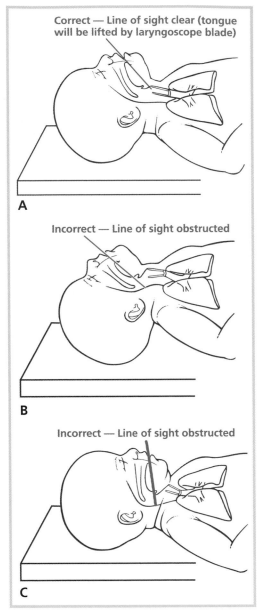

A Correct — Line of sight clear (tongue will be lifted by laryngoscope blade)

B Incorrect — Line of sight obstructed

C Incorrect — Line of sight obstructed

Figure 5.9. Correct (A) and incorrect (B and C) positioning for intubation

Both overextension and flexion of the neck will obstruct your view of the airway. If the shoulder roll is too large or the neck is overextended, the glottis will be raised above your line of sight. If the neck is flexed toward the chest, you will be viewing the posterior pharynx and will not be able to visualize the glottis (Figure 5.9).

Adjust the height of the bed, if possible, so that the baby's head is level with the operator's upper abdomen or lower chest to bring the head closer to the operator's eye level and improve her view of the airway.

Review

1 A newborn has been receiving face-mask ventilation, but is not improving. Despite performing the first 5 ventilation corrective steps, the heart rate is not rising and there is poor chest movement. An alternative airway, such as an endotracheal tube or laryngeal mask, (should)/(should not) be inserted immediately.

2 For babies weighing less than 1,000 g, the endotracheal tube size should be (2.5 mm)/(3.5 mm).

3 If using a stylet, the tip of the stylet (must)/(must not) extend beyond the endotracheal tube's side and end holes.

4 The preferred laryngoscope blade size for use in a term newborn is (No. 1)/(No. 0).

5 The vocal cord guide on an endotracheal tube (does)/(does not) reliably predict the correct insertion depth.

Answers

1 An alternative airway, such as an endotracheal tube or a laryngeal mask, should be inserted immediately.

2 For babies weighing less than 1,000 g, the endotracheal tube size should be 2.5 mm.

3 The tip of the stylet must not extend beyond the endotracheal tube's side and end holes.

④ The preferred laryngoscope blade size for use in a term newborn is No. 1.

⑤ The vocal cord guide on an endotracheal tube does not reliably predict the correct insertion depth.

How do you hold the laryngoscope?

Always hold the laryngoscope in your *left* hand with your thumb resting on the upper surface of the laryngoscope handle and the blade pointing away from you (Figure 5.10). The laryngoscope is designed to be held in the left hand by both right- and left-handed users. If held in the right hand, your view through the open, curved portion of the blade will be obstructed.

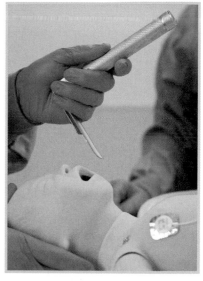

Figure 5.10. Hold the laryngoscope in your left hand.

How do you perform the intubation procedure?

The steps for tracheal intubation are briefly described as follows; however, proficiency requires considerable supervision and practice. Even if you are not performing the procedure, it is helpful to understand the steps so you can effectively assist the operator.

Get ready to insert the laryngoscope.

❶ Correctly position the baby. If possible, adjust the height of the warmer as needed. You may stabilize the baby's head with your right hand (Figure 5.11) while a team member ensures that the baby is lying straight and the head is in the "sniffing" position.

❷ Use your right index finger to gently open the baby's mouth.

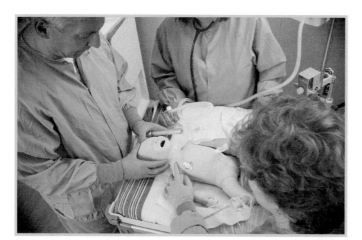

Figure 5.11. Positioning the baby for intubation

Insert the laryngoscope and identify key landmarks.

3 Insert the laryngoscope blade into the right side of the baby's mouth and slide the blade over the right side of the tongue toward the midline. Gently push the tongue toward the left side of the mouth and advance the blade until the tip lies just beyond the base of the tongue in the vallecula (Figure 5.12).

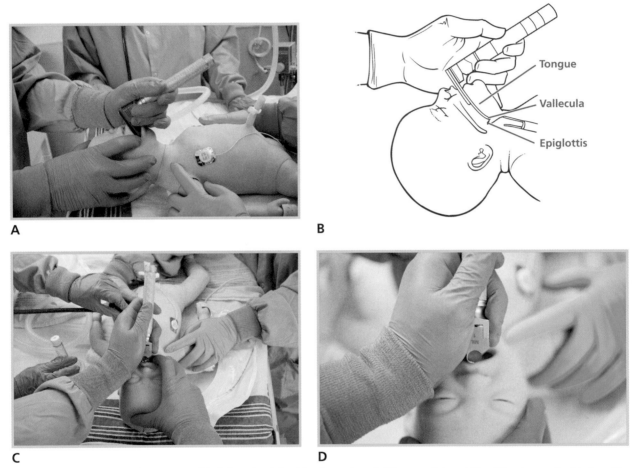

A

B

C

D

Tongue

Vallecula

Epiglottis

Figure 5.12. Insert the laryngoscope blade into the right side of mouth and slide toward the midline (A), advance the blade until the tip lies in the vallecua (B), and hold the laryngoscope in the midline (C) gently pushing the tongue toward the left side of the mouth (D) allowing you to identify landmarks.

4 Lift the entire laryngoscope in the direction that the handle is pointing, moving the tongue out of the way to expose the glottis. You may need to tilt the tip of the blade very slightly to lift the epiglottis.

When first learning the procedure, operators have a tendency to bend their wrist, pulling the top of the handle toward themselves in a "rocking" motion against the baby's upper gum. This will not produce the desired view of the glottis and may injure the baby's lips and gums (Figure 5.13).

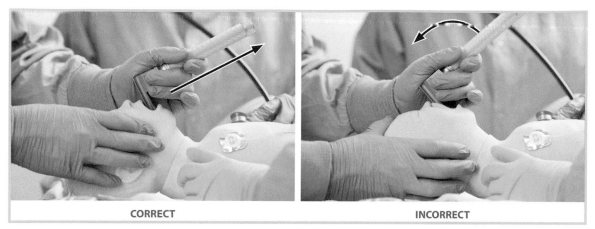

Figure 5.13. Correct (left) and incorrect (right) method for lifting the laryngoscope to expose the larynx. Lift the laryngoscope in the direction that the handle is pointed; do not rotate or "rock" the handle against the baby's upper gum.

Note: This lesson describes placing the tip of the blade in the vallecula to lift the epiglottis. In some cases, it may be necessary to use the blade tip to *gently* lift the epiglottis directly.

The glottis appears at the very top of your view as you look down the laryngoscope. An assistant can help bring the glottis into view by using his thumb and first finger to provide gentle pressure on the baby's thyroid and cricoid cartilage (Figure 5.14). The assistant should direct the pressure downward and toward the baby's right ear.

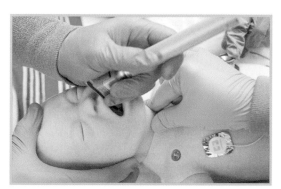

Figure 5.14. Thyroid and cricoid pressure provided by an assistant may improve visualization of the larynx. Press downward and toward the baby's right ear.

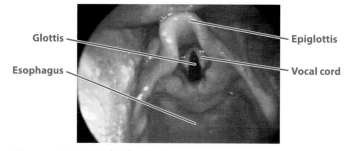

Glottis

Esophagus

Epiglottis

Vocal cord

Figure 5.15. Key landmarks

⑤ Identify the key landmarks (Figure 5.15). If the tip of the blade is correctly positioned in the vallecula, you should see the epiglottis hanging down from the top and the vocal cords directly below. The vocal cords appear as thin vertical stripes in the shape of an inverted letter "V".

If these structures are not immediately visible, adjust the blade until the structures come into view. You may need to insert or withdraw the blade slowly to see the vocal cords (Figure 5.16).

If the blade is not inserted far enough, you will see the base of the tongue and posterior pharynx (Figure 5.17). Advance the blade slightly until the epiglottis comes into view.

If the blade is inserted too far, you will see only the esophagus (Figure 5.18) and will need to withdraw the blade slightly until the epiglottis drops down from above.

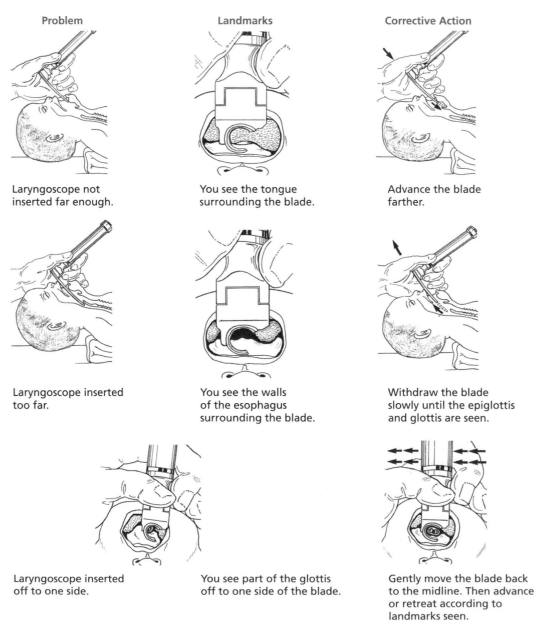

Problem	Landmarks	Corrective Action
Laryngoscope not inserted far enough.	You see the tongue surrounding the blade.	Advance the blade farther.
Laryngoscope inserted too far.	You see the walls of the esophagus surrounding the blade.	Withdraw the blade slowly until the epiglottis and glottis are seen.
Laryngoscope inserted off to one side.	You see part of the glottis off to one side of the blade.	Gently move the blade back to the midline. Then advance or retreat according to landmarks seen.

Figure 5.16. Corrective actions for poor visualization of the larynx during laryngoscopy

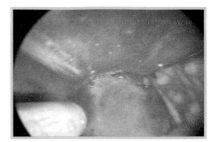

Figure 5.17. Laryngoscope not inserted far enough. Tongue and posterior pharynx obscure view.

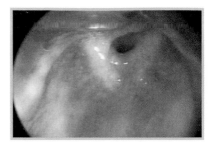

Figure 5.18. Laryngoscope inserted too far. Only the esophagus is visible.

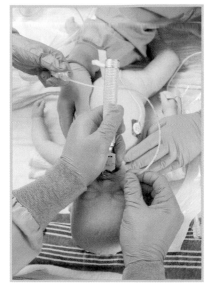

Figure 5.19. Suctioning secretions during laryngoscopy

If the anatomic landmarks are obstructed by secretions, use a size 10F or 12F catheter to remove secretions from the mouth and pharynx (Figure 5.19).

Insert the endotracheal tube.

6 Once you have identified the vocal cords, hold the laryngoscope steady, maintain your view of the vocal cords, and ask an assistant to place the endotracheal tube in your right hand. Insert the tube into the right side of the baby's mouth with the concave curve in the horizontal plane (Figure 5.20). Do not insert the tube through the laryngoscope's open channel. This will obstruct your view of the vocal cords.

After insertion, direct the tube into the hypopharynx and advance the tip toward the vocal cords. As the tip approaches the vocal cords, pivot the tube into the vertical plane so the tip is directed upward. When the

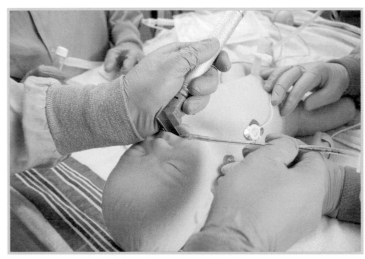

Figure 5.20. Insertion of the endotracheal tube into the right side of the mouth

vocal cords open, advance the tube until the vocal cords are positioned between the vocal cord guide lines. Your assistant may feel the tube pass beneath his fingers. Note the centimeter depth marking on the outside of the tube that aligns with the baby's upper lip.

If the vocal cords are closed, wait for them to open. Do not touch the closed cords with the tip of the tube and never try to force the tube between closed cords. If the cords do not open within 30 seconds, stop and resume ventilation with a mask until you are prepared to reattempt insertion.

Secure the endotracheal tube.

7 Use your right hand to hold the tube securely against the baby's hard palate. *Carefully remove the laryngoscope* without displacing the tube (Figure 5.21). If a stylet was used, an assistant should remove it from the endotracheal tube—again being sure that the operator is careful to hold the tube in place (Figure 5.22). Although it is important to hold the tube firmly, be careful not to squeeze the tube so tightly that the stylet cannot be removed.

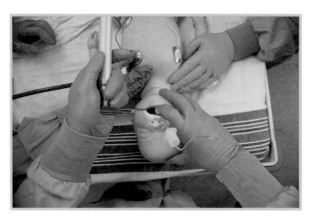

Figure 5.21. Stabilize the tube against the baby's palate or cheek while carefully removing the laryngoscope.

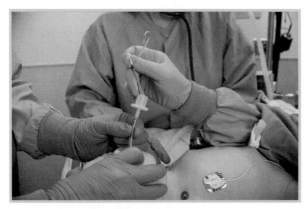

Figure 5.22. An assistant removes the optional stylet while the operator holds the tube in place.

Ventilate through the endotracheal tube.

8 An assistant should attach a CO_2 detector and PPV device to the endotracheal tube (Figure 5.23). Having the same person hold the endotracheal tube and the PPV device may help to avoid accidental extubation. Once the PPV device is attached, begin ventilation through the tube.

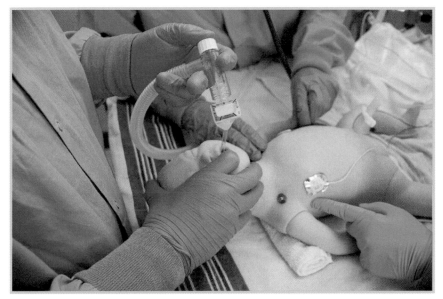

Figure 5.23. Attach a CO_2 detector and PPV device to the endotracheal tube and begin ventilation.

How much time should be allowed for an intubation attempt?

The steps of intubation should be completed within approximately **30** seconds. The baby is not being ventilated during the procedure, so rapid action is essential. If the baby's vital signs worsen during the procedure (severe bradycardia or decreased oxygen saturation), it is usually preferable to stop, resume PPV with a mask, and then try again.

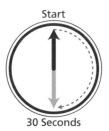

Start

30 Seconds

Repeated attempts at intubation are not advised because you will increase the likelihood of soft-tissue trauma and make subsequent airway management more difficult. If the initial attempts are unsuccessful, evaluate other options, including requesting assistance from another provider with intubation expertise (eg, anesthesiologist, emergency department physician, respiratory care practitioner, neonatal nurse practitioner), placing a laryngeal mask, or continuing face-mask ventilation.

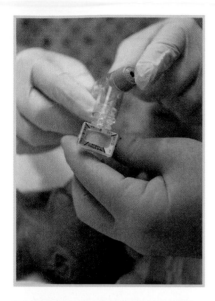

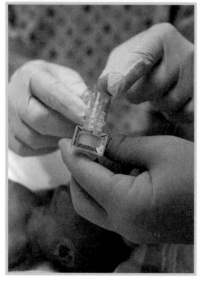

Figure 5.24. The colorimetric CO_2 detector is a purple or blue color before detecting exhaled CO_2 (top). The detector turns yellow in the presence of exhaled CO_2 (bottom).

How do you confirm that the endotracheal tube is in the trachea?

The primary methods of confirming endotracheal tube placement within the trachea are detecting exhaled CO_2 and a rapidly rising heart rate. As soon as you insert the endotracheal tube, connect a CO_2 detector (Figure 5.23) and confirm the presence of CO_2 during exhalation. If the tube is correctly placed and you are providing effective ventilation through the tube, you should detect exhaled CO_2 within 8 to 10 positive-pressure breaths.

There are 2 types of CO_2 detectors available. Colorimetric devices change color in the presence of CO_2 (Figure 5.24). These are the most commonly used devices in the delivery room. Capnographs are electronic monitors that display the CO_2 concentration with each breath.

Can the tube be in the trachea even though CO_2 is NOT detected?

Yes, there are limitations to the use of CO_2 detectors. If the tube is placed within the trachea, but the lungs are not adequately ventilated, there may not be enough exhaled CO_2 to be detected. This may occur if the endotracheal tube or trachea are obstructed by secretions, you are not using enough ventilating pressure, or there are large bilateral pneumothoraces and the lungs are collapsed. In addition, babies with a very low heart rate or decreased cardiac function (low cardiac output) may not carry enough CO_2 to their lungs to be detected.

Can the CO_2 detector change color when the tube is NOT in the trachea?

Although uncommon, it is possible for a colorimetric CO_2 device to change color even though the tube is not in the trachea (Table 5.3). If the detector has already changed color in the package and is yellow when you remove it, the device is defective and should not be used. If epinephrine is administered through the endotracheal tube and touches the paper inside the CO_2 detector, it will permanently change the screen yellow and make the detector unusable.

Table 5-3. Colorimetric CO_2 Detector Problems

False Negative (Tube IS IN trachea but NO color change)	False Positive (Tube IS NOT in trachea but color changes)
• Inadequate ventilating pressure • Collapsed lungs • Bilateral pneumothoraces • Low heart rate • Low cardiac output	• Defective device changed color in package before use • Epinephrine contamination

What are other indicators that the tube is in the trachea?

Demonstrating *exhaled CO_2* and observing a *rapidly increasing heart rate* are the *primary methods* of confirming endotracheal tube placement within the trachea.

If the tube is positioned correctly, you should also observe

- Audible and equal breath sounds near both axillae during PPV

- Symmetrical chest movement with each breath

- Little or no air leak from the mouth during PPV

- Decreased or absent air entry over the stomach

Be cautious when interpreting breath sounds in newborns because sounds are easily transmitted. When listening to breath sounds, use a small stethoscope and place it near the axilla. A large stethoscope, or one placed near the center of the chest, may transmit sounds from the esophagus or stomach.

What do you do if you suspect that the tube is not in the trachea?

The tube is not likely to be in the trachea if the CO_2 detector does not show the presence of exhaled CO_2 within 8 to 10 breaths. In most cases, you should remove the tube, resume ventilation with a face mask, ensure that your equipment is properly prepared, ensure that the baby is optimally positioned, and then repeat the procedure. Using an endotracheal tube that is placed in the esophagus provides no ventilation to the baby's lungs and continuing to use it only delays effective ventilation.

Remember that babies with a very low heart rate or decreased cardiac function may not carry enough CO_2 to their lungs to change the color on the CO_2 detector. If you believe that the tube is correctly placed in the trachea despite the lack of exhaled CO_2, you may choose to stabilize the tube, reinsert the laryngoscope, and attempt to confirm that the tube is passing between the vocal cords. This "second look" procedure can be difficult and may delay establishing effective ventilation if the tube is not correctly placed.

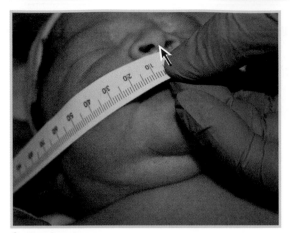

A. Nasal septum

How deeply should the tube be inserted within the trachea?

The goal is to place the endotracheal tube tip in the middle portion of the trachea. This generally requires inserting the tube so that the tip is only 1 to 2 centimeters below the vocal cords. It is important not to insert the tube too far so that the tip touches the carina or enters a main bronchus. Two methods may be used for estimating the insertion depth. Your team should determine which method is preferred in your practice setting.

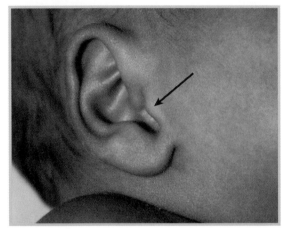

B. Ear tragus

The NTL is a method that has been validated in both full-term and preterm newborns. The NTL method uses a calculation based on the distance (cm) from the baby's nasal septum to the ear tragus (Figures 5.25A, 5.25B, and 5.25C). Use a measuring tape to measure the NTL. The estimated insertion depth (cm) is NTL + 1 cm. Place the endotracheal tube so that the marking on the tube corresponding to the estimated insertion depth is adjacent to the baby's lip.

Recent studies have shown that gestational age is also an accurate predictor of the correct insertion depth (Table 5-4) and has the advantage of being known before birth. This table could be placed near the radiant warmer or with your intubation supplies.

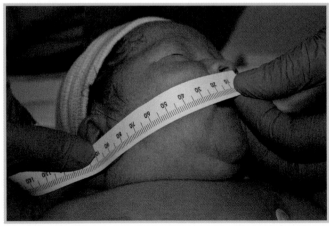

C. Measuring the NTL

Figure 5.25. Measuring the NTL. Measure from the middle of the nasal septum (arrow, A) to the ear tragus (arrow, B) and add 1 cm to the measurement.

Table 5-4. Initial endotracheal tube insertion depth ("tip to lip") for orotracheal intubation

Gestation (weeks)	Endotracheal tube insertion depth at lips (cm)	Baby's Weight (grams)
23-24	5.5	500-600
25-26	6.0	700-800
27-29	6.5	900-1000
30-32	7.0	1,100-1,400
33-34	7.5	1,500-1,800
35-37	8.0	1,900-2,400
38-40	8.5	2,500-3,100
41-43	9.0	3,200-4,200

Adapted from Kempley ST, Moreira JW, Petrone FL. Endotracheal tube length for neonatal intubation. *Resuscitation*. 2008;77(3):369-373.

Remember that both of these methods are estimates of the correct endotracheal tube depth. After placing the tube, use a stethoscope to listen for breath sounds in both axillae and over the stomach (Figure 5.26). If the tube is correctly placed, the breath sounds should be equal on both sides. If the tube is in too far, the breath sounds may be decreased on one side. Most often, if the tube is inserted too far, it will enter the right mainstem bronchus causing breath sounds to be louder on the right side and quieter on the left side. Slowly withdraw the tube while listening to the breath sounds on the quieter side. When the tube is correctly positioned, the breath sounds should improve and become equal.

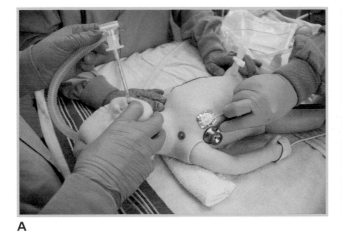
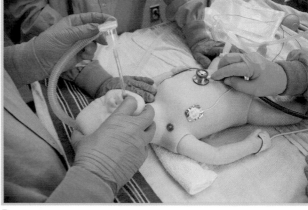

A   B

Figure 5.26. Listen for equal breath sounds in both axillae (A). Breath sounds should not be audible over the stomach (B).

If you plan to keep the tube in place, how do you secure it?

Several methods of securing the tube have been described. Either water-resistant tape or a device specifically designed to secure an endotracheal tube may be used.

One method is described as follows:

1 After you have correctly positioned the tube, note the centimeter marking on the side of the tube adjacent to the baby's upper lip (Figure 5.27).

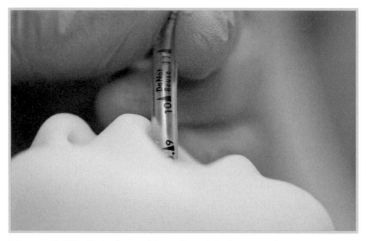

Figure 5.27. Note the marking adjacent to the upper lip.

2 Cut a piece of 3/4- or 1/2-inch tape so that it is long enough to extend from one side of the baby's mouth, across the upper lip, and about 2 cm onto the opposite cheek (Figure 5.28).

3 Split the tape along half its length so that it appears like a pair of pants (Figure 5.28A).

4 Place the uncut section of tape on the baby's cheek so that the beginning of the split is close to the corner of the baby's mouth. Place the upper "leg" of tape across the baby's upper lip (Figure 5.28B).

5 Carefully wrap the lower "leg" around the tube (Figures 5.28C and 5.28D). Be sure that the desired centimeter marking remains next to the baby's upper lip. It is easy to inadvertently push the tube in further than desired during the taping procedure.

6 At the end, turn the tape onto itself to leave a small "tab" that you can hold to unwind the tape when you want to remove the tube (Figure 5.28E).

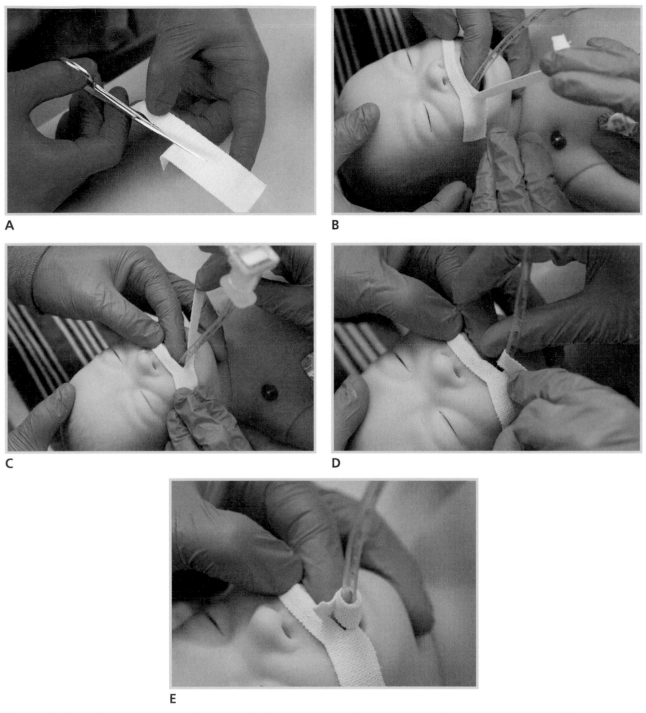

Figure 5.28. Split the tape along half its length (A). Place the uncut section on the baby's cheek close to the corner of the mouth and the upper "leg" of tape above the baby's lip (B). Wrap the lower "leg" of tape around the tube (C and D). Leave a small tab of tape folded over at the end to assist removal (E).

7 Listen with a stethoscope over both sides of the chest to be sure the tube has not been displaced.

8 If the tube will be left in place beyond the initial resuscitation, obtain a chest x-ray for final placement confirmation.

The tip of the tube should appear in the midtrachea *adjacent to the first **or** second thoracic vertebra* (Figure 5.29). The tip should be above the carina, which is generally adjacent to the third or fourth thoracic vertebra. Avoid using the clavicles as a landmark because their location varies depending upon the baby's position and the angle that the x-ray is taken. If the tube advanced too far, it may touch the carina or enter the right main bronchus and cause the right upper lobe or left lung to collapse (Figure 5.30).

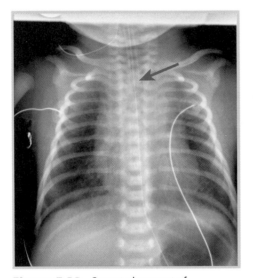

Figure 5.29. Correct placement of endotracheal tube with tip adjacent to the second thoracic vertebra

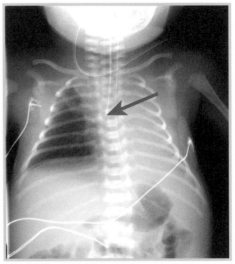

Figure 5.30. Incorrect placement. The tip of the endotracheal tube is in too far. It is touching the carina, approaching the right mainstem bronchus, and the left lung is collapsed.

What can an assistant do to help the operator during the intubation procedure?

❶ Check that suction is set at 80 to 100 mmHg.

❷ Ensure that the correct-sized laryngoscope blade and endotracheal tube are selected based on the newborn's expected gestational age or weight.

❸ Communicate with the operator about what method will be used to estimate the endotracheal tube insertion depth—the NTL or the estimated insertion depth table.

❹ Check that the stylet, if used, does not protrude beyond the tube's side or end hole.

5 Hold equipment so that the operator does not need to look away from anatomic landmarks to suction secretions or grasp the tube in preparation for insertion.

6 Monitor the newborn's heart rate and alert the operator if the intubation attempt lasts longer than 30 seconds.

7 Provide thyroid and cricoid pressure.

8 After endotracheal tube insertion, remove the stylet and attach the CO_2 detector.

9 Listen for increasing heart rate.

10 Check the tip-to-lip insertion depth.

11 Listen for breath sounds in both axillae.

12 Assist with securing the tube.

Special Consideration: Endotracheal intubation for suction

If a baby's condition has not improved and you have not been able to achieve chest movement despite all the ventilation corrective steps and a properly placed endotracheal tube, there may be thick secretions obstructing the airway. Thick secretions may be from blood, cellular debris, vernix, or meconium. You may attempt to clear the airway using a suction catheter inserted through the endotracheal tube (Table 5-2). If you cannot quickly clear the airway with the suction catheter, you may be able to clear the airway by applying suction directly to the endotracheal tube using a meconium aspirator. Although the device is called a meconium aspirator, it may be used for any thick secretion that is obstructing the airway.

Using a meconium aspirator to suction the trachea

Once the endotracheal tube has been inserted,

1 Connect a meconium aspirator, attached to a suction source (80-100 mmHg suction), directly to the endotracheal tube connector. Several types of meconium aspirators are commercially available. Some endotracheal tubes have an integrated suction port.

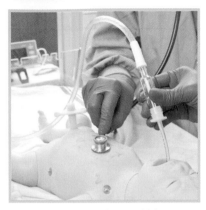

Figure 5.31. Suctioning thick secretions that obstruct ventilation using an endotracheal tube and meconium aspirator

Table 5-5. Sudden deterioration after intubation

The *DOPE* mnemonic	
D	**D**isplaced endotracheal tube
O	**O**bstructed endotracheal tube
P	**P**neumothorax
E	**E**quipment failure

Adapted from Kleinman ME, Chameides L, Schexnayder SM, et al. Part 14: Pediatric advanced life support: 2010 American Heart Association Guidelines for Cardiopulmonary Resuscitation and Emergency Cardiovascular Care. *Circulation. 2010;122(18 Suppl):S876-S908.*

❷ Occlude the suction-control port on the aspirator with your finger and gradually withdraw the tube over 3 to 5 seconds as you continue suctioning secretions in the trachea (Figure 5.31).

How many times should suctioning be repeated if thick secretions prevent you from achieving effective ventilation through an endotracheal tube?

If the airway is obstructed by secretions that have prevented you from achieving effective ventilation, you must repeat the procedure until you have cleared the airway sufficiently to achieve effective ventilation.

What problems should you consider if a baby's condition worsens after endotracheal intubation?

If a baby's condition suddenly worsens after intubation, the endotracheal tube may have been inadvertently advanced too far into the airway or pulled back into the pharynx and outside the trachea. The tube may be obstructed by blood, meconium, or other thick secretions. The baby may have developed a tension pneumothorax that collapses the lungs and prevents gas exchange. Additional information about this complication is discussed in Lesson 10. Finally, the device used to provide PPV may have become disconnected from the endotracheal tube or compressed gas source, or it may have developed a leak. The mnemonic *"DOPE"* has been used to help remember these potential problems (Table 5-5).

Laryngeal Masks

Case 2. Cannot ventilate and cannot intubate

Your resuscitation team is called to attend a birth complicated by fetal decelerations. You ask the obstetric provider about perinatal risk factors and complete a pre-resuscitation team briefing. The fluid is clear without meconium staining. A full-term baby is born and stimulated to breathe, but he remains limp and apneic. The umbilical cord is clamped and cut and he is brought to the radiant warmer. The initial steps of newborn care are performed, PPV is initiated, and a pulse oximeter sensor is attached to his right hand. The heart rate remains low and the team cannot achieve chest movement despite performing the ventilation corrective steps. A team member makes 2 attempts to place an endotracheal tube, but, each time, the tube enters the esophagus. The team leader notes that the baby has a small jaw and large tongue.

An assistant rapidly prepares a laryngeal mask. Team members insert the laryngeal mask, attach a PPV device and CO_2 detector, and begin PPV. Chest movement is noted with each PPV breath, the CO_2 detector changes color indicating ventilation that inflates the lungs, and the baby's heart rate increases. Although he begins to have spontaneous respiratory effort, the team suspects a congenital airway obstruction and the laryngeal mask is secured and left in place as he is transferred to the neonatal intensive care unit (NICU) for further evaluation and post-resuscitative care. Shortly afterward, the members of the care team conduct a debriefing to discuss their preparation, teamwork, and communication.

What is a laryngeal mask?

The laryngeal mask is an airway device that is an alternative to a face mask or endotracheal tube. There are several different designs, but one common example includes an airway tube attached to a small, flexible mask with an inflatable cuff (Figure 5.32). The mask is inserted into the baby's mouth and advanced until the tip nearly reaches the esophagus. Once the mask is fully inserted, the cuff is inflated. A small pilot balloon monitors the cuff's inflation. The mask covers the glottis (laryngeal opening) like a cap and the inflated cuff creates a seal against the hypopharynx (Figure 5.33). The mask opening is covered by small bars (aperture bars) that prevent the epiglottis from being drawn into the airway tube. The airway tube has a standard 15-mm connector that can be attached to any PPV device. When positive

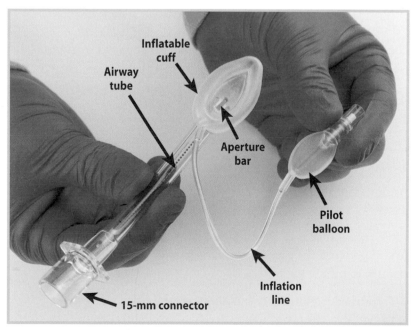

Figure 5.32. One example of a laryngeal mask

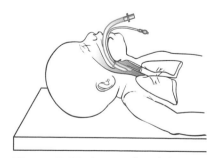

Figure 5.33. Laryngeal mask forming a seal over the glottis

pressure is applied to the airway tube, the pressure is transmitted through the tube and mask into the baby's trachea. No instruments are required to insert a laryngeal mask and you do not need to visualize the vocal cords during insertion. Several variations of the basic design are commercially available, including reusable and disposable versions, devices with a pre-curved airway tube and a gastric drain port, and a mask that creates a seal without an inflatable cuff. At this time, only the size-1 laryngeal mask is small enough for use in newborns weighing less than 5 kg.

When should you consider using a laryngeal mask?

Because the laryngeal mask does not require a tight seal against the face, bypasses the tongue, and does not require visualization of the vocal cords for placement, it may be an effective alternative when attempts at mask ventilation and endotracheal intubation are unsuccessful. When you "can't ventilate and can't intubate," a laryngeal mask may provide a successful rescue airway.

Common examples when a laryngeal mask should be considered during resuscitation include the following:

- Newborns with congenital anomalies involving the mouth, lip, tongue, palate or neck, where achieving a good seal with a face mask is difficult and visualizing the larynx with a laryngoscope is difficult or unfeasible

- Newborns with a small mandible or large tongue, where face-mask ventilation and intubation are unsuccessful. Common examples include the Robin sequence and Trisomy 21.

- When PPV provided with a face mask is ineffective and attempts at intubation are not feasible or are unsuccessful

What are the limitations of a laryngeal mask?

Laryngeal masks have several limitations to consider during neonatal resuscitation.

- The device has not been studied for suctioning secretions from the airway.

- If you need to use high ventilation pressures, air may leak through the seal between the pharynx and the mask, resulting in insufficient pressure to inflate the lungs.

- Few reports describe the use of a laryngeal mask during chest compressions. However, if endotracheal intubation is unsuccessful, it is reasonable to attempt compressions with the device in place.

- There is insufficient evidence to recommend using a laryngeal mask to administer intratracheal medications. Intratracheal medications may leak from the mask into the esophagus and not enter the lung.

- Laryngeal masks cannot be used in very small newborns. Currently, the smallest laryngeal mask is intended for use in babies who weigh more than approximately 2,000 g. Many reports describe its use in babies who weigh 1,500 to 2,000 g. Some reports have described using the size-1 laryngeal mask successfully in babies who weigh less than 1,500 g.

Remember to request help from a provider with expertise in airway management as soon as it becomes apparent that a small baby, or baby with a craniofacial anomaly, may require assisted ventilation.

How do you place a laryngeal mask?

The following instructions apply to one example of a disposable laryngeal mask with a pre-curved, anatomically shaped airway tube and a gastric drain port. Devices vary by manufacturer and you should refer to the manufacturer's instructions for the specific device used at your institution. If you are using a reusable laryngeal mask, refer to the manufacturer's instructions for proper cleaning and maintenance procedures.

Note: If you think that the stomach is distended in a baby in whom you have decided to place a laryngeal mask that does not have a gastric drain port, an orogastric tube should be placed and air in the stomach should be aspirated before inserting the laryngeal mask.

Prepare the laryngeal mask.

1. Wear gloves and follow standard precautions. Using clean technique, remove the size-1 device from the sterile package.

2. Quickly inspect the device to ensure that the mask, aperture bars, airway tube, 15-mm connector, and pilot balloon are intact without cuts, tears, or kinks.

3. Attach a syringe to the inflation port and completely deflate the cuff surrounding the mask, creating a vacuum inside the cuff, so that the mask achieves a wedge shape (Figure 5.34). Maintaining tension, disconnect the syringe from the inflation port.

4. Some clinicians lubricate the back of the laryngeal mask with a water-soluble lubricant. If you choose to do so, be careful to keep the lubricant away from the openings on the inside of the mask.

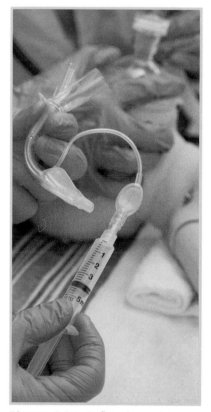

Figure 5.34. Deflate the mask to form a wedge shape and then remove the syringe.

Get ready to insert the laryngeal mask.

5 Stand at the baby's head and position the head in the "sniffing" position as you would for endotracheal intubation.

6 Hold the device as illustrated (Figure 5.35). You may hold the laryngeal mask in your right or left hand.

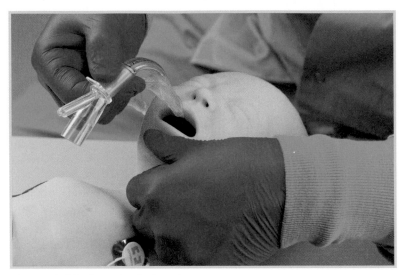

Figure 5.35. Preparing for insertion

Insert the laryngeal mask.

7 Gently open the baby's mouth and press the leading tip of the mask against the baby's hard palate (Figure 5.36).

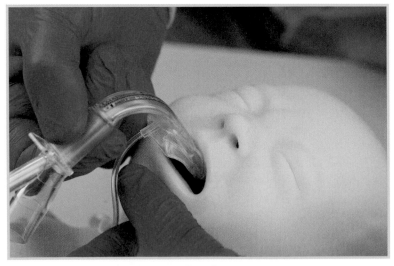

Figure 5.36. Press the tip against the palate.

⑧ While maintaining pressure against the palate, advance the device inward with a circular motion (Figure 5.37). The mask will follow the contour of the mouth and palate. Advance until you feel resistance.

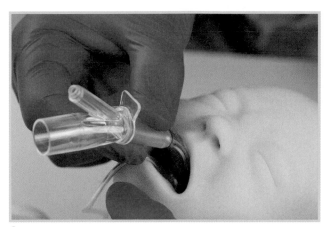 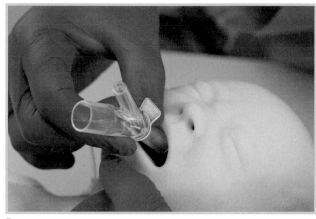

A   **B**

Figure 5.37. Advance the device following the contour of the mouth and palate.

Inflate the laryngeal mask.

⑨ Inflate the cuff by injecting just enough air into the inflation port to achieve a seal. After inflating the cuff, remove the syringe. Follow the manufacturer's recommendation for maximum inflation volume. The maximum inflation for the mask demonstrated is 5 mL (Figure 5.38). You can assess the inflation of the cuff by looking at the pilot balloon. The laryngeal mask will move slightly outward when it is inflated. **Never inflate the mask with more than the manufacturer recommended volume of air.**

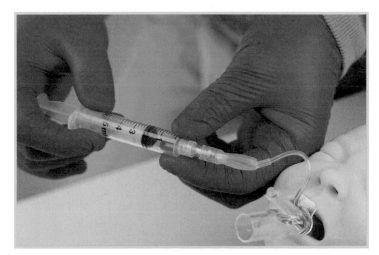

Figure 5.38. Inflate the cuff with air.

Ventilate through the laryngeal mask.

⑩ Attach a PPV device and CO_2 detector to the airway tube and begin PPV (Figure 5.39).

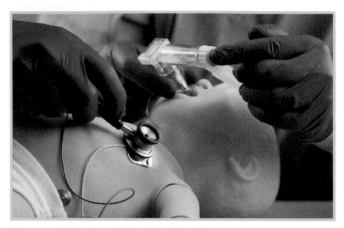

Figure 5.39. Start PPV and confirm placement.

Secure the laryngeal mask.

⑪ Press a piece of tape horizontally across the airway tube's fixation tab, pressing downward so that the tape adheres to the baby's cheeks and gently presses the device inward (Figure 5.40).

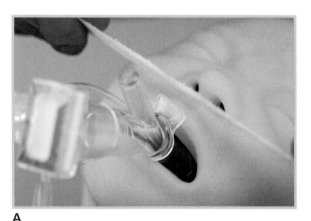
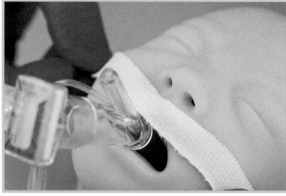

A   B

Figure 5.40. Press tape downward across the fixation tab and across the baby's cheeks.

How do you confirm that the laryngeal mask is properly placed?

As soon as you insert the laryngeal mask and begin PPV, connect a CO_2 detector and confirm the presence of CO_2 during exhalation (Figure 5.39). If the laryngeal mask is correctly placed and you are providing ventilation that inflates the lungs, you should detect exhaled CO_2 within 8 to 10 positive-pressure breaths. Similar to a properly placed endotracheal tube, you should notice a prompt increase in the baby's heart rate, chest wall movement, equal breath sounds when you listen with a stethoscope, and an increasing SpO_2. You should not hear a large leak of air coming from the baby's mouth or see a growing bulge in the baby's neck.

The laryngeal mask does not obstruct the vocal cords; therefore, you may hear grunting or crying through the device when the baby begins breathing spontaneously.

Insert a gastric drain tube (optional). You may lubricate a size 5F or 6F gastric tube and carefully insert it down the gastric drain port attached to the airway tube (Figure 5.41). Attach a syringe and gently aspirate air and stomach contents. Disconnect the syringe and leave the gastric tube open to air.

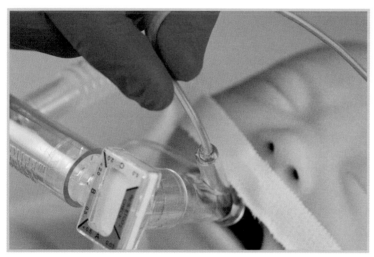

Figure 5.41. Insert a size 5F or 6F gastric tube through the gastric drain port.

When should you remove the laryngeal mask?

The laryngeal mask can be removed when the baby establishes effective spontaneous respirations or when an endotracheal tube can be inserted successfully. Babies can breathe spontaneously through the device. If necessary, the laryngeal mask can be attached to a ventilator or continuous positive airway pressure (CPAP) device during transport. When you decide to remove the laryngeal mask, suction secretions from the mouth and throat before you deflate and remove the device.

What complications may occur with a laryngeal mask?

The device may cause soft-tissue trauma, laryngospasm, or gastric distension from air leaking around the mask. Prolonged use over hours or days has been infrequently associated with oropharyngeal nerve damage or tongue swelling in adults; however, no information is available on the incidence of these complications in newborns.

Focus on Teamwork

Inserting an alternative airway highlights several opportunities for effective teams to use the Neonatal Resuscitation Program® (NRP®) Key Behavioral skills.

Behavior	Example
Call for additional help when needed.	If an alternative airway is required, you will likely need 3 to 4 or more health care providers to quickly perform all of the tasks, including preparing and testing several pieces of equipment, positioning the baby, holding the endotracheal tube, providing thyroid and cricoid pressure, monitoring the baby during the procedure, attaching a CO_2 detector, attaching a PPV device, auscultating breath sounds, securing the airway, and documenting events.
Communicate effectively. Maintain professional behavior.	When preparing to insert an alternative airway, clearly and calmly request the desired supplies. Confirm the insertion depth (endotracheal tube) or inflation volume (laryngeal mask) with your team members before securing the tube.
Delegate workload optimally.	Determine who will insert the endotracheal tube, who will provide thyroid and cricoid pressure, who will monitor the baby's heart rate, who will place the CO_2 detector, and who will auscultate breath sounds.
Allocate attention wisely.	Maintain situational awareness. At all times, a team member needs to be monitoring the baby's condition, the number of insertion attempts, the duration of insertion attempts, and alerting the operators to any important changes (eg, heart rate, oxygen saturation).
Use available resources.	If an alternative airway is needed, but initial intubation attempts are unsuccessful, do not make repeated intubation attempts. Use your other resources, such as another individual with intubation expertise or a laryngeal mask. Allow all team members to use their unique skills during the resuscitation process. For example, respiratory care practitioners (RCP) have valuable skills specific to intubation. Using the RCP's skills during intubation may allow another provider to focus attention on preparing equipment for vascular access and medications.

Frequently Asked Questions

Why should I place an endotracheal tube before starting chest compressions? Does that delay the initiation of chest compressions?

In most situations, this program recommends placing an endotracheal tube prior to starting chest compressions to ensure maximum ventilation efficacy both before and after chest compressions begin. In many cases, the baby's condition will improve during the 30 seconds of ventilation following intubation and compressions will not be necessary.

Can the provider with intubation skills be on call outside the hospital or in a distant location?

No. A person with intubation skills should be in the hospital and available to be called for immediate assistance if needed. If the need for resuscitation is anticipated, this person should be present at the time of birth. It is not sufficient to have someone "on call" at home or in a remote area of the hospital.

Should sedative premedication be used before intubation?

Prior to a non-emergent intubation in the NICU, premedication is recommended because it alleviates pain, decreases the number of attempts needed to complete the procedure, and minimizes the potential for intubation-related airway trauma. When emergency intubation is performed as part of resuscitation, there is generally insufficient time or vascular access to administer sedative premedication. This program focuses on resuscitation of the newly born baby and, therefore, the details of premedication are not included.

Can a nurse or respiratory care practitioner place a laryngeal mask?

Each health care provider's scope of practice is defined by his or her state licensing board, and each hospital determines the level of competence and qualifications required for licensed providers to perform clinical skills. Although laryngeal mask placement is consistent with the general guidelines for nurse and respiratory care practitioner practice, you must check with your state licensing board and institution.

Key Points

1 Insertion of an endotracheal tube or laryngeal mask should be considered

   a. If positive-pressure ventilation (PPV) with a face mask does not result in clinical improvement

   b. If PPV lasts more than a few minutes

2 Insertion of an endotracheal tube is strongly recommended

   a. If chest compressions are necessary. If intubation is not successful or feasible, a laryngeal mask may be used.

   b. In special circumstances, such as (1) stabilization of a newborn with a suspected diaphragmatic hernia, (2) for surfactant administration, and (3) for direct tracheal suction if the airway is obstructed by thick secretions.

3 A person with intubation skills should be in the hospital and available to be called for immediate assistance if needed. If the need for resuscitation is anticipated, this person should be present at the time of birth. It is not sufficient to have someone "on call" at home or in a remote area of the hospital.

4 The equipment necessary to place an alternative airway should be kept together and readily accessible. Anticipate the need for airway insertion and prepare the equipment before a high-risk delivery.

5 The appropriate endotracheal tube size is estimated from the baby's weight or gestational age.

6 The appropriate laryngoscope blade for a term newborn is size No. 1. The correct blade for a preterm newborn is size No. 0 (size No. 00 *optional* for very preterm newborn).

7 The intubation procedure ideally should be completed within 30 seconds. Effective teamwork is required to perform this procedure quickly.

8 For intubation, the baby should be placed on a flat surface with the head in the midline, the neck slightly extended, and the body straight. If possible, adjust the bed so the baby's head is level with the operator's upper abdomen or lower chest.

9 Demonstrating exhaled CO_2 and observing a rapidly increasing heart rate are the primary methods of confirming endotracheal tube placement within the trachea.

⑩ Endotracheal tube insertion depth (cm) can be estimated using the NTL + 1 cm (NTL = distance from nasal septum to ear tragus) or the baby's gestational age; however, the depth estimate should be confirmed by equal breath sounds. If the tube is to remain in place, obtain a chest x-ray for final confirmation.

⑪ If a baby's condition has not improved and you have not achieved chest movement with ventilation through a properly placed endotracheal tube, there may be thick secretions obstructing the airway. Clear the airway using a suction catheter inserted through the endotracheal tube. If you cannot quickly clear the airway with the suction catheter, you may be able to clear the airway by applying suction directly to the endotracheal tube using a meconium aspirator.

⑫ If a baby's condition worsens after endotracheal intubation, the tube may have become **D**isplaced or **O**bstructed, there may be a **P**neumothorax or positive-pressure ventilation **E**quipment failure (DOPE mnemonic).

⑬ Avoid repeated unsuccessful attempts at endotracheal intubation. A laryngeal mask may provide a rescue airway when PPV with a face mask fails to achieve effective ventilation and intubation is unsuccessful.

LESSON 5 REVIEW

1. A newborn has been receiving face-mask ventilation, but is not improving. Despite performing the first 5 ventilation corrective steps, the heart rate is not rising and there is poor chest movement. An alternative airway, such as an endotracheal tube or a laryngeal mask, (should)/(should not) be inserted immediately.

2. For babies weighing less than 1,000 g, the endotracheal tube size should be (2.5 mm)/(3.5 mm).

3. If using a stylet, the tip of the stylet (must)/(must not) extend beyond the endotracheal tube's side and end holes.

4. The preferred laryngoscope blade size for use in a term newborn is (No. 1)/(No. 0).

5. The vocal cord guide on an endotracheal tube (does)/(does not) reliably predict the correct insertion depth.

6. Which illustration shows the view of the oral cavity that you should see if you have the laryngoscope correctly placed for intubation?

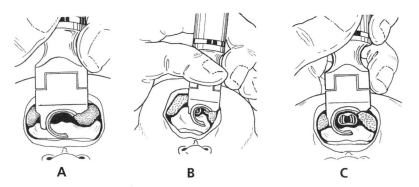

A   B   C

7. Both right- and left-handed people should hold the laryngoscope in their (right)/(left) hand.

8. You should try to take no longer than (30)/(60) seconds to complete the endotracheal intubation procedure.

9. If you have not completed endotracheal intubation within the recommended time limit, you should (continue the intubation attempt for another 30 seconds using free-flow oxygen to support the baby)/(stop, resume positive-pressure ventilation with a mask, then try again or insert a laryngeal mask).

10. Which image shows the correct way to lift the tongue out of the way and expose the larynx?

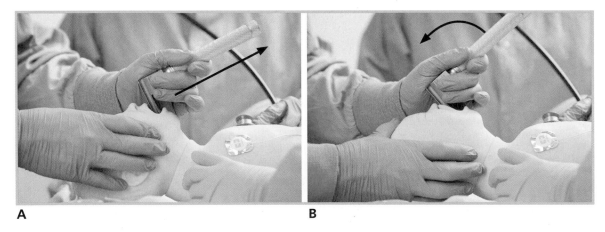

A   B

11. You have the glottis in view, but the vocal cords are closed. You (should)/(should not) wait until they are open to insert the tube.

12. You inserted an endotracheal tube and the CO_2 detector changed color when you gave positive-pressure breaths. You hear breath sounds with your stethoscope only on the right side of the chest. You should (withdraw)/(advance) the tube slightly and listen with the stethoscope again.

13. You have inserted an endotracheal tube and are giving positive-pressure ventilation through it. The CO_2 detector does not change color and the baby's heart rate is decreasing. The tube is most likely placed in the (esophagus)/(trachea).

14. Which x-ray shows the correct placement of the endotracheal tube?

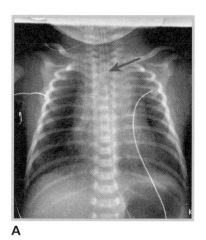
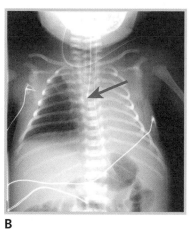

A   B

15. A baby is born at term with a bilateral cleft lip and palate and a very small mandible. She requires positive-pressure ventilation. You are unable to achieve a seal with bag and mask. You have tried to intubate twice but have not been successful. Insertion of a laryngeal mask (is)/(is not) indicated.

16. In the photograph, which arrow is pointing to the epiglottis?

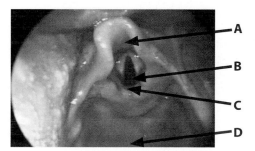

— A

— B

— C

— D

17. You have inserted a laryngoscope and are attempting intubation. You see the view depicted in the following illustration. The correct action is to (advance the laryngoscope farther/withdraw the laryngoscope).

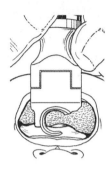

18. If a baby's condition worsens after endotracheal intubation, list 4 possible causes.

    1._____, 2. _____, 3. _____, 4. _____

Answers

1. An alternative airway, such as an endotracheal tube or a laryngeal mask, should be inserted immediately.

2. For babies weighing less than 1,000 g, the endotracheal tube size should be 2.5 mm.

3. The tip of the stylet must not extend beyond the endotracheal tube's side and end holes.

4. The preferred laryngoscope blade size for use in a term newborn is No. 1.

5. The vocal cord guide on an endotracheal tube does not reliably predict the correct insertion depth.

6. Image C shows the view of the oral cavity that you should see if you have the laryngoscope correctly placed for intubation.

7. Both right- and left-handed people should hold the laryngoscope in their left hand.

8. You should try to take no longer than 30 seconds to complete the endotracheal intubation procedure.

9. If you have not completed tracheal intubation within the recommended time limit, you should stop, resume positive-pressure ventilation with a mask, and then try again or insert a laryngeal mask.

10. Image A shows the correct way to lift the tongue out of the way and expose the larynx.

11. You should wait until they are open to insert the tube.

12. You should withdraw the tube slightly and listen with the stethoscope again.

13. The tube is most likely placed in the esophagus.

14. X-ray A shows the correct placement of the endotracheal tube.

15. Insertion of a laryngeal mask is indicated.

16. Arrow A is pointing to the epiglottis.

17. The correct action is to advance the laryngoscope farther.

18. Possible causes include (1) displaced endotracheal tube, (2) obstructed endotracheal tube, (3) pneumothorax, (4) equipment failure.

Additional Reading

Blayney MP, Logan DR. First thoracic vertebral body as reference for endotracheal tube placement. *Arch Dis Child Fetal Neonatal Ed.* 1994;71(1):F32-F35

Kempley ST, Moreiras JW, Petrone FL. Endotracheal tube length for neonatal intubation. *Resuscitation.* 2008;77(3):369-373

Mainie P, Carmichael A, McCullough S, Kempley ST. Endotracheal tube position in neonates requiring emergency interhospital transfer. *Am J Perinatol.* 2006;23(2):121-124

Rotschild A, Chitavat D, Puterman ML, Phang MS, Ling E, Baldwin V. Optimal positioning of endotracheal tubes for ventilation of preterm infants. *Am J Dis Child.* 1991;145(9):1007-1012

Shukla HK, Hendricks-Munoz KD, Atakent Y, Rapaport S. Rapid estimation of insertional length of endotracheal intubation in newborn infants. *J Pediatr.* 1997;131(4):561-564

Thayvil S, Nagakumar P, Gowers H, Sinha A. Optimal endotracheal tube tip position in extremely premature infants. *Am J Perinatol.* 2008; 25(1):13-16

Trevisanuto D, Doglioni N, Gottardi G, Nardo D, Micaglio M, Parotto M. Laryngeal mask: beyond neonatal upper airway malformations. *Arch Dis Child Fetal Neonatal Ed.* 2013;98(2):F185-F186

Whyte KL, Levin R, Powls A. Clinical audit: Optimal positioning of endotracheal tubes in neonates. *Scott Med J.* 2007;52(2):25-27

Lesson 5: Performance Checklist

Alternative Airways

The Performance Checklist Is a Learning Tool

The learner uses the checklist as a reference during independent practice or as a guide for discussion and practice with a Neonatal Resuscitation Program (NRP) instructor. When the learner and instructor agree that the learner can perform the skills correctly and smoothly without coaching and within the context of a scenario, the learner may move on to the next lesson's Performance Checklist.

Note: If the learner's institution uses a T-piece resuscitator or flow-inflating bag, the learner should also demonstrate proficiency with a self-inflating bag to be used in case of emergency (loss of compressed gas).

Knowledge Check

1. What are the indications for endotracheal intubation during resuscitation?

2. How do you determine what size of endotracheal tube should be used for various gestational ages and weights?

3. What 2 strategies can be used to determine depth of insertion of the endotracheal tube?

4. What indicators determine correct placement of the endotracheal tube?

5. What is the role of the assistant during intubation?

6. When should you consider using a laryngeal mask?

7. List at least 3 limitations of the laryngeal mask.

8. What indicators are used to determine correct placement of the laryngeal mask?

9. When and how should you remove the laryngeal mask?

Learning Objectives

1. Recognize the newborn that requires endotracheal intubation.

2 Demonstrate preparation for intubation, including choosing the correct-sized tube for the newborn's estimated weight.

3 Demonstrate correct technique for placing an endotracheal tube (operator).

4 Demonstrate the role of the assistant during intubation (assistant).

5 Demonstrate strategies to determine if the endotracheal tube is in the trachea.

6 Demonstrate how to use a suction catheter or meconium aspirator to suction thick secretions from the trachea.

7 Identify when placement of a laryngeal mask is indicated.

8 List the limitations of the laryngeal mask.

9 Demonstrate correct technique for placing and removing a laryngeal mask.

10 Practice behavioral skills to ensure clear communication and teamwork during this critical component of newborn resuscitation.

Endotracheal Intubation

Scenario

"You are called to attend a birth complicated by a Category III fetal heart rate pattern. The laboring mother is a 28-year-old primigravida at 39 weeks' gestation. Demonstrate how you would prepare for the birth of this baby. As you work, say your thoughts and actions aloud so I will know what you are thinking and doing."

✔	Critical Performance Steps
	Assesses perinatal risk (Learner asks 4 basic questions.)
	Gestational age? **"39 weeks' gestation."**
	Clear fluid? **"Amniotic fluid is clear."**
	How many babies? **"One baby is expected."**
	Additional risk factors? **"Mom has a fever."**
	Assembles team, identify leader, delegate tasks
	Performs equipment check

✔	Critical Performance Steps

"The baby has been born."

Rapid Evaluation

Term? Tone? Breathing or crying?

"Appears term, no tone, no breathing."

Initial Steps

Position, suction mouth and nose, dry, remove linen, stimulate

Vital Signs

Checks breathing

"Baby is apneic."

Positive-Pressure Ventilation

Positions head, applies mask, starts PPV at 20 to 25 cm H_2O; rate 40 to 60 breaths/min, requests pulse oximetry, requests ECG monitor (optional)

Within 15 seconds of beginning PPV, requests check to assess if heart rate is rising

"Heart rate about 40 bpm, not increasing."

Assesses chest movement

- If chest movement observed, continues PPV × 15 seconds

- If no chest movement observed, proceeds through corrective steps (MR. SOPA) until chest movement; then administers PPV × 30 seconds

- *If no chest movement with corrective steps, indicates need for alternative airway and proceeds directly to intubation*

Heart Rate

Checks heart rate

"Heart rate about 40 bpm, still not increasing."

Indicates need for alternative airway

Preparation for Intubation

Operator	Assistant
Prepares for intubation - Requests correct-sized tube - Requests correct-sized laryngoscope blade - Communicates preference for stylet usage	- Ensures suction set at 80 to 100 mm Hg - Selects correct-sized tube - Chooses correct laryngoscope blade (size 1 [term], size 0 [preterm]) - Checks laryngoscope light - Inserts stylet correctly *(stylet optional)* - Obtains CO_2 detector - Prepares tape or securing device - Places electronic cardiac (ECG) monitor leads and connects to monitor *(optional)*

✔ Critical Performance Steps

Intubating the Newborn

Operator	Assistant
• Holds laryngoscope correctly in left hand • Opens mouth with finger and inserts blade to base of tongue • Lifts blade correctly (no rocking motion) • Requests cricoid pressure if needed • Identifies landmarks, takes corrective action to visualize glottis if needed • Inserts tube from right side, not down center of laryngoscope blade • Aligns vocal cord guide with vocal cords • Removes laryngoscope • Holds tube against baby's palate	• Positions newborn in "sniffing" position, body straight, table at correct height • Monitors heart rate and announces if attempt lasts longer than 30 seconds • Applies cricoid pressure if requested • Hands endotracheal tube to operator • Removes stylet (if used) • Connects CO_2 detector and PPV device to endotracheal tube • Hands PPV device to operator

Positive-Pressure Ventilation and Confirming Endotracheal Tube Placement

• Administers PPV • Observes for symmetrical chest movement	• Assesses CO_2 detector color change • Listens for increasing heart rate and bilateral breath sounds and **reports breath sound findings**

If endotracheal tube not successfully placed,

"Color is not changing on the CO_2 detector and heart rate is not increasing."

• Removes endotracheal tube

• Resumes PPV by face mask

• Repeats intubation attempt or indicates need for laryngeal mask

If endotracheal tube successfully placed,

"Color is changing on the CO_2 detector and heart rate is increasing."

• Operator continues PPV × 30 seconds

• Assistant checks tip-to-lip depth using gestational age/weight table or NTL measurement.

   – If using NTL, measures distance from the nasal septum to the ear tragus. Insertion depth (cm) = NTL + 1 cm

• Assistant secures endotracheal tube

Vital Signs

Checks heart rate after 30 seconds of PPV through endotracheal tube

"Heart rate is >100 bpm; baby remains apneic. Oxygen saturation is 72%."

Continues PPV and adjust oxygen concentration per oximetry

Prepares for transport to nursery

Updates parents

Laryngeal Mask

Scenario

"A 17-year-old woman with no prenatal care has been admitted to the hospital in active labor. The woman believes she is at approximately 36 weeks' gestation.

You walk into the room a few minutes after the birth. The first responders could not achieve chest movement with face-mask ventilation. They have tried intubating twice without success. The newborn's heart rate is 40 bpm and not increasing. The newborn has a small mandible and large tongue and you suspect Robin sequence. You decide to insert a laryngeal mask."

✔	Critical Performance Steps
Laryngeal Mask Placement	
	Obtains size-1 laryngeal mask and 5-mL syringe
	Quickly inspects the device to ensure no cuts, tears, or kinks
	Attaches a syringe and completely deflates the cuff. Maintaining tension, disconnects syringe from inflation port.
	Lubricates back of the mask with water-soluble lubricant *(optional)*
	Places baby's head in sniffing position
	Opens mouth and presses the leading tip of the mask against the baby's hard palate
	Advances the device inward along palate with a circular motion until resistance is felt
	Attaches syringe, inflates cuff (2-5 mL air) per manufacturer's recommendation
	Assistant attaches PPV device and CO_2 detector to the adaptor
Positive-Pressure Ventilation and Confirming Laryngeal Mask Placement	
	Holds laryngeal mask in place, administers PPV
	Assistant confirms placement by color change on CO_2 detector, auscultating heart rate, bilateral breath sounds, and observing symmetrical chest movement.
	If laryngeal mask not successfully placed,
	"Color is not changing on the CO_2 detector and heart rate is not increasing."
	• Removes laryngeal mask
	• Resumes PPV by face mask
	• Repeats laryngeal mask insertion attempt
	If laryngeal mask successfully placed,
	"Color is changing on the CO_2 detector and heart rate is increasing."
	• Operator continues PPV × 30 seconds
	• Assistant secures laryngeal mask by pressing tape across the fixation tab and the baby's cheeks
Vital Signs	
	Checks heart rate after 30 seconds of PPV
	"Heart rate is >100 bpm; baby remains apneic. Oxygen saturation is 72%."
	Continues PPV and adjusts oxygen concentration per oximetry
	Prepares for transport to nursery
	Updates parents

Instructor asks the learner debriefing questions to enable self-assessment, such as

1 What went well during this resuscitation?

2 What will you do differently when faced with this situation in a future scenario?

3 Do you have additional comments or suggestions for your team?

4 Give me an example of how you used at least one of the NRP Key Behavioral Skills.

Neonatal Resuscitation Program Key Behavioral Skills

- Know your environment.
- Use available information.
- Anticipate and plan.
- Clearly identify a team leader.
- Communicate effectively.
- Delegate workload optimally.
- Allocate attention wisely.
- Use available resources.
- Call for additional help when needed.
- Maintain professional behavior.

Chest Compressions

What you will learn

- When to begin chest compressions
- How to administer chest compressions
- How to coordinate chest compressions with positive-pressure ventilation
- When to stop chest compressions

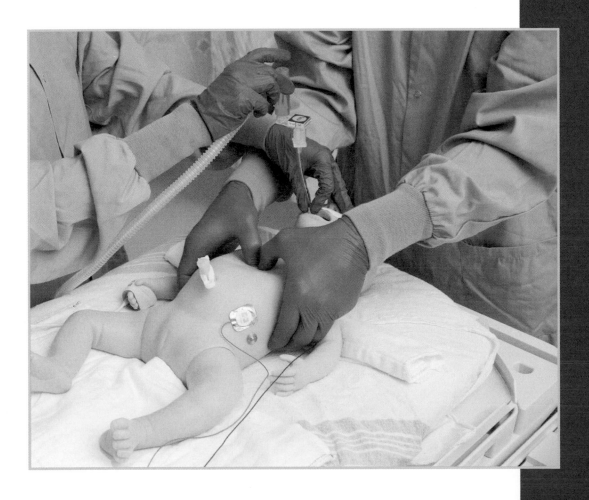

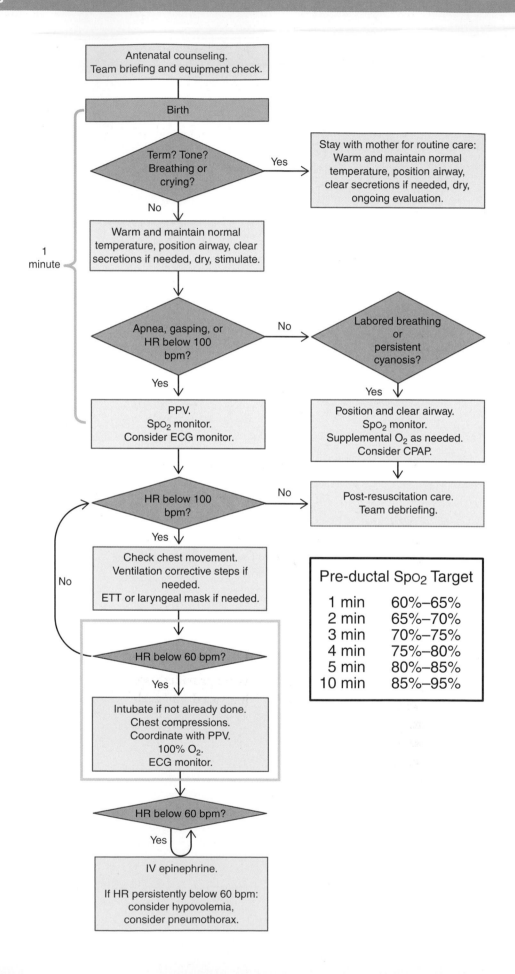

Antenatal counseling.
Team briefing and equipment check.

Birth

Term? Tone?
Breathing or
crying?

Yes → Stay with mother for routine care:
Warm and maintain normal
temperature, position airway,
clear secretions if needed, dry,
ongoing evaluation.

No

1 minute

Warm and maintain normal
temperature, position airway, clear
secretions if needed, dry, stimulate.

Apnea, gasping, or
HR below 100
bpm?

No → Labored breathing
or
persistent
cyanosis?

Yes

PPV.
SpO$_2$ monitor.
Consider ECG monitor.

Yes → Position and clear airway.
SpO$_2$ monitor.
Supplemental O$_2$ as needed.
Consider CPAP.

HR below 100
bpm?

No → Post-resuscitation care.
Team debriefing.

Yes

Check chest movement.
Ventilation corrective steps if
needed.
ETT or laryngeal mask if needed.

No

HR below 60 bpm?

Yes

Intubate if not already done.
Chest compressions.
Coordinate with PPV.
100% O$_2$.
ECG monitor.

HR below 60 bpm?

Yes

IV epinephrine.

If HR persistently below 60 bpm:
consider hypovolemia,
consider pneumothorax.

Pre-ductal SpO$_2$ Target

1 min	60%–65%
2 min	65%–70%
3 min	70%–75%
4 min	75%–80%
5 min	80%–85%
10 min	85%–95%

The following case is an example of how chest compressions are delivered during a more extensive resuscitation. As you read the case, imagine yourself as part of the resuscitation team.

Case: Late preterm newborn that does not respond to effective ventilation

Your team is called to attend an emergency cesarean birth at 36 weeks' gestation because of fetal distress. You perform a pre-resuscitation team briefing, assign roles and responsibilities, and complete an equipment check. After birth, the obstetrician stimulates the baby girl to breathe, but she remains limp and apneic. The umbilical cord is clamped and cut and she is moved to a radiant warmer. After performing the initial steps, she is still limp and apneic. You begin positive-pressure ventilation (PPV) with 21% oxygen, another team member listens to the baby's heart rate with a stethoscope, while a third team member places a sensor on her right hand and attaches it to a pulse oximeter. An assistant documents the events as they occur. The heart rate is 40 beats per minute (bpm), not increasing, and her chest is not moving with PPV. You proceed through the ventilation corrective steps, but the baby does not improve. A team member inserts an endotracheal tube and secures it, and ventilation is resumed. The carbon dioxide (CO_2) detector does not change color; however, there is good chest movement with PPV through the tube, and the breath sounds are equal in the axillae with each assisted breath. Electronic cardiac (ECG) monitor leads are placed on the chest and attached to an ECG monitor. Ventilation through the tube is continued for 30 seconds, but the heart rate remains 40 bpm. You increase the oxygen concentration to 100%, begin chest compressions coordinated with PPV, and call for additional help. During compressions and coordinated ventilation, the CO_2 detector changes color, and, within 60 seconds, the heart rate increases to 80 bpm. You stop compressions and continue PPV. Your team members frequently reevaluate the baby's condition and share their assessments with each other. The oxygen concentration is adjusted based on pulse oximetry. As the baby's tone improves, she begins to have intermittent spontaneous respiratory effort and her heart rate increases to 160 bpm. Her parents are updated and the baby is moved to the intensive care nursery for further evaluation. Shortly afterward, your team members conduct a debriefing to review their preparation, teamwork, and communication.

What are chest compressions?

Babies who do not respond to effective ventilation are likely to have very low blood oxygen levels, significant acidosis, and insufficient blood flow in the coronary arteries. As a result, cardiac muscle function is severely depressed. Improving coronary artery blood flow is crucial for restoring the heart's function.

The heart lies in the chest between the lower third of the sternum and the spine. Rhythmically depressing the sternum compresses the heart against the spine, pushes blood forward, and increases the diastolic blood pressure in the aorta. When pressure on the sternum is released, the heart refills with blood and blood flows into the coronary arteries (Figure 6.1). By compressing the chest and ventilating the lungs, you help to restore the flow of oxygenated blood to the heart muscle.

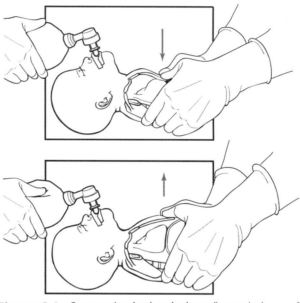

Figure 6.1. Compression (top) and release (bottom) phases of chest compressions

When do you begin chest compressions?

Chest compressions are indicated if the baby's heart rate remains **less than 60 bpm** after at least 30 seconds of PPV that inflates the lungs, as evidenced by chest movement with ventilation. In most cases, you should have given at least 30 seconds of ventilation through a properly inserted endotracheal tube or laryngeal mask.

If the lungs have been adequately ventilated, it is rare for a newborn to require chest compressions. Do not begin chest compressions unless you have achieved chest movement with your ventilation attempts. If the chest is not moving, you are most likely not providing effective ventilation. Focus your attention on the ventilation corrective steps, ensuring that you have an unobstructed airway, before starting compressions.

Apnea, gasping, or HR below 100 bpm?

Yes ↓

PPV.
SpO₂ monitor.
Consider ECG monitor.

↓

HR below 100 bpm?

Yes ↓

Check chest movement.
Ventilation corrective steps if needed.
ETT or laryngeal mask if needed.

↓

No ←

HR below 60 bpm?

Yes ↓

Intubate if not already done.
Chest compressions.
Coordinate with PPV.
100% O₂.
ECG monitor.

Indications for Chest Compressions

- Chest compressions are indicated when the heart rate remains **less than 60 bpm** after at least 30 seconds of PPV that inflates the lungs, as evidenced by chest movement with ventilation.

- In most cases, you should have given at least 30 seconds of ventilation through a properly inserted endotracheal tube or laryngeal mask.

Where do you stand to administer chest compressions?

When chest compressions are started, you may be standing at the side of the warmer. One of your team members, standing at the head of the bed, will be providing coordinated ventilations through an endotracheal tube.

If chest compressions are required, there is a high probability that you will also need to insert an emergency umbilical venous catheter for intravascular access. It is difficult to insert an umbilical venous catheter if the person administering compressions is standing at the side of the warmer with his arms encircling the chest. Once intubation is completed and the tube is secure, the compressor should move to the head of the bed while the person operating the PPV device moves to the side (Figure 6.2). In addition to providing space for umbilical venous catheter insertion, this position has mechanical advantages that result in less fatigue for the compressor.

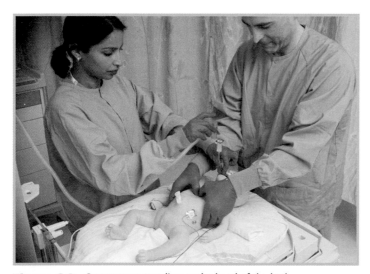

Figure 6.2. Compressor standing at the head of the bed

Where do you position your hands during chest compressions?

During chest compressions, pressure should be applied to the lower third of the sternum (Figure 6.3). Place your thumbs on the sternum just below an imaginary line connecting the baby's nipples. Your thumbs should be placed either side-by-side or one on top of the other in the center of the sternum. Do not place your thumbs on the ribs or on the xiphoid. The xiphoid is the small, pointed projection where the lower ribs meet at the midline.

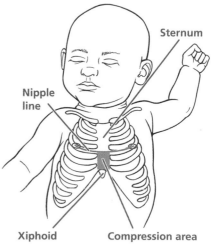

Figure 6.3. Landmarks for chest compressions

167

Encircle the baby's chest with your hands. Place your fingers under the baby's back to provide support (Figure 6.4). Your fingers do not need to touch.

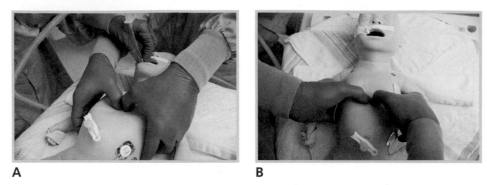

A
B

Figure 6.4. Chest compressions using 2 thumbs from the head of the bed (A) and side of the bed (B). Thumbs are placed over the lower third of the sternum, hands encircling the chest.

How deeply do you compress the chest?

Using your thumbs, press the sternum downward to compress the heart between the sternum and the spine. Do not squeeze the chest with your encircling hands. With your thumbs correctly positioned, use enough pressure to depress the sternum *approximately one-third of the anterior-posterior (AP) diameter of the chest* (Figure 6.5), and then release the pressure to allow the heart to refill. One compression consists of the downward stroke plus the release. The actual distance compressed will depend on the size of the baby.

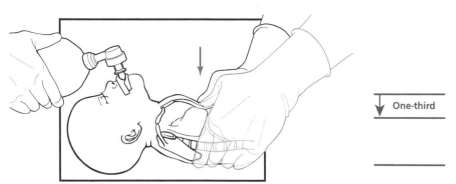

One-third

Figure 6.5. Compression depth is approximately one-third of the anterior-posterior diameter of the chest.

Your thumbs should remain in contact with the chest during both compression and release. Allow the chest to fully expand by lifting your thumbs sufficiently during the release phase to permit the chest to expand; however, do not lift your thumbs completely off the chest between compressions.

Review

1. A newborn is apneic. She does not improve with initial steps, and PPV is started. The first assessment of heart rate is 40 beats per minute. After 30 seconds of positive-pressure ventilation that moves the chest, her heart rate is 80 beats per minute. Chest compressions (should)/(should not) be started. Positive-pressure ventilation (should)/(should not) continue.

2. A newborn is apneic. She does not improve with the initial steps or positive-pressure ventilation. Her heart rate remains 40 beats per minute. An endotracheal tube is placed properly, the chest is moving, bilateral breath sounds are present, and ventilation has continued for another 30 seconds. Her heart rate is still 40 beats per minute. Chest compressions (should)/(should not) be started. Positive-pressure ventilation (should)/(should not) continue.

3. Mark the area on this baby where you would apply chest compressions.

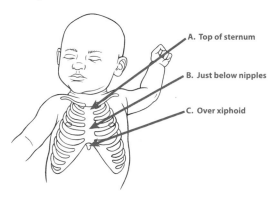

A. Top of sternum

B. Just below nipples

C. Over xiphoid

4. The correct depth of chest compressions is approximately

    a. One-fourth of the anterior-posterior diameter of the chest

    b. One-third of the anterior-posterior diameter of the chest

    c. One-half of the anterior-posterior diameter of the chest

    d. Two inches

Answers

1. Chest compressions should not be started. Positive-pressure ventilation should continue.

2. Chest compressions should be started. Positive-pressure ventilation should continue.

3 Compression area (B) just below the nipples.

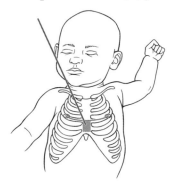

4 The correct depth of chest compressions is approximately one-third of the anterior-posterior diameter of the chest.

What is the compression rate?

The compression rate is 90 compressions per minute. To achieve this rate, you will give 3 rapid compressions and 1 ventilation during each 2-second cycle.

How are compressions coordinated with positive-pressure ventilation?

During neonatal cardiopulmonary resuscitation, chest compressions are always accompanied by coordinated PPV. Give 3 rapid compressions followed by 1 ventilation.

> **Coordinated Compressions and Ventilations**
> 3 compressions + 1 ventilation every 2 seconds

To assist coordination, the person doing compressions should count the rhythm out loud. The goal is to give 90 compressions per minute and 30 ventilations per minute (90 + 30 = 120 "events" per minute). This is a rapid rhythm, and achieving good coordination requires practice.

Learn the rhythm by counting out loud: "*One-and-Two-and-Three-and-Breathe-and*; *One-and-Two-and-Three-and-Breathe-and*; *One-and-Two-and-Three-and-Breathe-and...*".

• Compress the chest with each counted number ("*One, Two, Three*").

• Release the chest between each number ("*-and-*").

• Pause compressions and give a positive-pressure breath when the compressor calls out "*breathe-and*".

Inhalation occurs during the "breathe-and" portion of the rhythm, and exhalation occurs during the downward stroke of the next compression. Note that during chest compressions, the ventilation rate is slower than you used when giving only assisted ventilation. This slower rate is used to provide an adequate number of compressions and avoid simultaneous compressions and ventilation.

3:1 Compression:Ventilation Rhythm

One-and-Two-and-Three-and-__Breathe-and__ ;

One-and-Two-and-Three-and-__Breathe-and__ ;

One-and-Two-and-Three-and-__Breathe-and__ ...

What oxygen concentration should be used with positive-pressure ventilation during chest compressions?

When chest compressions are started, increase the oxygen concentration to 100%.

During chest compressions, circulation may be so poor that the pulse oximeter will not give a reliable signal. Once the heart rate is greater than 60 bpm and a reliable pulse oximeter signal is achieved, adjust the oxygen concentration to meet the target oxygen saturation.

When should you check the baby's heart rate after starting compressions?

Wait *60 seconds* after starting coordinated chest compressions and ventilation before pausing briefly to reassess the heart rate.

Studies have shown that it may take a minute or more for the heart rate to increase after chest compressions are started. When compressions are stopped, coronary artery perfusion is decreased and requires time to recover once compressions are resumed. It is, therefore, important to avoid unnecessary interruptions in chest compressions because each time you stop compressions, you may delay the heart's recovery.

How should you assess the baby's heart rate response during compressions?

Briefly pause compressions and, if necessary, pause ventilation. An electronic cardiac (ECG) monitor is the preferred method for assessing heart rate during chest compressions. You may assess the baby's heart rate by listening with a stethoscope or using a pulse oximeter. There are limitations to each of these methods.

- During resuscitation, auscultation can be difficult, prolonging the interruption in compressions and potentially giving inaccurate results.

- If the baby's perfusion is very poor, a pulse oximeter may not reliably detect the baby's pulse.

- An electronic cardiac (ECG) monitor displays the heart's electrical activity and may shorten the interruption in compressions, but slow electrical activity may be present without the heart pumping blood ("pulseless electrical activity"). In the newborn, pulseless electrical activity is treated the same as an absent pulse (asystole).

When do you stop chest compressions?

Stop chest compressions when the heart rate is **60 bpm or higher.**

Once compressions are stopped, return to giving PPV at the faster rate of 40 to 60 breaths per minute.

What do you do if the heart rate is *not* improving after 60 seconds of compressions?

While continuing to administer chest compressions and coordinated ventilation, your team needs to quickly assess the quality of your ventilation and compressions. In most circumstances, endotracheal intubation or laryngeal mask insertion should have been performed. If not, this procedure should be performed now.

Quickly ask each of the following questions out loud and confirm your assessment as a team:

- Is the chest moving with each breath?

- Are bilateral breath sounds audible?

- Is 100% oxygen being administered through the PPV device?

- Is the depth of compressions adequate (one-third of the AP diameter of the chest)?

- Is the compression rate correct?

- Are chest compressions and ventilations well-coordinated?

If the baby's heart rate remains less than 60 bpm despite 60 seconds of good quality, coordinated chest compressions and effective ventilation, epinephrine administration is indicated. Emergency vascular access will be needed. If compressions are being administered from the side of the bed, the team member providing chest compressions should move to the head of the bed to continue compressions and allow space for an operator to safely place an umbilical venous catheter or intraosseous needle.

Focus on Teamwork

Providing chest compressions highlights several opportunities for effective teams to use the Neonatal Resuscitation Program® (NRP®) Key Behavioral Skills.

Behavior	Example
Anticipate and plan.	Ensure that you have enough personnel present at the time of delivery based on the risk factors you identified. If there is evidence of severe fetal distress, be prepared for the possibility of a complex resuscitation, including chest compressions.
	If chest compressions are required, there is a high likelihood of also needing epinephrine. Plan for this possibility during your team briefing. If compressions are started, a team member should immediately start preparing the equipment necessary for emergency vascular access (umbilical venous catheter or intraosseous needle) and epinephrine.
Call for help when needed. Delegate workload optimally.	If chest compressions are required, you may need 4 or more health care providers. Performing all of the tasks quickly, including PPV, auscultation, placing a pulse oximeter, intubating the airway, administering compressions, monitoring the quality of compressions and ventilations, monitoring the baby's response, placing ECG monitor leads, preparing emergency vascular access, and documenting events as they occur, requires multiple team members.
Clearly identify a team leader. Allocate attention wisely.	The team leader needs to maintain situational awareness, paying attention to the entire situation, and not becoming distracted by any single activity or procedure. This means that leadership may need to shift to another person if the team leader is performing a procedure that occupies her attention.
	It is important for someone to monitor the quality of ventilation and compressions while also monitoring the baby's response (heart rate and oxygen saturation).
Use available resources.	If the compressor becomes fatigued, have another team member take over compressions. A respiratory care practitioner can administer PPV and monitor oxygen saturation, enabling a nurse or physician to prepare for emergency vascular placement and medication administration.
Communicate effectively. Maintain professional behavior.	During compressions, the compressor and ventilator need to coordinate their activity and maintain correct technique. If a correction is required, make a clear, calm, and directed statement.
	Share information with the individual documenting events so they can be accurately noted.

Frequently Asked Questions

What are the potential complications of chest compressions?

Chest compressions can cause trauma to the baby. Two vital organs lie within the rib cage—the heart and lungs. As you perform chest compressions, you must apply enough pressure to compress the heart between the sternum and spine without damaging underlying organs. The liver lies in the abdominal cavity partially under the ribs. Pressure applied directly over the xiphoid could cause laceration of the liver.

Chest compressions should be administered with the force directed straight down on the middle of the sternum. Do not become distracted and allow your thumbs to push on the ribs connected to the sternum. By following the procedure outlined in this lesson, the risk of injuries can be minimized.

Why does the Neonatal Resuscitation Program Flow Diagram follow A-B-C (Airway-Breathing-Compressions) when other programs follow C-A-B (Compressions-Airway-Breathing)?

The NRP focuses on establishing effective ventilation, rather than starting chest compressions because the vast majority of newborns who require resuscitation have a healthy heart. The underlying problem is respiratory failure with impaired gas exchange; therefore, ventilation of the baby's lungs is the single most important and effective action during neonatal resuscitation. Very few babies will require chest compressions once effective ventilation has been established. Other programs focus on chest compressions because adults are more likely to have a primary cardiac problem causing cardiorespiratory collapse, and teaching a single approach for children and adults simplifies the educational process.

Why does the Neonatal Resuscitation Program use a 3:1 compression-to-ventilation ratio instead of the 15:2 ratio used in other programs?

Neonatal animal studies have shown that the 3:1 ratio shortens the time to return of spontaneous circulation.

In the case at the beginning of the lesson, the CO_2 detector did not change color even though the endotracheal tube was correctly placed. Why?

If a baby has a very low heart rate or very poor cardiac function, there may not be enough CO_2 carried to the lungs to change the detector's color. In this case, you will need to use other indicators (chest movement and breath sounds) to determine if the endotracheal tube is correctly placed. If the CO_2 detector begins to change color during compressions, this may be an indication of improving cardiac function.

Key Points

1 Chest compressions are indicated when the heart rate remains below 60 beats per minute (bpm) despite at least 30 seconds of positive-pressure ventilation (PPV) that inflates the lungs (chest movement). In most cases, you should have given ventilation through a properly inserted endotracheal tube or laryngeal mask.

2 If the chest is not moving with PPV, the lungs have not been inflated and chest compressions are not yet indicated. Continue to focus on achieving effective ventilation.

3 If the heart rate is below 60 bpm, the pulse oximeter may stop working. You should continue ventilation with 100% oxygen until the heart rate is at least 60 bpm and the pulse oximeter has a reliable signal.

4 Once the endotracheal tube or laryngeal mask is secure, move to the head of the bed to give chest compressions. This provides space for safe insertion of an umbilical venous catheter and has mechanical advantages that result in less compressor fatigue.

5 To administer chest compressions, place your thumbs on the sternum, in the center, just below an imaginary line connecting the baby's nipples. Encircle the torso with both hands. Support the back with your fingers.

6 Use enough downward pressure to depress the sternum approximately one-third of the anterior-posterior (AP) diameter of the chest.

7 The compression rate is 90 compressions per minute and the breathing rate is 30 breaths per minute. This equals 3 compressions and 1 breath every 2 seconds, or 120 "events" per minute. *This is a slower ventilation rate than used during assisted ventilation without compressions.*

8 To achieve the correct rate, use the rhythm: "One-and-Two-and-Three-and-**Breathe-and**..."

9 After 60 seconds of chest compressions and ventilation, briefly stop compressions and check the heart rate. If necessary, briefly stop ventilation. An electronic cardiac (ECG) monitor is the preferred method for assessing heart rate during chest compressions. You may assess the baby's heart rate by listening with a stethoscope.

   a. If the heart rate is 60 bpm or greater, discontinue compressions and resume PPV at 40 to 60 breaths per minute.

b. If the heart rate is less than 60 bpm, check the quality of ventilation and compressions. If ventilation and compressions are being correctly administered, epinephrine administration is indicated.

LESSON 6 REVIEW

1. A newborn is apneic. She does not improve with initial steps, and PPV is started. The first assessment of heart rate is 40 beats per minute. After 30 seconds of positive-pressure ventilation that moves the chest, her heart rate is 80 beats per minute. Chest compressions (should)/(should not) be started. Positive-pressure ventilation (should)/(should not) continue.

2. A newborn is apneic. She does not improve with the initial steps or positive-pressure ventilation. Her heart rate remains 40 beats per minute. An endotracheal tube is placed properly, the chest is moving, bilateral breath sounds are present, and ventilation has continued for another 30 seconds. Her heart rate is still 40 beats per minute. Chest compressions (should)/(should not) be started. Positive-pressure ventilation (should)/(should not) continue.

3. Mark the area on this baby where you would apply chest compressions.

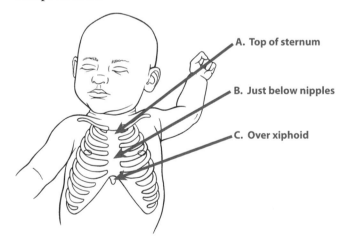

A. Top of sternum

B. Just below nipples

C. Over xiphoid

4. The correct depth of chest compressions is approximately

   a. One-fourth of the anterior-posterior diameter of the chest

   b. One-third of the anterior-posterior diameter of the chest

   c. One-half of the anterior-posterior diameter of the chest

   d. Two inches

5. The ratio of chest compressions to ventilation is (3 compressions to 1 ventilation)/(1 compression to 3 ventilations).

6. What phrase is used to achieve the correct rhythm for coordinating chest compressions and ventilation? _____
_____.

7. You should briefly stop compressions to check the baby's heart rate response after (30 seconds)/(60 seconds) of chest compressions with coordinated ventilations.

8. A baby has received chest compressions and coordinated ventilation. You briefly stop compressions and the electronic cardiac (ECG) monitor shows the baby's heart rate is 80 beats per minute. You should (continue)/(stop) chest compressions. You should (continue)/(stop) positive-pressure ventilation.

Answers

1. Chest compressions should not be started. Positive-pressure ventilation should continue.

2. Chest compressions should be started. Positive-pressure ventilation should continue.

3. Compression area (B) just below the nipples.

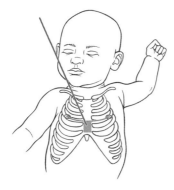

4. The correct depth of chest compressions is approximately one-third of the anterior-posterior diameter of the chest.

5. The ratio of chest compressions to ventilation is 3 compressions to 1 ventilation.

6. "One-and-Two-and-Three-and-Breathe-and ..."

7. You should briefly stop compressions to check the baby's heart rate response after 60 seconds of chest compressions with coordinated ventilations.

8. You should stop chest compressions. You should continue positive-pressure ventilation.

Additional Reading

Hemway RJ, Christman C, Perlman J. The 3:1 is superior to a 15:2 ratio in a newborn manikin model in terms of quality of chest compressions and number of ventilations. *Arch Dis Child Fetal Neonatal Ed.* 2013;98(1):F42-F45

Kapadia V, Wyckoff MH. Chest compressions for bradycardia or asystole in neonates. *Clin Perinatol.* 2012;39(4):833-842

Mildenhall LF, Huynh TK. Factors modulating effective chest compressions in the neonatal period. *Semin Fetal Neonatal Med.* 2013;18(6):352-356

Saini SS, Gupta N, Kumar P, Bhalla AK, Kaur H. A comparison of two-fingers technique and two-thumbs encircling hands technique of chest compression in neonates. *J Perinatol.* 2012;32(9):690-694

Lesson 6: Performance Checklist

Chest Compressions

The Performance Checklist Is a Learning Tool

The learner uses the checklist as a reference during independent practice or as a guide for discussion and practice with a Neonatal Resuscitation Program (NRP) instructor. When the learner and instructor agree that the learner can perform the skills correctly and smoothly without coaching and within the context of a scenario, the learner may move on to the next lesson's Performance Checklist.

Knowledge Check

1 What procedure is highly recommended before beginning chest compressions?

2 What are the indications for chest compressions?

3 What oxygen concentration is used when chest compressions are required?

4 Where are thumbs and fingers placed during chest compressions?

5 What is the correct compression depth?

6 What is the compression rate? What is the call-out rhythm to help ensure coordination between compressions and ventilation?

7 How long are chest compressions administered before checking a heart rate?

8 When can chest compressions be discontinued?

Learning Objectives

1 Identify the newborn that requires chest compressions.

2 Demonstrate the correct technique for performing chest compressions.

3 Identify the sign that indicates chest compressions should be discontinued.

4 Demonstrate behavioral skills to ensure clear communication and teamwork during this critical component of newborn resuscitation.

Scenario

"You are called to attend a birth due to fetal bradycardia. How would you prepare for the resuscitation of the baby? As you work, say your thoughts and actions aloud so I will know what you are thinking and doing."

✔	Critical Performance Steps
	Assesses perinatal risk (Learner asks 4 basic questions.)
	Gestation? **"Term."**
	Fluid clear? **"Fluid is clear."**
	How many babies? **"One baby is expected."**
	Additional risk factors? **"Fetal bradycardia for the last 3 minutes."**
	Assembles team, identifies leader, delegates tasks
	Performs equipment check
	**"The baby has been born."**

Rapid Evaluation

	Term? Tone? Breathing or crying?
	"Appears term, no tone, no breathing."

Initial Steps

	Positions, suctions, dries, removes linen, stimulates

Vital Signs

	Checks breathing
	"Baby is apneic."

Positive-Pressure Ventilation

	Begins PPV
	Within 15 seconds of beginning PPV, requests check to assess if heart rate is rising
	Asks assistant to place ECG leads and connect to cardiac monitor *(optional)*
	"Heart rate is about 40 bpm, not increasing."
	Assesses chest movement
	• If chest movement observed, continues PPV × 15 seconds
	• If no chest movement observed, proceeds through corrective steps (MR. SOPA) until chest movement; then administers PPV × 30 seconds
	• *If no chest movement with corrective steps, indicates need for alternative airway and proceeds directly to intubation or laryngeal mask placement*

Heart Rate

	Checks heart rate
	"Heart rate about 40 bpm, still not increasing."
	Indicates need for alternative airway

✔	Critical Performance Steps

Alternative Airway

- Intubates (size-1 blade and 3.5-mm endotracheal tube) or inserts laryngeal mask (size 1)
- Checks carbon dioxide (CO_2) detector color change, bilateral breath sounds, chest movement, and rising heart rate
- For endotracheal tube, checks tip-to-lip insertion depth using nasal-tragus length (NTL) or insertion depth chart
- Asks assistant to secure endotracheal tube or laryngeal mask
- Asks assistant to place ECG leads and connect to monitor *(optional)*

If device not successfully placed,

"Color is not changing on the CO_2 detector and heart rate is not increasing."

- Removes device
- Resumes PPV by face mask
- Repeats insertion attempt

If device successfully placed,

"Color is changing on the CO_2 detector. Pulse oximetry is not detecting a signal."

- Continues PPV × 30 seconds
- Assistant checks tip to lip depth (endotracheal tube) and secures device

Heart Rate

Checks heart rate after 30 seconds of PPV

"Heart rate is 40 bpm and not increasing, pulse oximetry is not detecting a signal."

Chest Compressions

Calls for additional help if necessary

Asks assistant to increase oxygen concentration to 100%

Asks assistant to place ECG leads and attach to monitor *(recommended)*

Compressor moves to head-of-bed position, ventilator to side of bed

Places thumbs on sternum (lower one-third, below imaginary line connecting nipples), fingers under back supporting spine (fingers do not need to touch)

Compresses sternum one-third of the AP diameter of chest, straight up and down

- Compressor counts cadence "One-and-two-and-three-and-breathe-and"
- Positive-pressure ventilation administered during compression pause ("breathe-and")
- 3 compressions and 1 breath every 2 seconds

Heart Rate

Checks heart rate after 60 seconds of compressions and ventilations

"The heart rate is 70 bpm and rising. Pulse oximetry is starting to detect a signal. No spontaneous respirations."

Positive-Pressure Ventilation Without Compressions

- Discontinues chest compressions
- Continues PPV with higher ventilation rate (40-60 breaths/min)
- Adjusts oxygen concentration per oximetry

"The heart rate is >100 bpm. Oxygen saturation is 78%. No spontaneous respirations."

✔	Critical Performance Steps
Vital Signs	
	Continues PPV and adjusts oxygen concentration per oximetry
	"Heart rate is >100 bpm. Oxygen saturation is 90%. Tone is improving, beginning to have some spontaneous respirations."
	Continues PPV and adjusts oxygen concentration per oximetry
	Prepares for transport to nursery
	Updates parents

Instructor asks the learner debriefing questions to enable self-assessment, such as

① What went well during this resuscitation?

② What will you do differently when faced with chest compressions in a future scenario?

③ Do you have additional comments or suggestions for your team?

④ Give me an example of how you used at least one of the NRP Key Behavioral Skills.

If significant errors were made, consider asking the learners,

⑤ What happened? What should have happened? What could you have done to make the right things happen?

⑥ What NRP Key Behavioral Skills might have been helpful in this situation?

Neonatal Resuscitation Program Key Behavioral Skills

- Know your environment.
- Use available information.
- Anticipate and plan.
- Clearly identify a team leader.
- Communicate effectively.
- Delegate workload optimally.
- Allocate attention wisely.
- Use available resources.
- Call for additional help when needed.
- Maintain professional behavior.

Medications

What you will learn

- When to give epinephrine during resuscitation
- How to administer epinephrine
- When to give a volume expander during resuscitation
- How to administer a volume expander
- What to do if the baby is not improving after giving intravenous epinephrine and volume expander
- How to insert an emergency umbilical venous catheter
- How to insert an intraosseous needle

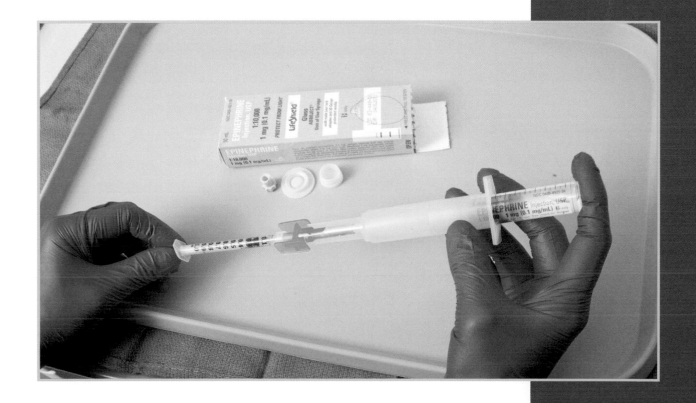

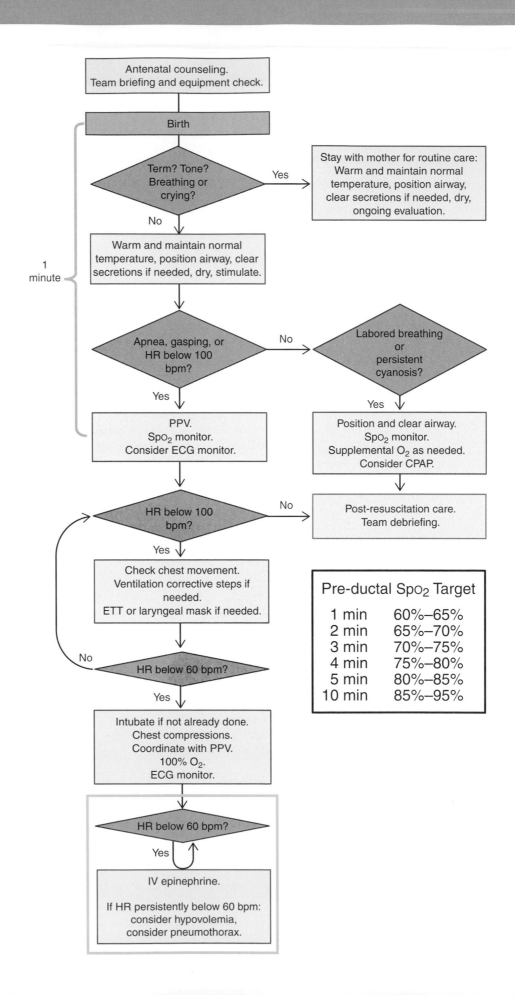

Antenatal counseling.
Team briefing and equipment check.

Birth

Term? Tone?
Breathing or
crying?

Yes → Stay with mother for routine care:
Warm and maintain normal
temperature, position airway,
clear secretions if needed, dry,
ongoing evaluation.

No

Warm and maintain normal
temperature, position airway, clear
secretions if needed, dry, stimulate.

1 minute

Apnea, gasping, or
HR below 100
bpm?

No → Labored breathing
or
persistent
cyanosis?

Yes

PPV.
SpO₂ monitor.
Consider ECG monitor.

Yes → Position and clear airway.
SpO₂ monitor.
Supplemental O₂ as needed.
Consider CPAP.

HR below 100
bpm?

No → Post-resuscitation care.
Team debriefing.

Yes

Check chest movement.
Ventilation corrective steps if
needed.
ETT or laryngeal mask if needed.

No

HR below 60 bpm?

Yes

Intubate if not already done.
Chest compressions.
Coordinate with PPV.
100% O₂.
ECG monitor.

HR below 60 bpm?

Yes

IV epinephrine.

If HR persistently below 60 bpm:
consider hypovolemia,
consider pneumothorax.

Pre-ductal SpO₂ Target

1 min	60%–65%
2 min	65%–70%
3 min	70%–75%
4 min	75%–80%
5 min	80%–85%
10 min	85%–95%

The following case is an example of how medications may be used during an extensive resuscitation. As you read the case, imagine yourself as part of the resuscitation team.

Case: Resuscitation with positive-pressure ventilation, chest compressions, and medications

A pregnant woman at 36 weeks' gestation is brought to the emergency department after an automobile accident. Fetal bradycardia is noted on the monitor. Your resuscitation team quickly assembles in the delivery room, completes a pre-resuscitation team briefing, and prepares equipment. An endotracheal tube, umbilical venous catheter, epinephrine, and volume replacement are prepared because an extensive resuscitation is anticipated. An emergency cesarean birth is performed, the umbilical cord is immediately clamped and cut, and a limp, pale baby boy is handed to the resuscitation team. A team member begins documenting the resuscitation events as they occur.

You perform the initial steps under a radiant warmer; however, the baby remains limp without spontaneous respirations. You begin positive-pressure ventilation (PPV) with 21% oxygen, a pulse oximeter sensor is placed on his right hand, and electronic cardiac (ECG) monitor leads are placed on his chest. The baby's heart rate is 40 beats per minute (bpm) by ECG and auscultation. The pulse oximeter does not register a signal. Although PPV appears to achieve good chest movement, his heart rate does not increase. You quickly perform the ventilation corrective steps without improvement. The baby is successfully intubated and PPV through the endotracheal tube is continued for 30 seconds, but his heart rate remains 40 bpm. Chest compressions are performed with coordinated PPV using 100% oxygen. A team member confirms the quality of compressions and ventilation, but, after 60 seconds, the baby's heart rate has slowed to 30 bpm.

One team member quickly inserts the umbilical venous catheter. With the assistance of another team member, a dose of epinephrine is administered through the catheter followed by a normal saline flush. Ventilation and compressions are continued, and, 1 minute later, the baby's heart rate has increased to 50 bpm. Because the baby has persistent bradycardia and a history of probable blood loss, a 30-mL infusion of normal saline is begun through the umbilical catheter. The heart rate increases and chest compressions are stopped when it rises above 60 bpm. As the heart rate continues to increase, the oximeter begins to detect a reliable signal and shows oxygen saturation 70% and rising. Assisted ventilation continues and the oxygen concentration is adjusted to maintain the baby's oxygen saturation within the target range. By 10 minutes after birth, the baby makes an initial gasp. He is transferred to the nursery for post-resuscitation care. Shortly afterward, your team members conduct a debriefing to discuss their preparation, teamwork, and communication.

A very small number of newborns will require emergency medication.

Most newborns requiring resuscitation will improve without emergency medications. Before administering medications, you should check the effectiveness of ventilation and compressions. In most cases, you should have inserted an endotracheal tube or laryngeal mask to improve the efficacy of ventilation.

Despite inflating the lungs and augmenting cardiac output with chest compressions, a very small number of newborns (approximately 1-3 per 1,000 term and late preterm births) will still have a heart rate below 60 bpm. This occurs when blood flow into the coronary arteries is severely decreased, resulting in such low oxygen delivery to the newborn's heart that it cannot contract effectively. These newborns should receive epinephrine to improve coronary artery perfusion and oxygen delivery (Figure 7.1). Newborns with shock from acute blood loss (eg, bleeding vasa previa, fetal trauma, cord disruption, severe cord compression) may also require emergency volume expansion.

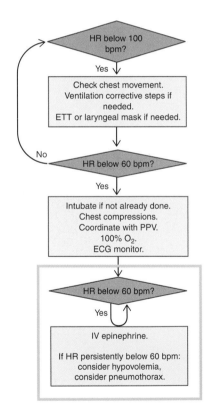

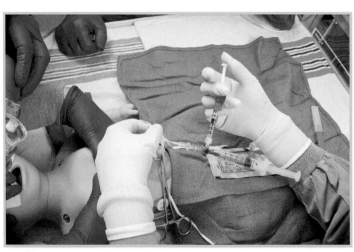

Figure 7.1. Few newborns require emergency medication to regain cardiac function.

What is epinephrine and what does it do?

Epinephrine is a cardiac and vascular stimulant. It causes constriction of blood vessels outside of the heart, which increases blood flow into the coronary arteries. Blood flowing into the coronary arteries carries the oxygen required to restore cardiac function. In addition, epinephrine increases the rate and strength of cardiac contractions.

When is epinephrine indicated and how should it be administered?

Indication

Epinephrine is indicated if the baby's heart rate remains **below 60 bpm after**

- At least 30 seconds of PPV that inflates the lungs (moves the chest), **and**

- Another 60 seconds of chest compressions coordinated with PPV using 100% oxygen.

In most cases, 30 seconds of ventilation should have been provided through a properly inserted endotracheal tube or laryngeal mask. Epinephrine **is not** indicated before you have established ventilation that effectively inflates the lungs.

Concentration

Epinephrine is available in 2 concentrations.

Only the 1:10,000 preparation (0.1 mg/mL) should be used for neonatal resuscitation.

Route

<u>Intravenous *(preferred)* or Intraosseous:</u> Epinephrine needs to rapidly reach the central venous circulation. Medications reach the central venous circulation quickly when administered into either an umbilical venous catheter or an intraosseous needle. Attempting insertion of a peripheral intravenous catheter is not recommended for emergency medication administration in the setting of cardiovascular collapse because it is likely to be unsuccessful, result in epinephrine extravasation into the tissue, and delay the administration of potentially lifesaving therapy.

<u>Endotracheal *(less effective)*:</u> Some clinicians may choose to give a dose of epinephrine into the endotracheal tube while vascular access is established. Although it may be faster to give endotracheal epinephrine, studies suggest that absorption is unreliable and the endotracheal route is less effective. For this reason, the intravenous and intraosseous routes are recommended.

Preparation

Use a sterile connector or stopcock to transfer epinephrine from the glass vial injector to a syringe (Figure 7.2).

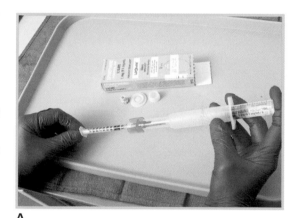

A

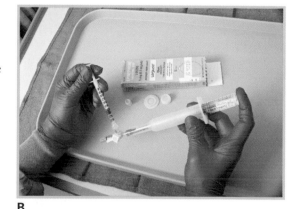

B

Figure 7.2. Use a connector or stopcock to transfer epinephrine.

<u>Intravenous/Intraosseous:</u> Prepare intravenous or intraosseous epinephrine in a labeled **1-mL syringe.** Clearly label the syringe: *"Epinephrine-IV."*

<u>Endotracheal:</u> Prepare endotracheal epinephrine in a 3- to 5-mL syringe. Clearly label the syringe: *"Epinephrine-ET ONLY."* Be certain not to use this larger syringe for intravenous or intraosseous administration.

Dose

<u>Intravenous or intraosseous:</u> The recommended **intravenous or intraosseous dose** is **0.1 to 0.3 mL/kg** (equal to 0.01 to 0.03 mg/kg). You will need to estimate the baby's weight after birth.

<u>Endotracheal:</u> If you decide to give an endotracheal dose while vascular access is being established, the recommended dose is 0.5 to 1 mL/kg (equal to 0.05 to 0.1 mg/kg). This higher dose is **only** recommended for endotracheal administration. **DO NOT give the higher dose via the intravenous or intraosseous route.**

Administration

Epinephrine is given rapidly.

<u>Intravenous or intraosseous:</u> Follow the drug with a 0.5- to 1-mL flush of normal saline.

<u>Endotracheal:</u> When giving endotracheal epinephrine, be sure to give the drug directly into the tube, being careful not to leave it deposited in the tube connector. Because you will be giving a large fluid volume into the endotracheal tube, you should follow the drug with several positive-pressure breaths to distribute the drug into the lungs.

What should you expect to happen after giving epinephrine?

Assess the heart rate 1 minute after epinephrine administration. As you continue PPV with 100% oxygen and chest compressions, the heart rate should increase to 60 bpm or higher within approximately 1 minute of intravenous or intraosseous epinephrine administration.

If the heart rate is less than 60 bpm after the first dose of intravenous or intraosseous epinephrine, you can repeat the dose every 3 to 5 minutes. If you started at the lower end of the dosage range, you should consider increasing subsequent doses. Do not exceed the maximum recommended dose. If there is not a satisfactory response after intravenous or intraosseous epinephrine, consider other problems such as hypovolemia and tension pneumothorax.

The response may take longer, or may not occur, if you give endotracheal epinephrine. If the first dose is given by the endotracheal route and there is not a satisfactory response, a repeat dose should be given as soon as an umbilical venous catheter or intraosseous needle is inserted. All subsequent doses, if necessary, should be given by the intravenous or intraosseous route.

In addition, check to be certain that

- The lungs are being adequately ventilated as indicated by chest movement. Insertion of an endotracheal tube or laryngeal mask should be strongly considered if not already done. If PPV is provided through an endotracheal tube or laryngeal mask, there should be equal breath sounds.

- The endotracheal tube is not displaced, bent, or obstructed by secretions.

- Chest compressions are being given at the correct depth (one-third of the anterior-posterior [AP] diameter of the chest) and correct rate (90/min).

- Interruptions in chest compressions are minimized because each interruption decreases coronary artery perfusion.

Epinephrine Summary

Concentration
1:10,000 epinephrine (0.1 mg/mL)

Route
Intravenous (preferred) or Intraosseous
Option: Endotracheal only while intravenous or intraosseous access is being obtained

Preparation
Intravenous or Intraosseous = 1-mL syringe labeled "Epinephrine-IV"
Endotracheal = 3- to 5-mL syringe labeled "Epinephrine-ET only"

Dose
Intravenous or Intraosseous = 0.1 to 0.3 mL/kg
Endotracheal = 0.5 to 1 mL/kg

Administration
Rapidly—as quickly as possible
Intravenous or Intraosseous: Flush with 0.5 to 1 mL normal saline
Endotracheal: PPV breaths to distribute into lungs
Repeat every 3 to 5 minutes if heart rate remains less than 60 bpm.

When should you consider administering a volume expander?

If there has been an acute fetal-maternal hemorrhage, bleeding vasa previa, extensive vaginal bleeding, a placental laceration, fetal trauma, an umbilical cord prolapse, a tight nuchal cord, or blood loss from the umbilical cord, the baby may be in hypovolemic shock. The baby may have a persistently low heart rate that does not respond to effective ventilation, chest compressions, and epinephrine. Babies with hypovolemic shock may appear pale, have delayed capillary refill, and/ or have weak pulses. In some cases, there will be signs of shock with no obvious evidence of blood loss. Administration of a volume expander is indicated if the baby is not responding to the steps of resuscitation **and** there are signs of shock or a history of acute blood loss.

Volume expanders should not be given routinely during resuscitation in the absence of shock or a history of acute blood loss. Giving a large volume load to a heart that is already injured may actually worsen cardiac output and further compromise the newborn.

> Emergency volume expansion is indicated if the baby is not responding to the steps of resuscitation AND has signs of shock or a history of acute blood loss.

What volume expanders should be considered and how should they be administered?

Crystalloid fluid

The recommended crystalloid solution for acutely treating hypovolemia is 0.9% NaCl (normal saline).

Red blood cells

Packed red blood cells should be considered for volume replacement when severe fetal anemia is suspected. If fetal anemia was diagnosed before birth, the donor unit can be cross-matched to the mother to ensure compatibility with any maternal antibodies transferred to the baby. If cross-matched blood is not immediately available, use *emergency, non–cross-matched, type-O, Rh-negative packed red blood cells.*

Dose

The initial dose of the selected volume expander is 10 mL/kg. If the baby does not improve after the first dose, you may need to give an additional 10 mL/kg. In unusual cases of large blood loss, administration of additional volume may be considered.

Route

Options for emergency access to the vascular system during hypovolemic shock include placing an umbilical venous catheter or inserting an intraosseous needle. Attempting insertion of a peripheral intravenous catheter is not recommended for emergency volume administration in the setting of cardiovascular collapse.

Preparation

Fill a large syringe (30-60 mL) with the selected volume expander. If using saline, label the syringe.

Administration

In most cases, acute hypovolemia resulting in a need for resuscitation should be corrected fairly quickly. No clinical trials have established a preferred infusion rate, but, in most cases, a steady infusion over 5 to 10 minutes is reasonable.

In preterm newborns less than 30 weeks' gestation, rapid administration of a volume expander may increase the risk of intracranial hemorrhage.

Volume Expander Summary

Solution
Normal saline (0.9% NaCl)
Suspected anemia: O-negative packed red blood cells

Route
Intravenous or Intraosseous

Preparation
30- to 60-mL syringe (labeled)

Administration
Over 5 to 10 minutes
(Use caution with preterm newborns less than 30 weeks' gestation.)

What do you do if the baby is not improving after giving intravenous epinephrine and volume expander?

While continuing to administer chest compressions and ventilation, your team needs to quickly reassess the quality of your ventilation and compressions. Intravenous epinephrine may be repeated every 3 to 5 minutes.

If you have not inserted an alternative airway, this procedure should be performed now. In addition, obtaining a STAT chest x-ray may provide valuable information. If necessary, call for additional expertise.

Quickly ask each of the following questions out loud and confirm your assessment as a team:

- Is the chest moving with each breath?

- Are equal breath sounds present?

- Is the airway device or trachea obstructed by secretions?

- Is 100% oxygen being administered through the PPV device?

- Is the compression depth adequate (one-third of the AP diameter of the chest)?

- Was the correct dose of epinephrine given intravenously? If epinephrine has been given only by the endotracheal route, quickly insert an umbilical venous catheter or intraosseous needle and repeat epinephrine.

- Is a pneumothorax present?

You have followed the Neonatal Resuscitation Program® (NRP®) Flow Diagram, but the newly born baby still has no detectable heart rate (Apgar 0). For how long should you continue?

The persistent absence of a detectable heart rate (Apgar 0) at 10 minutes is a strong, but not absolute, predictor of mortality and serious morbidity in late preterm and term newborns. If there is a confirmed absence of heart rate after 10 minutes of resuscitation, it is reasonable to stop resuscitative efforts; however, the decision to continue or discontinue should be individualized.

When making the decision to continue resuscitation beyond 10 minutes, variables to be considered may include uncertainty about the duration of asystole, whether the resuscitation interventions were considered to have been optimized, the availability of advanced neonatal care such as therapeutic hypothermia, the baby's gestational age, the specific circumstances prior to birth such as the presumed etiology and timing of the perinatal events leading to cardiorespiratory arrest, and the family's previously expressed feelings about acceptable risk of morbidity.

There are other situations, such as prolonged bradycardia without improvement, where, after complete and adequate resuscitation efforts, discontinuation of resuscitation may be appropriate. However, there is not enough information on outcomes in these situations to make specific recommendations. Decisions on how to proceed in these circumstances have to be made on a case-by-case basis. If possible, emergency consultation with a colleague or individual with additional expertise may be helpful.

Review

① Epinephrine (increases)/(decreases) coronary artery blood flow and (increases)/(decreases) the strength and rate of cardiac contractions.

② Ventilation that moves the chest has been performed through an endotracheal tube for 30 seconds and coordinated with chest compressions and 100% oxygen for an additional 60 seconds. If the baby's heart rate remains below (60 beats per minute)/(80 beats per minute), you should give epinephrine while continuing chest compressions and ventilation.

③ The preferred route for epinephrine is (intravenous)/(endotracheal).

④ In the absence of shock or a history of acute blood loss, routine administration of a volume expander (is)/(is not) recommended.

⑤ If an emergency volume expander is indicated, the initial dose is (1 mL/kg)/(10 mL/kg).

Answers

① Epinephrine increases coronary artery blood flow and increases the strength and rate of cardiac contractions.

② If the baby's heart rate remains below 60 beats per minute, you should give epinephrine while continuing chest compressions and ventilation.

③ The preferred route for epinephrine is intravenous.

④ In the absence of shock or a history of acute blood loss, routine administration of a volume expander is not recommended.

⑤ The initial dose is 10 mL/kg.

How do you establish rapid intravascular access during resuscitation?

The umbilical vein

The umbilical vein is a rapidly accessible, direct intravenous route in the newborn (Figure 7.3). If the use of epinephrine can be anticipated because the baby is not responding to PPV, one member of the resuscitation team should prepare to place an umbilical venous catheter while others continue to provide PPV and chest compressions.

Emergency Umbilical Venous Catheter Insertion

1. Put on gloves and quickly prepare an area for your equipment (Figure 7.4). Although you should attempt to use sterile technique, you must balance the need to rapidly secure emergency venous access with the risk of possibly introducing infection. If central venous access will be needed after stabilization, the emergency umbilical venous catheter will be removed and a new catheter placed using full sterile technique.

2. Fill a 3.5F or 5F single lumen umbilical catheter with normal saline using a syringe (3-10 mL) connected to a stopcock. Once filled, close the stopcock to the catheter to prevent fluid loss and air entry (Figure 7.4). Be certain that you know which direction is "off" on the stopcock used in your practice setting.

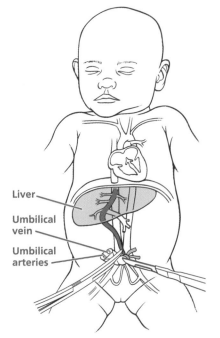

Liver

Umbilical vein

Umbilical arteries

Figure 7.3. The umbilical vein travels through the liver to join the central venous circulation.

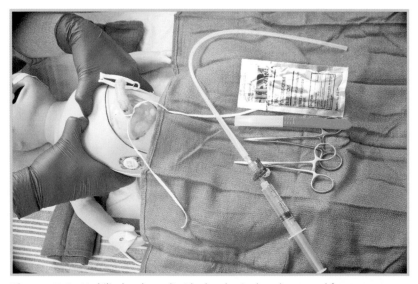

Figure 7.4. Umbilical catheter (inside the plastic sleeve) prepared for emergency insertion

③ Quickly clean the umbilical cord with an antiseptic solution. Place a loose tie at the base of the umbilical cord (Figure 7.5) around Wharton's jelly or the skin margin. This tie can be tightened if there is excessive bleeding after you cut the cord. If the tie is placed around the skin, be sure that it does not compromise skin perfusion.

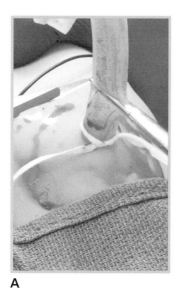 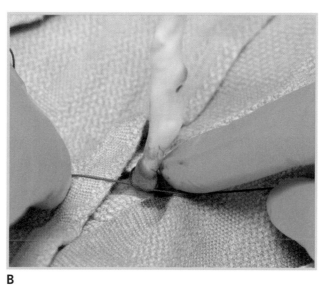

A   **B**

Figure 7.5. Tie placed around Wharton's jelly (A) or the skin margin (B). (Figure 7.5B used with permission of Mayo Foundation for Medical Education and Research.)

④ Briefly stop chest compressions and caution the team that a scalpel is entering the field. Cut the cord with a scalpel below the umbilical clamp and about 1 to 2 cm above the skin line (Figure 7.6). Attempt to cut straight across the cord rather than at an angle.

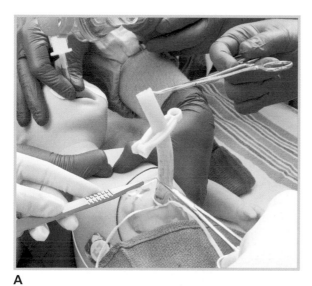 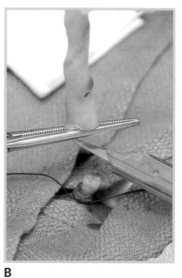

A   **B**

Figure 7.6. Cut the umbilical cord 1 to 2 cm above the skin line. (Figure 7.6B used with permission of Mayo Foundation for Medical Education and Research.)

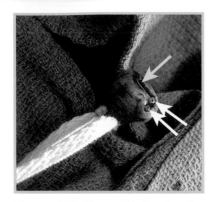

Figure 7.7. The umbilical cord ready for catheter insertion. The umbilical vein is shown by the yellow arrow. The 2 umbilical arteries are shown by the white arrows.

⑤ The umbilical vein will be seen as a larger, thin-walled structure, often near the 12-o'clock position. The 2 umbilical arteries are smaller, have thicker walls, and frequently lie close together (Figure 7.7). The arteries coil within the cord and their position will vary depending on where you cut the cord.

⑥ Insert the catheter into the umbilical vein (Figures 7.8 and 7.9).

    a. Continue inserting the catheter 2 to 4 cm (less in preterm babies) until you get free flow of blood when you open the stopcock between the baby and the syringe and gently aspirate.

    b. For emergency use, the tip of the catheter should be located only a short distance into the vein—only to the point at which blood can be aspirated. If the catheter is inserted farther, there is risk of infusing medication directly into the liver, which may cause hepatic injury (Figure 7.10).

    c. Continue to hold the catheter securely in place with 1 hand until it is either secured or removed.

⑦ Attach the syringe containing either epinephrine or volume expander to the available stopcock port, turn the stopcock so that it is open between the syringe and the catheter, ensure that there are no air bubbles in the syringe or catheter, administer the appropriate dose, and flush the catheter (Figure 7.11). It may be helpful to ask an assistant to infuse the medication while the operator holds the catheter in place.

⑧ After medications have been administered, either remove the catheter or secure it for temporary intravenous access as the baby

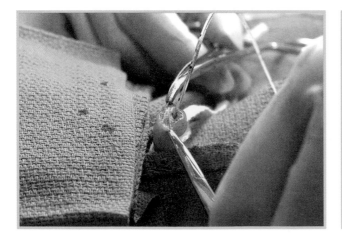

Figure 7.8. Saline-filled catheter inserted into the umbilical vein. Note the black centimeter markings on the catheter.

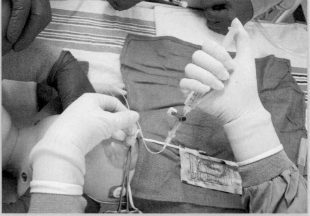

Figure 7.9. Advance the catheter until blood can be aspirated and the catheter can be easily flushed.

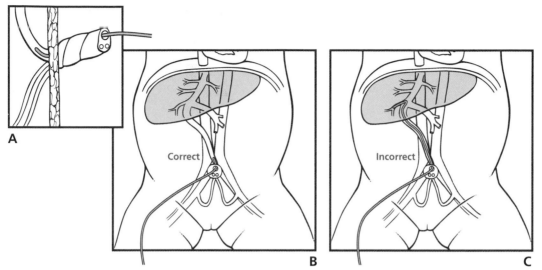

Figure 7.10. Correct (A and B) and incorrect (C) umbilical vein catheter placement

is transported to the nursery. If you decide to leave the catheter in place during stabilization or transport, it should be secured. A clear adhesive dressing can be used to temporarily secure the line to the newborn's abdomen (Figure 7.12). Suturing and "goal post" tape are effective methods for securing the catheter for prolonged use, but they take time and may not be the best choice during resuscitation.

9. If you remove the catheter, do it slowly and be prepared to control bleeding by tightening the cord tie, squeezing the umbilical stump, or applying pressure above the umbilicus.

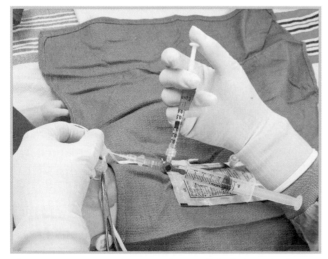

Figure 7.11. Open the stopcock toward the baby and infuse the medication.

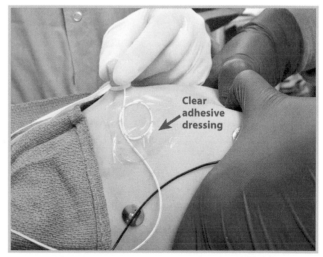

Figure 7.12. Temporarily secure the umbilical catheter with a clear adhesive dressing.

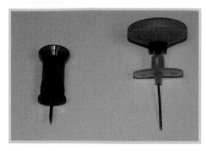

Figure 7.13. Examples of intraosseous needles. Some needles are inserted with a drill (left) and others are inserted manually (right).

The intraosseous needle

Although an umbilical venous catheter is typically the preferred method of obtaining emergency vascular access in the delivery room, an intraosseous needle is a reasonable alternative and is frequently used for emergency access in pre-hospital settings and emergency departments. An intraosseous needle (Figure 7.13) is inserted through the skin into the flat portion of a large bone and advanced into the bone marrow cavity (Figure 7.14). When medications and fluids are infused, they quickly reach the central venous circulation and have the same hemodynamic effect as intravenous administration. All medications and fluids that can be infused into an umbilical venous catheter can be infused into an intraosseous needle. Small studies have shown that intraosseous needles are feasible to place in term and preterm newborns, have similar efficacy to intravenous routes, and can be inserted quickly. Health care providers with limited neonatal intensive care experience may find an intraosseous needle easier to insert than an umbilical venous catheter.

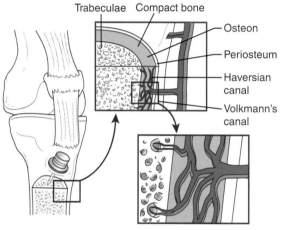

Figure 7.14. Intraosseous needle in the bone marrow cavity. Infused medications and fluids reach the central venous circulation quickly. (Adapted from Teleflex Incorporated. © 2016 Teleflex Incorporated. All rights reserved.)

Several different types of intraosseous needles are commercially available. Some are intended to be manually inserted using a twisting motion to penetrate the skin and bone. Other needles are inserted using a battery operated drill. Consult the manufacturer's literature to identify the correct-sized needle for your patient. The intraosseous needle will have a stylet that is used during insertion and must be removed before infusion.

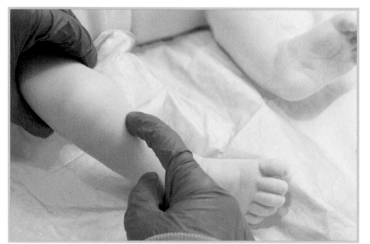

Figure 7.15. Needle insertion site along the flat anteromedial surface of the tibia

Intraosseous Needle Insertion Procedure

1. Identify the insertion site. For term newborns, the preferred site is the flat surface of the lower leg, approximately 2 cm below and 1 to 2 cm medial to the tibial tuberosity (the bony bulge below the knee cap) (Figure 7.15).

② Clean the insertion site with antiseptic solution (Figure 7.16).

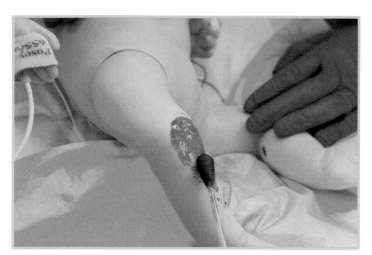

Figure 7.16. Quickly clean the insertion site.

③ Hold the intraosseous needle perpendicular to the skin and advance the needle through the skin to the surface of the bone (periosteum) (Figure 7.17).

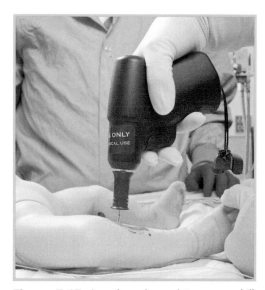

Figure 7.17. Insertion using an intraosseous drill

④ Direct the needle perpendicular to the bone and advance the needle through the bone cortex into the marrow space. If advancing the needle by hand, use strong downward pressure with a twisting motion. If advancing the needle with an electric drill, press the trigger while holding downward pressure as described in the manufacturer's instructions. When the needle enters the marrow space, a distinct change in resistance ("pop") is noticeable.

⑤ Follow the manufacturer's instructions for removing the stylet and securing the needle (Figure 7.18).

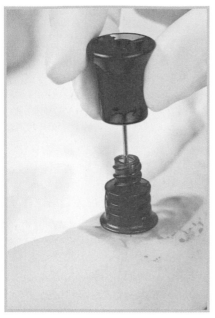

Figure 7.18. Remove the intraosseous needle stylet.

⑥ Connect an infusion set to the needle's hub, open the stopcock toward the needle, flush the needle, and administer the medication or fluid (Figure 7.19).

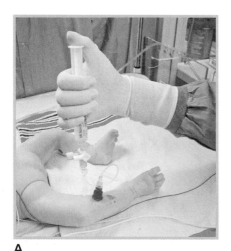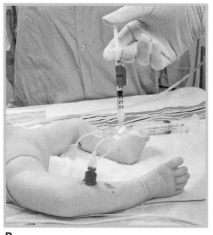

A   B

Figure 7.19. Connect an infusion set to the intraosseous needle, open the stopcock toward the needle, flush the needle (A), and infuse the medication or fluid (B).

⑦ Monitor the insertion site for evidence of swelling or fluid extravasation.

Focus on Teamwork

The administration of epinephrine and volume during resuscitation highlights several opportunities for effective teams to use the NRP Key Behavioral skills.

Behavior	Example
Anticipate and plan. Use available information.	If perinatal risk factors suggest that the fetus may have experienced acute blood loss or have severe cardiorespiratory compromise (eg, prolonged fetal bradycardia), prepare an umbilical venous catheter or an intraosseous needle, epinephrine, and fluid for volume expansion.
	Emergency insertion of an umbilical venous catheter or intraosseous needle and blood administration are infrequently used skills, and teams must practice them frequently to be certain that they can be performed correctly and efficiently during an emergency.
	If a baby requires chest compressions, it is likely that epinephrine also will be required. Once compressions are started, a team member should begin preparing epinephrine and an umbilical venous catheter or an intraosseous needle so that intravascular epinephrine can be administered without delay.
Know your environment.	Your team needs to know where emergency type O-negative blood is stored, how it will be obtained when needed, and what additional equipment will be needed to prepare and infuse it without delay.
	Your team needs to know where the emergency vascular access equipment is stored.
Call for help when needed.	If epinephrine or volume expansion is required, you will need additional help. It will likely take more than 4 team members to continue effective ventilation and compressions, quickly insert and secure emergency vascular access, prepare and administer epinephrine or fluid, monitor the passage of time, monitor the quality of compressions and ventilations, document events as they occur, and provide support for the baby's family.
Allocate attention wisely. Clearly identify a team leader.	If the team leader becomes involved in umbilical catheter placement, her attention is focused primarily on that task and she may not be able to pay full attention to the baby's condition, the passage of time, or the adequacy of ventilation and compressions.
	Any team member who has mastered the NRP Flow Diagram and has strong leadership skills can become the team leader. Clearly announce the change in leadership when it occurs.
Use available resources.	If you have difficulty placing an emergency umbilical venous catheter, use an intraosseous needle.
Communicate effectively. Maintain professional behavior.	Use efficient, directed, closed-loop communication when epinephrine or volume expanders are requested.
	When you give an instruction, direct the request to a specific individual, call the team member by name, make eye contact, and speak clearly.
	After giving an instruction, ask the receiver to report back as soon as the task is completed.
	After receiving an instruction, repeat the instruction back to the sender.
	During a complex resuscitation, it is easy for the quality of communication to deteriorate. It is critically important for the leader to establish and maintain calm and professional behavior.

Frequently asked questions

The epinephrine box says "1:10,000", but the dose in the lesson is described as mL/kg. What does 1:10,000 mean? Can we use the 1:1,000 preparation?

The description "1:10,000" is an older method of describing a drug concentration that persists on the labeling for epinephrine. A 1:10,000 concentration means that 1 g of epinephrine is dissolved in 10,000 mL of fluid. This is equivalent to 0.1 mg per mL. In the lesson, the dose is described as mL/kg so that health care providers do not have to convert milligrams to milliliters during an emergency and risk making a decimal point error.

Do not use the 1:1,000 preparation. It is 10 times more concentrated and not appropriate for neonatal resuscitation.

Why is the intravenous route for epinephrine administration preferred over the endotracheal route? Isn't the endotracheal route easier and faster?

Epinephrine given into the endotracheal tube may be absorbed by the lungs and enter blood that drains directly into the heart. Although it may be faster to give epinephrine to an intubated baby through the endotracheal tube, the process of absorption by the lungs makes the response time slower and more unpredictable than if epinephrine is given directly into the blood. Data from both animal models and clinical studies suggest that the standard intravenous dose is ineffective if given via the endotracheal tube. There is some evidence in animal models that giving a higher dose can compensate for the delayed absorption from the lungs; however, no studies have confirmed the efficacy or safety of this practice in newborns. If the need for medications is anticipated, advance preparation of an umbilical venous catheter, before delivery, allows rapid administration of intravenous epinephrine without delay.

After intraosseous needle insertion, is it necessary to aspirate the syringe before infusing fluid?

No. In the newborn, aspiration of the intraosseous needle is not a reliable indicator of correct needle placement and is not necessary. If the needle is correctly placed, it should feel firmly secured in the bone and not "wiggle." When fluid is infused, the soft tissue surrounding the bone should not swell.

Ethical Considerations
How do you tell parents that their baby is dying?
How do you take care of a baby that is dying?
These questions are explored in detail in Lesson 11.

Key Points

1 Epinephrine is indicated if the baby's heart rate remains **below 60 beats per minute (bpm) after**

- At least 30 seconds of positive-pressure ventilation (PPV) that inflates the lungs as evidenced by chest movement **and**
- Another 60 seconds of chest compressions with PPV using 100% oxygen.
- In most cases, ventilation should have been provided through a properly inserted endotracheal tube or laryngeal mask.

2 Epinephrine is not indicated before you have established ventilation that effectively inflates the lungs, as evidenced by chest movement.

3 Epinephrine recommendations

   a. Concentration: 1:10,000 (0.1 mg/mL)

   b. Route:

   Intravenous (preferred) or Intraosseous

   The central venous circulation may be rapidly accessed using either an umbilical venous catheter or an intraosseous needle.

   One endotracheal dose may be considered while vascular access is being established.

   c. Preparation:

   Intravenous or Intraosseous: 1-mL syringe (labeled *Epinephrine-IV)*

   Endotracheal: 3- to 5-mL syringe (labeled *Epinephrine-ET ONLY)*

   d. Dose: Intravenous or Intraosseous = 0.1 to 0.3 mL/kg. May repeat every 3 to 5 minutes.

   Consider higher dose (0.5 to 1 mL/kg) ONLY for endotracheal route.

   e. Rate: *Rapidly*—as quickly as possible

4 Administration of a volume expander is indicated if the baby is not responding to the steps of resuscitation AND there are signs of shock or a history of acute blood loss.

5 Volume expansion recommendations

   a. Solution: Normal saline (0.9% NaCl) or type-O Rh-negative blood

   b. Route: Intravenous or intraosseous

    c. Preparation: Volume drawn into a 30- to 60-mL syringe (labeled)

    d. Dose: 10 mL/kg

    e. Administration: Over 5 to 10 minutes

6 The persistent absence of a detectable heart rate (Apgar 0) at 10 minutes is a strong, but not absolute, predictor of mortality and serious morbidity in late preterm and term newborns. If there is a confirmed absence of heart rate after 10 minutes of resuscitation, it is reasonable to stop resuscitative efforts; however, the decision to continue or discontinue should be individualized.

LESSON 7 REVIEW

1. Epinephrine (increases)/(decreases) coronary artery blood flow and (increases)/(decreases) the strength and rate of cardiac contractions.

2. Ventilation that moves the chest has been performed through an endotracheal tube for 30 seconds and continued with chest compressions and 100% oxygen for an additional 60 seconds. If the baby's heart rate remains below (60 beats per minute)/(80 beats per minute), you should give epinephrine while continuing chest compressions and ventilation.

3. The preferred route for epinephrine is (intravenous)/(endotracheal).

4. In the absence of shock or a history of acute blood loss, routine administration of a volume expander (is)/(is not) recommended.

5. If an emergency volume expander is indicated, the initial dose is (1 mL/kg)/(10 mL/kg).

6. The recommended concentration of epinephrine for newborns is (1:1,000)/(1:10,000).

7. Using the correct concentration of epinephrine, the recommended intravenous dose is (0.1 to 0.3 mL/kg)/(0.5 to 1 mL/kg).

8. Epinephrine should be administered (slowly)/(as quickly as possible).

9. If the baby's heart rate remains below 60 beats per minute, you can repeat the dose of epinephrine every (3 to 5 minutes)/(8 to 10 minutes).

10. In a full-term baby, insert an emergency umbilical venous catheter (at least 8 to 10 cm or until it reaches the liver)/ (approximately 2 to 4 cm or until blood can be aspirated).

11. Your team is resuscitating a baby born at term. His heart rate is 40 beats per minute after ventilation through an endotracheal tube and coordinated chest compressions. You determine that epinephrine is indicated. Your team should (quickly attempt to place a peripheral intravenous catheter in his right hand)/(insert an umbilical venous catheter or an intraosseous needle).

Answers

1. Epinephrine increases coronary artery blood flow and increases the strength and rate of cardiac contractions.

2. If the baby's heart rate remains below 60 beats per minute, you should give epinephrine while continuing chest compressions and ventilation.

3. The preferred route for epinephrine is intravenous.

4. In the absence of shock or a history of acute blood loss, routine administration of a volume expander is not recommended.

5. The initial dose is 10 mL/kg.

6. The recommended concentration of epinephrine for newborns is 1:10,000 (0.1 mg/mL).

7. Using the correct concentration of epinephrine, the recommended intravenous dose is 0.1 to 0.3 mL/kg.

8. Epinephrine should be administered as quickly as possible.

9. If the baby's heart rate remains below 60 beats per minute, you can repeat the dose of epinephrine every 3 to 5 minutes.

10. In a full-term baby, insert an emergency umbilical venous catheter approximately 2 to 4 cm or until blood can be aspirated.

11. Your team should insert an umbilical venous catheter or an intraosseous needle. During cardiopulmonary collapse, a peripheral intravenous catheter is unlikely to be successful and attempts at insertion may delay appropriate therapy.

Additional Reading

Barber CA, Wyckoff MH. Use and efficacy of endotracheal versus intravenous epinephrine during neonatal cardiopulmonary resuscitation in the delivery room. *Pediatrics.* 2006;118(3):1028-1034

Weiner GM, Niermeyer S. Medications in neonatal resuscitation: epinephrine and the search for better alternative strategies. *Clin Perinatol.* 2012;39(4):843-855

Wyckoff MH, Perlman JM, Laptook AR. Use of volume expansion during delivery room resuscitation in near-term and term infants. *Pediatrics.* 2005;115(4):950-955

Yamada NK, Fuerch JH, Halamek LP. Impact of standardized communication techniques on errors during simulated neonatal resuscitation. *Am J Perinatol.* 2015 [Epub ahead of print]

Yamada NK, Halamek LP. On the need for precise, concise communication during resuscitation: a proposed solution. *J Pediatr.* 2015;166(1):184-187

Lesson 7: Performance Checklist

Emergency Medications

The Performance Checklist Is a Learning Tool

The learner uses the checklist as a reference during independent practice or as a guide for discussion and practice with a Neonatal Resuscitation Program (NRP) instructor. When the learner and instructor agree that the learner can perform the skills correctly and smoothly without coaching and within the context of a scenario, the learner may move on to the next lesson's Performance Checklist.

Knowledge Check

1. What are the indications for epinephrine during neonatal resuscitation?

2. What epinephrine concentration is used during neonatal resuscitation?

3. What is the preferred route of administration? What is the alternative route?

4. What is the correct dose range for each route? Where is the drug dosage chart our hospital uses during a neonatal code?

5. How quickly should you expect to see a rising heart rate after giving intravenous epinephrine? How often can you repeat epinephrine?

6. If the heart rate does not respond to intravenous epinephrine, what clinical conditions might be considered?

7. What are signs of shock in a newborn, indicating the need for volume expander?

8. What volume expanders are used? What is the dose of the selected volume expander?

9. What is the route of the volume expander and how fast is it administered?

Learning Objectives

1. Identify when the newborn requires epinephrine and volume expander during resuscitation.

2. Demonstrate preparation and administration of epinephrine and volume expander.

3. Demonstrate preparation and insertion of an emergency umbilical venous catheter.

4. Demonstrate how to secure an emergency umbilical venous catheter.

5. Practice NRP Key Behavioral Skills to ensure effective communication and teamwork during this critical component of neonatal resuscitation.

Scenario

"You are called to attend a birth due to umbilical cord prolapse with fetal bradycardia. How would you prepare for the resuscitation of the baby? As you work, say your thoughts and actions aloud so I will know what you are thinking and doing."

✔	Critical Performance Steps
	Assesses perinatal risk (learner asks 4 basic questions)
	Gestation? **"Term."**
	Fluid clear? **"Fluid is clear."**
	How many babies? **"One baby is expected."**
	Additional risk factors? **"Cord prolapse and fetal bradycardia for the last 3 minutes."**
	Assembles team, identifies leader, delegates tasks
	Performs Equipment Check
	"The baby has been born."
Rapid Evaluation	
	Term? Tone? Breathing or crying?
	"Appears term, no tone, no breathing."
Initial Steps	
	Positions, suctions, dries, removes linen, stimulates
Vital Signs	
	Checks breathing
	"Baby is apneic."

✔	**Critical Performance Steps**

Positive-Pressure ventilation

Begins PPV. Within 15 seconds of beginning PPV, requests heart rate check to assess if heart rate is rising

Asks assistant to place ECG leads and connect to cardiac monitor *(optional)*

"Heart rate is 30 bpm, not increasing."

Chest Movement

- If chest movement observed, continues PPV × 15 seconds
- If no chest movement observed, proceeds through corrective steps (MR. SOPA) until chest movement; then administers PPV × 30 seconds
- *If no chest movement with corrective steps, indicates need for alternative airway and proceeds directly to intubation or laryngeal mask placement*

Heart Rate

Checks heart rate

"Heart rate is 30 bpm, still not increasing."

Indicates need for alternative airway

Alternative Airway (endotracheal tube or laryngeal mask)

- Intubates (size-1 blade and 3.5-mm endotracheal tube) or insert laryngeal mask (size 1)
- Checks carbon dioxide (CO_2) detector color change, bilateral breath sounds, chest movement, and rising heart rate
- For endotracheal tube: checks tip-to-lip insertion depth using nasal-tragus length or insertion depth chart
- Asks assistant to secure endotracheal tube or laryngeal mask
- Asks assistant to place ECG leads and connect to cardiac monitor *(optional)*

If device not successfully placed,

"Color is not changing on the CO_2 detector, chest is not moving, and heart rate is not increasing."

- Removes device
- Resumes PPV by face mask
- Repeats insertion attempt

If device successfully placed,

"Color is faintly changing on the CO_2 detector, chest is moving, breath sounds are equal, pulse oximetry is not detecting a signal."

- Continues PPV × 30 seconds
- Assistant checks tip-to-lip depth (endotracheal tube) and secures device

Heart Rate

Checks heart rate after 30 seconds of PPV

"Heart rate is 30 bpm and not increasing, pulse oximetry is not detecting a signal."

Chest Compressions

- Calls for additional help
- Asks assistant to increase oxygen to 100%
- Asks assistant to place ECG leads and attach to cardiac monitor *(recommended)*
- Administers compressions from head of bed with coordinated ventilation (thumbs on lower one-third of sternum, compressions one-third of the AP diameter of the chest, 3 compressions: 1 ventilation every 2 seconds)

✔	Critical Performance Steps

Heart Rate

	Checks heart rate after 60 seconds of compressions and ventilations using ECG monitor
	"The heart rate is 30 bpm and not increasing. Pulse oximetry is not detecting a signal."
	Indicates need for emergency vascular access

Medication Administration via Endotracheal Tube (optional)

	Requests 1:10,000 epinephrine via endotracheal tube while umbilical venous catheter is prepared
	• Requests estimated weight **"Estimated weight is 3.5 kg."**
	• Orders epinephrine (1:10,000) 1.7 mL to 3.5 mL (0.5-1 mL/kg) via the endotracheal tube using closed-loop communication with confirmation of medication, dose, and route
	• Assistant checks medication label, opens medication, attaches stopcock or Luer lock syringe connector and 5-mL syringe
	• Assistant prepares correct volume, labels syringe with medication name and intended route
	• Correct dose of epinephrine administered per endotracheal tube
	• Announces, "endotracheal epinephrine given"
	Requests heart rate check after 60 seconds using ECG monitor
	"Heart rate is 30 bpm and not increasing. Pulse oximetry is not detecting a signal."
	Continues PPV and compressions

Preparing Emergency Umbilical Venous Catheter (may be performed by assistant or operator)

	• Obtains syringe with normal saline flush
	• Attaches 3-way stopcock to umbilical venous catheter
	• Flushes umbilical venous catheter and stopcock with normal saline
	• Closes stopcock to catheter

Inserting Emergency Umbilical Venous Catheter

	• Cleans lower segment of umbilical cord with antiseptic solution
	• Ties umbilical tape loosely at base of cord
	• Cuts cord approximately 1 to 2 cm above base (may request compressions pause)
	• Inserts catheter into vein, opens stopcock and gently aspirates syringe, advances catheter approximately 2 to 4 cm until blood return is detected
	• Flushes catheter and closes stopcock to catheter

Medication Administration via Umbilical Venous Catheter

	Requests 1:10,000 epinephrine via umbilical venous catheter
	• Requests estimated weight **"Estimated weight is 3.5 kg."**
	• Orders epinephrine (1:10,000) 0.35 mL to 1 mL (0.1-0.3 mL/kg) via the umbilical venous catheter using closed-loop communication with confirmation of medication, dose, and route
	• Assistant checks medication label, opens medication, attaches stopcock or Luer lock syringe connector and 1-mL syringe
	• Assistant prepares correct volume, labels syringe with medication name and intended route
	Administers umbilical venous catheter epinephrine (can be performed by assistant or operator)
	• Ensures that catheter is being held in place; attaches syringe to stopcock, opens stopcock to catheter and syringe, administers epinephrine rapidly without air bubbles
	• Flushes umbilical venous catheter with .5 to 1 mL of normal saline
	• Announces, *"Intravenous epinephrine given."*

✔	Critical Performance Steps
Heart Rate	
	• Continues PPV and compressions
	• Checks heart rate 60 seconds after umbilical venous catheter epinephrine using ECG.
	"The heart rate is 50 bpm, pulse oximetry is not detecting a signal, he appears pale."
	• Continues PPV and compressions
Administration of Volume Expander	
	Requests 35 mL (10 mL/kg) of normal saline per umbilical venous catheter over 5 to 10 minutes using closed-loop communication
	• Draws up correct volume or uses prefilled syringes. Numbers more than one syringe (#1, #2).
	• Ensures that catheter is being held in place; attaches syringe to stopcock, opens stopcock to catheter and syringe, administers volume in slow infusion over 5 to 10 minutes without air bubbles.
	• Announces *"35 mL of normal saline given."*
Heart Rate	
	• Continues PPV and compressions
	• Monitors heart rate while volume administered
	"Heart rate is 100 bpm and increasing. Spo_2 is 68%."
Discontinue Compressions – Continue PPV	
	• Discontinues chest compressions.
	• Continues PPV with higher ventilation rate (40-60 breaths/min)
	"The heart rate is >100 bpm. Oxygen saturation is 80%. No spontaneous respirations."
Vital Signs	
	Continues PPV and adjusts oxygen concentration per oximetry
	"Heart rate is >100 bpm. Oxygen saturation is 90%. He is beginning to have tone and some spontaneous respirations."
	Continues PPV and adjusts oxygen concentration per oximetry
	Prepares for transport to nursery
	Updates parents

Instructor asks the learner Debriefing Questions to enable
self-assessment such as

1 What went well during this resuscitation?

2 What will you do differently when faced with this complex
resuscitation in a future scenario?

3 Do you have additional comments or suggestions for your team?

4 Give me an example of how you used at least one of the NRP Key
Behavioral Skills.

Neonatal Resuscitation Program Key Behavioral Skills

- Know your environment.
- Use available information.
- Anticipate and plan.
- Clearly identify a team leader.
- Communicate effectively.
- Delegate workload optimally.
- Allocate attention wisely.
- Use available resources.
- Call for additional help when needed.
- Maintain professional behavior.

Post-resuscitation Care

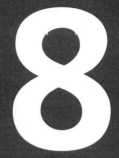

What you will learn

- What to do after neonatal resuscitation
- Medical conditions that may occur following neonatal resuscitation
- Management considerations following neonatal resuscitation
- The role of therapeutic hypothermia in post-resuscitation care

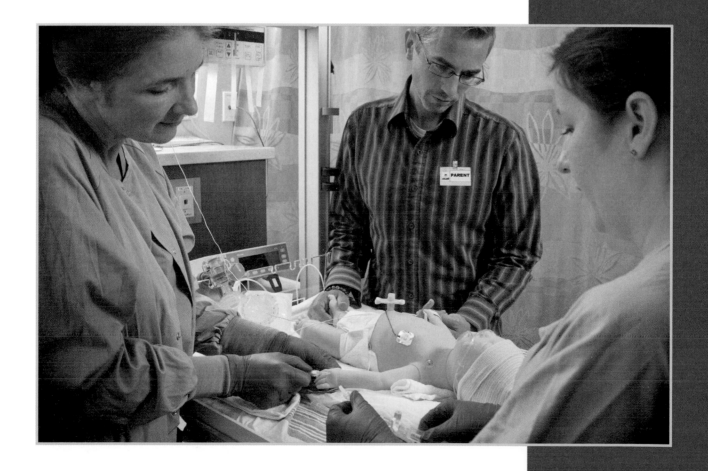

Case: An early term pregnancy with fetal distress

A baby girl was born at 37 weeks' gestation by emergency cesarean section because of maternal fever and fetal distress during labor. After birth, she was limp and apneic and did not respond to the initial steps of newborn care. She received positive-pressure ventilation (PPV) for 3 minutes until effective spontaneous respiratory effort was established. During the next several minutes, she developed labored breathing and required supplemental oxygen to maintain her saturation within the target range. The team leader updated her parents, explained her condition, and described the post-resuscitation care plan.

The newborn arrives in the nursery where vital signs, including temperature, oxygen saturation, and blood pressure, are recorded. She continues to require supplemental oxygen, and a chest x-ray is requested. A team member obtains a blood sample for glucose, culture, and blood gas testing. An intravenous catheter is inserted and the baby receives fluids and parenteral antibiotics. The health care providers discuss their plan for close monitoring and frequent assessment. Her father arrives at the bedside where he touches and comforts his baby. The medical provider gives the father an interval update and explains the treatment plan. Shortly afterward, the team members conduct a debriefing to review their preparation, teamwork, and communication.

Postnatal Care

The physiologic transition to extrauterine life continues for several hours after birth. Babies who required resuscitation may have problems making this transition even after their vital signs appear to return to normal. Medical complications after resuscitation may involve multiple organ systems. Many of these complications can be anticipated and promptly addressed by appropriate monitoring.

This program refers to 2 broad categories of postnatal care. The intensity of monitoring and the interventions required for individual babies will vary within these categories.

- **Routine Care**

Nearly 90% of newborns are vigorous term babies with no risk factors and they should remain with their mothers to promote bonding, initiate breastfeeding, and receive routine newborn care (Figure 8.1). Similarly, a baby with certain prenatal or intrapartum risk factors, who responded well to the initial steps of newborn care, may only need close observation and does not need to be separated from the mother. Ongoing observation of breathing, thermoregulation, feeding, and activity are important to determine if additional interventions are required. The frequency of these evaluations will be determined by the specific perinatal risk factors and the baby's condition.

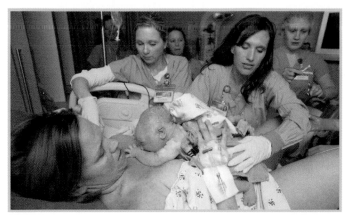

Figure 8.1. Routine care. (Used with permission of Mayo Foundation for Medical Education and Research.)

- **Post-resuscitation Care**

Babies who required supplemental oxygen or PPV after delivery will need closer assessment. They may develop problems associated with abnormal transition and should be evaluated frequently during the immediate newborn period. They often require ongoing respiratory support, such as supplemental oxygen, nasal continuous positive airway pressure (CPAP), or mechanical ventilation. Many will require admission to a nursery environment where continuous cardiorespiratory monitoring is available and vital signs can be measured frequently (Figure 8.2). Some will require transfer to a neonatal intensive care unit. If a newborn requires post-resuscitation care in a location outside of the mother's room, the parents should be encouraged to see and touch their baby as soon as it is feasible. The period of time needed for post-resuscitation care is dependent on the newborn's condition, progress toward normal transition, and the presence of identifiable risk factors.

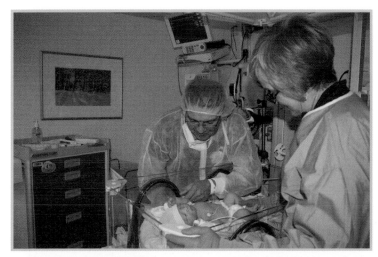

Figure 8.2. Post-resuscitation care in a setting where continuous cardiorespiratory monitoring is available and vital signs can be taken frequently

What medical conditions may occur in babies who required resuscitation?

Abnormalities in multiple organ systems may occur following neonatal resuscitation. Anticipated clinical signs, laboratory findings, and management considerations are summarized in Table 8-1. Individual circumstances will determine which of these management considerations are appropriate.

Table 8-1. Clinical signs, laboratory findings, and management

Organ System	Clinical Signs and Laboratory Findings	Management Considerations
Neurologic	Apnea, seizures, irritability, poor tone, altered neurologic examination, poor feeding coordination	Monitor for apnea. Support ventilation as needed. Monitor glucose and electrolytes. Avoid hyperthermia. Consider anticonvulsant therapy. Consider therapeutic hypothermia. Consider delayed initiation of feedings and use of intravenous fluids.
Respiratory	Tachypnea, grunting, retractions, nasal flaring, low oxygen saturation, pneumothorax	Maintain adequate oxygenation and ventilation. Avoid unnecessary suctioning. Cluster care to allow periods of rest. Consider antibiotics. Consider x-ray and blood gas. Consider surfactant therapy. Consider delayed initiation of feedings and use of intravenous fluids.
Cardiovascular	Hypotension, tachycardia, metabolic acidosis	Monitor blood pressure and heart rate. Consider volume replacement or inotrope administration if baby is hypotensive.
Renal	Decreased urine output, edema, electrolyte abnormalities	Monitor urine output. Monitor serum electrolytes as indicated. Monitor weight. Restrict fluids if baby has decreased urine output and vascular volume is adequate.
Gastrointestinal	Feeding intolerance, vomiting, abdominal distention, abnormal liver function tests, gastrointestinal bleeding	Consider abdominal x-ray. Consider delayed initiation of feedings and use of intravenous fluids. Consider parenteral nutrition.
Endocrine-Metabolic	Metabolic acidosis, hypoglycemia (low glucose), hypocalcemia (low calcium), hyponatremia (low sodium), hyperkalemia (high potassium)	Monitor blood glucose. Monitor serum electrolytes as indicated. Consider intravenous fluids. Replace electrolytes as indicated.
Hematologic	Anemia, thrombocytopenia, delayed clotting, pallor, bruising, petechiae	Monitor hematocrit, platelets and coagulation studies as indicated.
Constitutional	Hypothermia	Delay bathing.

Pneumonia and other respiratory problems

The need for resuscitation may be an early sign that a newborn has pneumonia, a perinatal infection, or an aspiration event. Neonatal pneumonia (Figure 8.3) may present with tachypnea and other signs of respiratory distress such as grunting, nasal flaring, and retracting. It can be difficult to differentiate between respiratory distress syndrome, retained fetal lung fluid, and neonatal pneumonia by chest x-ray. If a baby who required resuscitation continues to show signs of respiratory distress or requires supplemental oxygen, consider evaluating the baby for pneumonia and perinatal infection. Obtain appropriate laboratory tests and begin parenteral antibiotics.

If acute respiratory deterioration occurs during or after resuscitation, consider the possibility that the baby has a pneumothorax (Figure 8.4). Lesson 10 includes details about managing a pneumothorax. If the baby is intubated, ensure that the endotracheal tube has not become dislodged or obstructed by secretions.

Pulmonary hypertension

As described previously, blood vessels in the fetal lungs are tightly constricted. After birth, the pulmonary vessels relax and blood flows into the lungs where hemoglobin can be saturated with oxygen for delivery to the tissues and organs.

The pulmonary blood vessels may remain constricted after birth. This condition is called persistent pulmonary hypertension of the newborn (PPHN) and is most often seen in babies greater than or equal to 34 weeks' gestational age. PPHN usually is managed with supplemental oxygen and, in many cases, mechanical ventilation. Severe PPHN may require special therapies such as inhaled nitric oxide and extracorporeal membrane oxygenation (ECMO).

After resuscitation, the baby's pulmonary vascular tone can be labile and may increase in response to sudden decreases in oxygen saturation or unintentional hypothermia; therefore, avoid unnecessary suction, excessive stimulation, and immediate bathing. While avoiding sudden decreases in saturation may be beneficial, intentionally maintaining very high blood levels of oxygen is not likely to be helpful and may cause additional complications. A pulse oximeter should be used to guide oxygen therapy. In the setting of suspected PPHN, an arterial blood gas provides additional useful information that cannot be determined from pulse oximetry alone.

Hypotension

Hypotension during the post-resuscitation phase may occur for multiple reasons. Low oxygen levels around the time of birth can

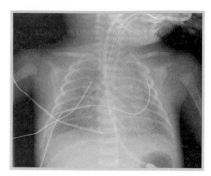

Figure 8.3. Neonatal pneumonia

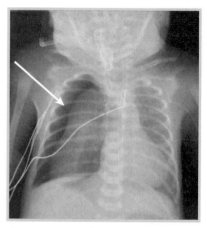

Figure 8.4. Right pneumothorax

decrease both cardiac function and blood vessel tone. If the baby had significant blood loss, the circulating blood volume may be low and contribute to hypotension. Babies with sepsis may have normal or high cardiac output, but they may become hypotensive because of dilation of peripheral blood vessels.

Babies who require significant resuscitation should have their blood pressure monitored until it is stable within an acceptable range. If there is evidence of hypovolemia, volume expansion with a crystalloid solution, or blood transfusion, may be indicated. Routine volume expansion without evidence of hypovolemia is not recommended. Some babies may require a medication, such as dopamine or dobutamine, to improve cardiac output and increase systemic blood flow.

Hypoglycemia

Glucose consumption is increased when metabolism occurs without adequate oxygen (anaerobic metabolism). Hypoglycemia may occur because glucose stores are depleted rapidly during perinatal stress. A transiently high glucose level may occur in some stressed newborns before the blood glucose level begins to fall. Glucose is an essential fuel for brain function in newborns and prolonged hypoglycemia may contribute to brain injury after resuscitation.

Babies who require resuscitation need to have their blood glucose level checked soon after resuscitation and then at regular intervals until it remains stable and within normal limits. Intravenous dextrose is often necessary to maintain normal blood glucose levels until oral feedings are established.

Feeding problems

The newborn's gastrointestinal tract is very sensitive to decreased oxygen and blood flow. Feeding intolerance, poor motility, inflammation, bleeding, and perforation of the intestinal wall can occur after resuscitation. In addition, sucking patterns and oral feeding coordination may be affected for several days because of neurologic dysfunction. Alternative methods for providing nutrition may be required during this interval.

Ideally, feedings should be initiated with breast milk. If the baby is born very preterm or is unable to start breastfeeding, work with the mother's health care provider to develop a plan that supports expressing, pumping, and storing breast milk shortly after birth.

Renal failure

Hypotension, hypoxia, and acidosis can decrease blood flow to the kidneys and cause either temporary or permanent renal failure. Acute tubular necrosis (ATN) is usually a temporary form of renal failure that may occur after resuscitation. It can cause fluid retention and significant electrolyte abnormalities. Babies initially may have low urine output and require fluid restriction for several days. During the recovery phase, they may develop very high urine output and require additional fluid.

Babies who require significant resuscitation should have their urine output, body weight, and serum electrolyte levels checked frequently. Adjust fluid and electrolyte intake based on the baby's urine output, body weight changes, and laboratory results.

Metabolic acidosis

Metabolic acidosis is a common finding after resuscitation because acids are produced when tissues receive insufficient oxygen and blood flow. Severe acidosis may interfere with heart function and worsen pulmonary hypertension. In most cases, the acidosis will gradually resolve as the baby's respiratory and circulatory systems recover. The most important intervention is to identify and correct the underlying cause of the metabolic acidosis.

Seizures or apnea

Newborns with hypotension, hypoxemia, and acidosis may develop signs of brain injury. This injury is called hypoxic-ischemic encephalopathy (HIE). Initially, the baby may have depressed muscle tone, lethargy, poor respiratory effort, or apnea. Seizures may appear after several hours. Babies who have required extensive resuscitation should be carefully examined for signs of HIE. A standardized neurologic assessment is a useful tool. Consultation with a specialist should be considered.

Lethargy, apnea, and seizures may be signs of other conditions such as exposure to a maternal narcotic or anesthetics, an infection, electrolyte disturbances, or a metabolic abnormality.

Hypothermia and hyperthermia

After resuscitation, babies may become too cold (hypothermic) or too warm (hyperthermic). Premature newborns are at high risk of hypothermia and this has been associated with increased mortality. Special techniques for maintaining body temperature in preterm newborns are addressed in Lesson 9. Babies may become hyperthermic if their mother has a fever or chorioamnionitis, if the baby has an infection, or if the radiant warmer is not adjusted properly. Among babies with HIE, hyperthermia has been associated with worsened outcomes and should be avoided.

When should therapeutic hypothermia (cooling) be considered?

Recent studies have demonstrated that therapeutic hypothermia after resuscitation reduces the risk of death and improves neurologic outcomes in some late preterm and term babies with moderate to severe HIE.

If your hospital does not have a neonatal hypothermia program, you should contact the closest referral center that provides this therapy as soon as you suspect that a baby may be a candidate. Work with your referral center to develop an organized plan to identify candidates for therapy and quickly arrange for transport. Delay in the recognition or referral of a baby that qualifies for cooling could mean that treatment cannot be initiated because the baby is outside of the therapeutic window. If the decision is made to transport the baby to another center, take steps to avoid unintentional hyperthermia while awaiting transport.

Focus on Teamwork

Post-resuscitation care highlights several opportunities for effective teams to use the Neonatal Resuscitation Program® (NRP®) Key Behavioral skills.

Behavior	Example
Anticipate and plan.	Plan where post-resuscitation care will take place at your institution.
	Discuss what type of post-resuscitation care will be provided in the mother's room and when care should be transferred to a transitional area or intensive care nursery.
	Plan who will be responsible for ongoing monitoring and who to contact if the baby's condition changes.
	Develop a plan to rapidly recognize babies who may qualify for therapeutic hypothermia and who to contact if you believe that this therapy is indicated.
	Practice how to initiate therapeutic hypothermia or the process for promptly transferring the baby to a tertiary center with the required expertise.
Know your environment.	Know what equipment is available in your institution to obtain a blood gas, electrolytes, and serum glucose.
	Know how to use the temperature sensor on your radiant warmer.
Delegate workload optimally.	Many procedures need to be performed during the first hour after a successful resuscitation. Plan who will perform each task to avoid unnecessary delays.
Communicate effectively.	Bring the care team together for a post-resuscitation debriefing to reinforce good teamwork habits and identify areas for improvement.
	Identifying a series of small changes may result in significant improvements in your team's performance and patient safety.

Frequently asked questions

Can post-resuscitation care and monitoring be performed in the mother's room?

The location of post-resuscitation care is less important than ensuring that appropriate monitoring occurs, medical conditions that require intervention are promptly recognized, and the necessary treatment is initiated. In many institutions, this will require transfer to a transitional nursery or intensive care setting.

Should sodium bicarbonate routinely be given to babies with metabolic acidosis?

No. Infusing a chemical buffer, like sodium bicarbonate, initially may appear to be a helpful intervention; however, there is currently no evidence to support this routine practice. Sodium bicarbonate infusion has several potential side effects. When sodium bicarbonate mixes with acid, carbon dioxide (CO_2) is formed. If the baby's lungs cannot rapidly exhale the additional CO_2, the acidosis will worsen. Although the blood measurement of acid (pH) may appear to improve, sodium bicarbonate may interfere with other acid-buffering systems and actually worsen the acidosis inside of cells. In addition, rapid administration of sodium bicarbonate may increase the risk of intraventricular hemorrhage in preterm newborns.

Ethical Considerations

Once you have resuscitated a baby, are you obligated to continue critical care interventions?

This question will be explored in detail in Lesson 11.

Key Points

1. A baby who required resuscitation must have close monitoring and frequent assessment of respiratory effort, oxygenation, blood pressure, blood glucose, electrolytes, urine output, neurologic status, and temperature during the immediate neonatal period.

2. Be careful to avoid overheating the baby during or after resuscitation.

3. If indicated, therapeutic hypothermia must be initiated promptly; therefore, every birth unit should have a system for identifying potential candidates and contacting appropriate resources.

LESSON 8 REVIEW

1. A baby born at 36 weeks' gestation received positive-pressure ventilation and oxygen supplementation in the delivery room. This baby (does)/(does not) need frequent evaluation of her respiratory effort and oxygenation during the immediate neonatal period.

2. If a newborn requires admission to a neonatal intensive care unit, the parent(s) (should)/(should not) be encouraged to see and touch the baby.

3. A full-term newborn had significant birth depression and required a complex resuscitation. He has continued respiratory failure with CO_2 retention and a metabolic acidosis. Sodium bicarbonate (should)/(should not) be infused immediately after resuscitation.

4. Among babies with moderate to severe hypoxic-ischemic encephalopathy, aggressive warming and hyperthermia (improves)/(worsens) the baby's outcome and should be (encouraged)/(avoided).

5. Babies at risk of pulmonary hypertension should routinely receive sufficient supplemental oxygen to achieve a target oxygen saturation of 100%. (True/False)

Answers

1. This baby does need frequent evaluation of her respiratory effort and oxygenation during the immediate neonatal period.

2. The parent(s) should be encouraged to see and touch the baby.

3. Sodium bicarbonate should not be infused immediately after resuscitation.

4. Aggressive warming and hyperthermia worsens the baby's outcome and should be avoided.

5. False. Babies at risk of pulmonary hypertension should NOT routinely receive sufficient supplemental oxygen to achieve a target oxygen saturation of 100%.

Additional Reading

Akinloye O, O'Connell C, Allen AC, El-Naggar W. Post-resuscitation care for neonates receiving positive pressure ventilation at birth. *Pediatrics.* 2014;134(4):e1057-e1062

Aschner JL, Poland RL. Sodium bicarbonate: basically useless therapy. *Pediatrics.* 2008;122(4):831-835

Committee on Fetus and Newborn, Papile LA, Baley JE, et al. Clinical Report: Hypothermia and neonatal encephalopathy. *Pediatrics.* 2014;133(6):1146-1150

Committee on Fetus and Newborn. Postnatal glucose homeostasis in late-preterm and term infants. *Pediatrics.* 2011;127(3):575-579

Resuscitation and Stabilization of Babies Born Preterm

What you will learn

- Why babies born preterm are at higher risk of medical complications

- The additional resources needed to prepare for a preterm birth

- Additional strategies to maintain the preterm baby's body temperature

- How to assist ventilation when a preterm baby has difficulty breathing

- Additional considerations for oxygen management in a preterm baby

- Ways to decrease the chances of lung and brain injury in preterm babies

- Special precautions to take after the initial stabilization period

- How to present information to parents before the birth of an extremely premature baby

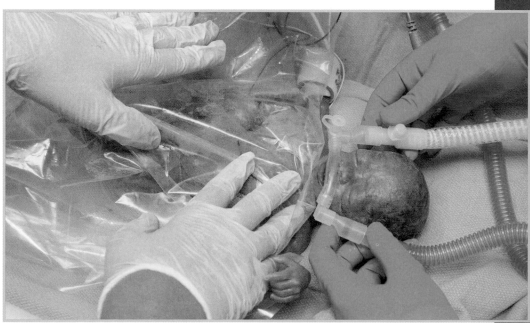

(Used with permission of Mayo Foundation for Medical Education and Research.)

The following 2 cases describe the birth and resuscitation of preterm babies. As you read the cases, imagine yourself as part of the team from the anticipation of the delivery through the resuscitation, stabilization, and transfer to an intensive care nursery.

Case 1: Stabilization of a baby born preterm

A woman is admitted to the hospital at 29 weeks' gestation with ruptured membranes and premature labor. Despite tocolysis, she has progressive cervical dilation and a vaginal birth is anticipated. The resuscitation team leader meets with the obstetrician and parents to discuss the care plan. Anticipating the possibility of a complex resuscitation, your resuscitation team is assembled and reviews each team member's role. You identify who will be responsible for leading the team, managing the airway, starting positive-pressure ventilation (PPV) if needed, monitoring the baby's heart rate and oxygen saturation, performing endotracheal intubation and umbilical catheterization if necessary, and documenting the events as they occur. Using a written checklist, your team ensures that all equipment and supplies needed to resuscitate and stabilize a preterm baby are ready for use. One team member attaches a preterm-sized mask to the T-piece resuscitator. The peak inspiratory pressure (PIP) is adjusted to 20 cm H_2O and positive end-expiratory pressure (PEEP) is set at 5 cm H_2O. Next, he prepares a laryngoscope with a size-0 blade, and a 3.0-mm endotracheal tube. The oxygen blender is adjusted to deliver 30% oxygen. Additional team members increase the delivery room temperature, turn on the radiant warmer, obtain polyethylene plastic wrap, activate a thermal mattress, and cover the mattress with a cotton blanket. The obstetrician prepares a warm blanket.

At the time of birth, the baby girl has flexed extremities, but does not cry. The obstetrician holds her on the warm blanket and provides gentle tactile stimulation. Secretions are carefully suctioned from her mouth and nose. After 15 seconds, she begins to take spontaneous breaths. By 30 seconds, she has sustained respirations and is actively moving. An assistant clamps and cuts the umbilical cord 60 seconds after birth and the baby is handed to your resuscitation team. She is carried to the radiant warmer where she is placed on the blanket-covered thermal mattress and covered with plastic wrap. A hat is placed on her head. She is breathing regularly and her heart rate is greater than 100 beats per minute (bpm), but she has labored breathing and decreased breath sounds. A team member attaches a pulse oximeter sensor to her right hand and electronic cardiac (ECG) monitor leads to her chest. Continuous positive airway pressure (CPAP) with 30% oxygen is administered using the face mask and T-piece resuscitator. Her breath sounds and work of breathing improve, but her oxygen saturation is below the minute-specific target range. The oxygen concentration is gradually increased and her Spo_2 begins to rise. Nasal CPAP prongs are placed. Your team continues to adjust the oxygen blender based on pulse oximetry and, by 10 minutes of age, the oxygen concentration has been decreased to 21%.

The parents are updated on her progress, they have an opportunity to see and touch her, and she is moved to the intensive care nursery in a pre-warmed transport incubator for additional care. Shortly afterward, your team members conduct a debriefing to review their preparation, teamwork, and communication.

Case 2: Resuscitation and stabilization of a baby born extremely preterm

A woman is admitted to the hospital at 24 weeks' gestation with ruptured membranes and premature labor. Your resuscitation team leader meets with the obstetrician, the mother, and her partner. They discuss the procedures that may be required to resuscitate and stabilize an extremely premature newborn and current outcome data. After the discussion, they develop a care plan based on the parents' assessment of their baby's best interest. The parents and health care providers agree to provide intensive medical care, including endotracheal intubation, chest compressions, and emergency medication if necessary. Despite tocolysis, labor progresses and a vaginal birth is anticipated. Your resuscitation team is assembled for a pre-resuscitation team briefing to review each member's roles and responsibilities. Using a written checklist, they prepare the necessary equipment and supplies.

At the time of birth, the baby girl is flaccid and does not cry. The obstetrician holds her on a warm towel and provides gentle tactile stimulation. Clear secretions are carefully suctioned from her mouth and nose, but her tone remains poor and she is not breathing. The umbilical cord is clamped and cut and the baby is handed to a member of your resuscitation team. She is carried to the radiant warmer where she is placed on the blanket-covered thermal mattress and covered with plastic wrap, and a hat is placed on her head. The baby remains limp without respiratory effort. You administer PPV using the T-piece resuscitator and 30% oxygen. A team member attaches a pulse oximeter sensor to her right wrist and ECG monitor leads to her chest. Her heart rate is 60 bpm and her chest is not moving with PPV. Each of the ventilation corrective steps are performed, including carefully increasing the pressure to 30 cm H_2O, but her heart rate still does not improve. A 2.5-mm endotracheal tube is inserted and placement is confirmed with a carbon dioxide (CO_2) detector. Positive-pressure ventilation is continued with the T-piece resuscitator, breath sounds are equal bilaterally, and her heart rate promptly increases. The nasal-tragus length (NTL) is 4.5 cm and the endotracheal tube is secured with the 5.5-cm mark adjacent to the baby's lip. The oxygen concentration is gradually adjusted to meet the minute-specific saturation target. A short time later, surfactant is administered through the endotracheal tube and the T-piece PIP is adjusted to maintain gentle chest rise with each breath. By 30 minutes, the oxygen concentration has been decreased to 25%.

The parents are updated on her progress, they have an opportunity to see and touch her, and she is moved to the intensive care nursery in a pre-warmed transport incubator with blended oxygen and continuous monitoring. Shortly afterward, your team members conduct a debriefing to discuss their preparation, teamwork, and communication.

Preterm birth

In the previous lessons, you learned a systematic approach to neonatal resuscitation. When birth occurs before term, additional challenges make the transition to extrauterine life more difficult. The likelihood that a preterm newborn will need help making this transition is related to gestational age. Babies born at lower gestational ages are more likely to require additional interventions. Because preterm newborns are also more vulnerable to injury from resuscitation procedures, it is important to find the correct balance between initiating resuscitation without delay and avoiding unnecessarily invasive procedures. Your management during these first minutes may decrease the risk of both short- and long-term complications. This lesson focuses on the additional problems associated with preterm birth and the actions you can take to prevent or manage them.

Why do babies born preterm have a higher risk of complications?

Some complications result from the underlying problem that caused the preterm birth while others reflect the baby's anatomic and physiologic immaturity.

- Thin skin, decreased subcutaneous fat, large surface area relative to body mass, and a limited metabolic response to cold lead to rapid heat loss.

- Weak chest muscles and flexible ribs decrease the efficiency of spontaneous breathing efforts.

- Immature lungs that lack surfactant are more difficult to ventilate and are at greater risk of injury from PPV.

- Immature tissues are more easily damaged by oxygen.

- Infection of the amniotic fluid and placenta (chorioamnionitis) may initiate preterm labor, and the baby's immature immune system increases the risk of developing severe infections such as pneumonia, sepsis, and meningitis.

- A smaller blood volume increases the risk of hypovolemia from blood loss.

- Immature blood vessels in the brain cannot adjust to rapid changes in blood flow, which may cause bleeding or damage from insufficient blood supply.

- Limited metabolic reserves and immature compensatory mechanisms increase the risk of hypoglycemia after birth.

What additional resources do you need for resuscitating a preterm newborn?

The chance that a preterm baby will require resuscitation is significantly higher than for a baby born at full term. This is true even for late preterm babies born at 34 through 36 weeks' gestation. If the baby is anticipated to be less than 32 weeks' gestation, prepare a polyethylene bag/wrap and a thermal mattress as described in the next section. A servo-controlled radiant warmer with a temperature sensor helps to maintain the baby's temperature within the normal range. An oxygen blender and oximeter with an appropriate-sized sensor should be available for all preterm births. An ECG monitor with 3 chest leads or limb leads provides a rapid and reliable method of continuously displaying the baby's heart rate if the pulse oximeter has difficulty acquiring a stable signal. A resuscitation device capable of providing PEEP and CPAP, such as a T-piece resuscitator or flow-inflating bag, is preferred. A preterm-sized resuscitation mask, size-0 laryngoscope blade (size 00 optional), and appropriate-sized endotracheal tubes (3.0 mm and 2.5 mm) should be prepared. Consider having surfactant available if the baby is expected to be less than 30 weeks' gestation. A pre-warmed transport incubator with blended oxygen and a pulse oximeter is important for maintaining the baby's temperature and oxygenation within the target range if the baby will be moved after the initial stabilization.

How do you keep the preterm newborn warm?

Preterm newborns have a high risk of developing hypothermia (body temperature below 36.5°C) and complications from cold stress. While drying with warm towels, skin-to-skin contact, and early breastfeeding may be sufficient to maintain normal temperature for term newborns and some vigorous late preterm newborns, additional measures are required for more premature newborns and those requiring assistance after birth. When a preterm birth is expected, anticipate that temperature regulation will be challenging and prepare for it.

- Increase the temperature in the room where the baby will receive initial care. Set the room temperature to approximately 23°C to 25°C (74°F to 77°F).

- Preheat the radiant warmer well before the time of birth.

- Place a hat on the baby's head.

- For babies born at less than 32 weeks' gestation,*

  – *Place a thermal mattress under the blanket on the radiant warmer* (Figure 9.1).
  Portable thermal mattresses release heat when a chemical gel inside the mattress is activated to form crystals. Following the manufacturer's recommendations, squeeze the pad to activate the gel at least 5 minutes before the baby is born. Cover the thermal mattress with a blanket so the heated surface is not in direct contact with the baby's skin. The mattress should be stored and activated at room temperature (19°C to 28°C or 66°F to 82°F) to reach the target surface temperature within 5 minutes and maintain that temperature for 1 hour after activation.

  – *Wrap the baby in a polyethylene plastic bag or wrap.*
  Drying and placing the baby under a radiant warmer are not sufficient measures to prevent heat loss in very premature newborns. Instead of drying the body with towels, very premature newborns should be covered or wrapped up to their neck in polyethylene plastic immediately after birth. Drying the body is not necessary.

    ◦ You may use a food-grade reclosable 1-gallon plastic bag, a large plastic surgical bag, food wrap, or sheets of commercially available polyethylene plastic (Figure 9.2). If using a reclosable bag, you may cut the bottom open, slide the baby into the bag through the cut side, and close the bag below the baby's feet. If using a plastic sheet or food wrap, you may either wrap the baby in a single sheet or use 2 sheets and place the baby between the sheets.

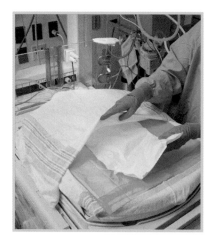

Figure 9.1. Thermal mattress placed under a blanket on the radiant warmer

---

*Note: Depending on the baby's birth weight and environmental conditions, some babies up to 35 weeks' gestation may benefit from the use of a thermal mattress and occlusive wrap.

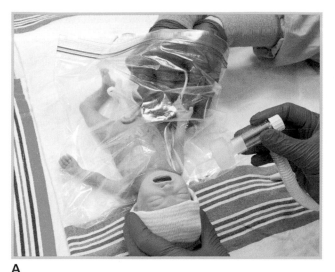 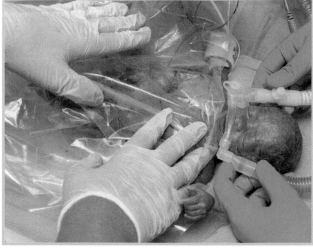

A **B**

Figure 9.2. Polyethylene plastic bag (A) and wrap (B) for reducing heat loss. (Figure 9.2B used with permission of Mayo Foundation for Medical Education and Research.)

- It is important to keep the newborn fully covered during resuscitation and stabilization. If the newborn requires insertion of an umbilical catheter, cut a small hole in the plastic and pull the umbilical cord through the hole rather than uncovering the newborn.

- Monitor the baby's temperature frequently because *overheating* has been described while using a combination of warming methods. Consider placing a temperature sensor and sensor cover on the newborn and using the warmer's servo-control mode to adjust the radiant heat.

- Use a pre-warmed transport incubator if the baby will be moved after initial care is completed.

- Maintain the baby's axillary temperature between 36.5°C and 37.5°C.

How do you assist ventilation?

Preterm babies have immature lungs that may be difficult to ventilate and are more susceptible to injury from PPV. Use the same criteria for initiating PPV with a preterm baby that you have learned for a term baby (apnea, gasping, or heart rate <100 bpm within 60 seconds of birth despite the initial steps). If the baby is breathing spontaneously and the heart rate is at least 100 bpm, PPV is not required. If the baby has labored respirations or oxygen saturation remains below the target range, CPAP may be helpful.

The following are special considerations for assisting ventilation of preterm babies:

- **If the baby is *breathing spontaneously*, consider using CPAP rather than intubating.**

  If the baby is breathing spontaneously and has a heart rate at least 100 bpm, but has labored respirations or oxygen saturation below the target range, administration of CPAP may be helpful. Using early CPAP, you may be able to avoid the need for intubation and mechanical ventilation. CPAP alone is **NOT** appropriate therapy for a baby who is not breathing **or** whose heart rate is less than 100 bpm.

- **If PPV is required, use the lowest inflation pressure necessary to achieve and maintain a heart rate greater than 100 bpm.**

  The baby's heart rate response is the best indicator of effective ventilation. An initial inflation pressure of 20 to 25 cm H_2O is adequate for most preterm newborns. The volume of air required to ventilate a preterm baby's lungs is very small and may not result in perceptible chest rise.

  Use the lowest inflation pressure necessary to maintain a heart rate of at least 100 bpm and gradually improve oxygen saturation. During face-mask ventilation for a baby born at term, the maximum recommended inspiratory pressure is 40 cm H_2O (Lesson 4). This may be too high for a preterm baby. Use your judgment when increasing ventilation pressure; however, it is reasonable to limit face-mask ventilation to an inspiratory pressure of 30 cm H_2O. If face-mask ventilation at this pressure does not result in clinical improvement, providing ventilation through an endotracheal tube may improve the efficacy of PPV and allow you to decrease the ventilating pressure.

  Airway obstruction and face-mask leak are common problems during face-mask ventilation with preterm newborns, and very small changes in the head and neck position may lead to significant improvements in ventilation. A CO_2 detector placed between the mask and PPV device may provide a visual cue to help identify when you have achieved the correct mask and neck position. The CO_2 detector will change color when ventilation successfully exchanges gas within the baby's lungs and CO_2 is exhaled through the mask.

- **If PPV is required, it is preferable to use a device that can provide PEEP.**

  Using PEEP (5 cm H_2O) helps the baby's lungs to remain inflated between positive-pressure breaths. This is particularly important if you are using an endotracheal tube for ventilation. Both the

T-piece resuscitator and flow-inflating bag can provide PEEP during ventilation through either a face mask or an endotracheal tube. If a PEEP valve is attached, a self-inflating bag may provide PEEP during endotracheal tube ventilation. It is difficult to maintain PEEP during face-mask ventilation with a self-inflating bag.

- **Consider administering surfactant if the baby requires intubation for respiratory distress or is extremely preterm.**

Preterm babies who need intubation and mechanical ventilation because of severe respiratory distress syndrome should be given surfactant after initial stabilization.

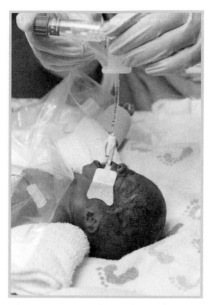

Figure 9.3. Intubation for surfactant administration. (Used with permission of Mayo Foundation for Medical Education and Research.)

Studies completed prior to the common use of antenatal steroids and early CPAP concluded that babies born at less than approximately 30 weeks' gestation would benefit from intubation and prophylactic surfactant treatment before they developed respiratory distress. Recent studies indicate that CPAP used immediately after birth should be considered as an alternative to routine intubation and prophylactic surfactant administration. Many preterm babies can be treated with early CPAP and avoid the risks of intubation and mechanical ventilation. Surfactant can be selectively administered to babies who fail a trial of CPAP (Figure 9.3). In some cases, you may be able to remove the endotracheal tube immediately after surfactant administration and return to CPAP for ongoing respiratory support ("INtubate-SURfactant-Extubate" or "*INSURE*"). Some experts, however, still recommend prophylactic surfactant for extremely premature newborns (less than 26 weeks' gestation) because the likelihood of CPAP failure in this subgroup is relatively high. Criteria for CPAP failure and the administration of prophylactic surfactant should be developed in coordination with local experts.

Surfactant administration is not a component of the initial resuscitation and it should be delayed until the baby has a stable heart rate. Appropriate endotracheal tube placement should be confirmed by auscultation of bilateral breath sounds or a chest radiograph prior to surfactant administration. If the resuscitation team has not had expertise in surfactant administration, it may be preferable to wait for the arrival of more experienced providers.

How much oxygen should you use?

You have learned in previous lessons that injury during transition may result from inadequate blood flow and oxygen delivery and that restoring these factors are important goals during resuscitation. However, research indicates that administering excessive oxygen after

Table 9-1. Oxygen saturation target range

Targeted Pre-ductal Spo$_2$ After Birth	
1 min	60%-65%
2 min	65%-70%
3 min	70%-75%
4 min	75%-80%
5 min	80%-85%
10 min	85%-95%

perfusion has been restored can result in additional injury. Preterm babies may be at higher risk for this reperfusion injury because fetal tissues normally develop in a low oxygen environment and the mechanisms that protect the body from oxygen-associated injury have not yet fully developed. Nevertheless, many preterm newborns will require supplemental oxygen to achieve the gradual increase in oxygen saturation that occurs after a healthy term birth.

When resuscitating a preterm baby, it is important to balance the desire to rapidly correct low oxygen saturation against avoiding exposure to excessive levels of oxygen. The current recommendation is to initiate resuscitation of preterm newborns (less than 35 weeks' gestational age) with 21% to 30% oxygen and use a pulse oximeter and oxygen blender to maintain oxygen saturation within the same target range described for full-term newborns (Table 9-1).

What can you do to decrease the chances of neurologic injury in preterm newborns?

Before approximately 32 weeks' gestation, preterm newborns have a fragile network of capillaries in their brain that are prone to rupture and bleeding. Obstruction of venous drainage from the head or rapid changes in blood CO_2 levels, blood pressure, or blood volume may increase the risk of rupturing these capillaries. Bleeding in the brain may cause tissue damage and lead to lifelong disability. Inadequate blood flow and oxygen delivery may cause damage to other areas of the brain even in the absence of hemorrhage, while excessive oxygen administration may cause damage to the developing retina, leading to visual loss.

Consider the following precautions when resuscitating a preterm newborn:

- **Handle the baby gently.**

  While this may seem obvious, this aspect of care may be forgotten when members of the resuscitation team are trying to perform many steps quickly.

- **Do not position the baby's legs higher than the head (Trendelenburg position).**

- **Avoid delivering excessive pressure during PPV or CPAP.**

  Excessive inflation pressure or too much CPAP can create a pneumothorax or interfere with venous return from the head. Both of these complications have been associated with an increased risk of brain hemorrhage.

- **Use a pulse oximeter and blood gases to monitor and adjust ventilation and oxygen concentration.**

  Continuously monitor Spo_2 until you are confident that the baby can maintain normal oxygenation while breathing room air. If the baby requires continued assistance with ventilation, a blood gas should be obtained to guide therapy. Rapid changes in CO_2 levels can increase the risk of bleeding. If your hospital does not have the resources to manage preterm babies who require ongoing assisted ventilation, arrange transfer to an appropriate facility.

- **Do not rapidly infuse intravenous fluids.**

  If volume expansion is needed, infuse the fluid slowly over at least 5 to 10 minutes. Hypertonic intravenous solutions should be avoided or given very slowly.

What special precautions should be taken after the initial stabilization period?

During the last trimester of pregnancy, the fetus undergoes physiologic changes in preparation for extrauterine survival. If a baby is born prematurely, many of these adaptations have not occurred. In addition to the steps described in Lesson 8, consider the following:

- **Monitor the baby's temperature.**

  Continue to carefully monitor the baby's temperature after the initial resuscitation and stabilization period. A servo-controlled warmer or incubator that uses a skin sensor to adjust the heat output based on the baby's skin temperature may be helpful. Very premature babies should remain wrapped in polyethylene plastic until they have been moved to a warmed and humidified incubator. Even moderate and late preterm newborns remain at risk for hypothermia and should be carefully monitored.

- **Monitor blood glucose.**

  Babies born very prematurely have lower amounts of stored glucose than babies born at term. If resuscitation is required, it is more likely that these stores will be depleted quickly and the baby may become hypoglycemic. Promptly secure intravenous access, initiate a dextrose infusion, and monitor the baby's blood glucose.

- **Monitor the baby for apnea and bradycardia.**

  Respiratory control is often unstable in preterm babies. Significant apnea and bradycardia during the stabilization period may be the first clinical sign of an abnormality in body temperature, oxygen, CO_2, electrolytes, blood glucose, or blood acid levels.

Focus on Teamwork

The resuscitation and stabilization of babies born preterm highlights several opportunities for effective teams to use the Neonatal Resuscitation Program® (NRP®) Key Behavioral skills.

Behavior	Example
Anticipate and plan. Delegate workload optimally.	Multiple procedures may need to be performed in a brief period of time. Work with a multidisciplinary team to develop and practice a systematic approach to the first hours of care by predefining roles and responsibilities.
Use available information. Clearly identify a team leader.	Complete a pre-resuscitation team briefing to review the prenatal and intrapartum history, identify a team leader, and review roles and responsibilities of each team member and the planned approach to respiratory support.
Know your environment.	Know where polyethylene plastic bags/wrap and thermal mattresses are stored. Know how to use the temperature sensor on your radiant warmer. Know how to set up a device to administer CPAP.
Allocate attention wisely.	If the team leader becomes involved in endotracheal intubation, her attention is focused primarily on that task and she may not be able to pay full attention to the baby's condition or the passage of time.
Communicate effectively. Maintain professional behavior.	Share your assessments aloud so that all members of the team are aware of the baby's condition and response to treatment.
	The importance of effective communication continues after the resuscitation is completed. A post-resuscitation team debriefing is an important opportunity to review the team's performance, identify areas for improvement, practice effective communication skills, and improve teamwork.
	If the baby will be transferred to another hospital after birth, develop a plan for efficiently communicating the maternal and newborn history.

Frequently Asked Questions

Should delayed cord clamping be considered for preterm newborns?

Among preterm newborns, delayed cord clamping has been associated with improved cardiovascular stability, increased blood pressure, decreased need for blood transfusions, decreased incidence of intraventricular hemorrhage, and decreased incidence of necrotizing enterocolitis. For vigorous preterm newborns with intact placental circulation, umbilical cord clamping should be delayed for 30 to 60 seconds after birth. By carefully coordinating with the obstetric providers, the initial steps of newborn care, including clearing the airway if necessary and providing gentle stimulation, can be performed with the umbilical cord intact.

If the placental circulation is not intact, such as after a placental abruption, bleeding placenta previa, bleeding vasa previa, or cord avulsion, the cord should be clamped immediately after birth.

There is not enough evidence to make a definitive recommendation whether umbilical cord clamping should be delayed in preterm newborns who are not vigorous after birth. If the placental circulation is intact, it may be reasonable to briefly delay cord clamping while the obstetric provider clears the airway and gently stimulates the baby to breathe. If the baby does not begin to breathe during this time, additional treatment is required. The cord should be clamped and the baby brought to the radiant warmer. Other situations where safety data for delayed cord clamping are limited are discussed in lesson 3.

Before birth, establish the plan for the timing of umbilical cord clamping with the obstetric providers.

How do you counsel parents before the birth of an extremely preterm baby?

Meeting with parents before the birth of an extremely preterm baby is important for both the parents and the neonatal care providers. Prenatal discussions are an opportunity to provide parents with important information, discuss goals, and establish a trusting relationship that will support the goal of shared decision making for their baby. These discussions can be difficult because of the challenges inherent in communicating a large amount of complex information during a stressful time. You should be prepared with accurate information about available treatment options and the anticipated short- and long-term outcomes for the specific situation. You should be familiar with both national and local outcome data and understand the limitations of each. If necessary, consult with specialists at your regional referral center to obtain up-to-date information. Ideally, both the obstetric provider and the neonatal provider should be present to talk with the parents. The obstetric and neonatal perspectives may be different. These differences should be discussed before meeting with the parents so that the information presented is consistent.

If possible, meet with both parents (or the mother and her chosen support person) at the same time and allow enough time for them to consider the content of your discussion and ask questions. Try to meet with the parents before the mother has received medications that might make it difficult for her to understand or remember your conversation and before the final stages of labor. If you are called when the woman is in active labor, there may not be time for an extended discussion, but it is still helpful to introduce yourself and briefly describe potential issues and your preliminary treatment plan. Use clear language without medical abbreviations or jargon. Be cautious about describing outcomes in terms of risk ratios, proportions, or percentages because parents may have limited understanding of mathematical concepts. In addition, quoting these data may give the impression that your estimates are more precise than they actually are. It is important to present a balanced and objective picture of the range of possible outcomes while avoiding excessively negative or unrealistically positive descriptions. Use an appropriately trained medical interpreter if the family is not proficient in English or includes someone with a hearing disability. Visual aids and written materials, including pictures and graphs, can supplement your discussion and help the parents remember the topics that you discussed. Offer to give the parents time alone to discuss what you have told them. Some parents may want to consult with other family members or clergy. If time allows, offer to make a return visit to confirm both their understanding of what may occur and your understanding of their wishes.

After you meet with the parents, document a summary of your conversation in the mother's chart. Review what you discussed with the obstetric care providers and the other members of your nursery's resuscitation team. If it was decided that resuscitation would not be initiated, ensure that all members of your team, including on-call personnel and the obstetric care providers, are informed and in agreement with this decision. If disagreements occur, discuss them in advance and consult additional professionals, including legal and ethics consultants, if necessary.

Ethical Considerations

What are the ethical considerations involved in deciding whether or not to resuscitate a newborn at the threshold of viability?

What should you do if you are uncertain about the chances of survival or serious disability when you examine the baby immediately after birth?

These questions are explored in detail in Lesson 11.

Key Points

1 Preterm newborns are at increased risk for requiring resuscitation and assistance with transition after birth.

2 Preterm newborns are at increased risk of complications because of

- Rapid heat loss
- Immature lungs
- Vulnerability to injury from excessive oxygen
- Vulnerability to severe infection
- Small blood volumes
- Immature brains that are prone to bleeding
- Vulnerability to hypoglycemia

3 Additional resources for a preterm birth include

- Enough skilled personnel to perform a complex resuscitation and document events as they occur

- Additional supplies for maintaining temperature, including polyethylene plastic wrap or bag, hat, thermal mattress, temperature sensor and cover for a servo-controlled radiant warmer

- Oxygen blender, compressed air source, pulse oximeter, appropriate-sized oximeter sensor

- Electronic cardiac (ECG) monitor with chest or limb leads

- Resuscitation device capable of providing PEEP and CPAP

- Preterm-sized mask, size-0 laryngoscope blade (size 00 optional), preterm-sized endotracheal tubes (2.5 mm and 3.0 mm)

- Surfactant

- Pre-warmed transport incubator (if baby will be moved)

4 Preterm newborns are more susceptible to heat loss.

- Increase room temperature to approximately 23°C to 25°C (74°F-77°F).

- Preheat radiant warmer.

- If less than 32 weeks' gestation, consider using polyethylene plastic wrap/bag and thermal mattress.

- Pre-warm a transport incubator if baby will be moved after birth.

5 When assisting ventilation in preterm babies,

- Consider using CPAP immediately after birth if the baby is breathing spontaneously with a heart rate of at least 100 bpm, but has labored respirations or low oxygen saturation.

- Use the same criteria for initiating PPV as with term babies.

- If PPV is required, use the lowest inflation pressure necessary to achieve an adequate heart rate response.

- If positive-pressure ventilation (PPV) is required, it is preferable to use a device that can provide PEEP.

- Consider administering surfactant if the baby requires intubation and mechanical ventilation for respiratory distress or is extremely premature.

- Criteria for CPAP failure and the administration of prophylactic surfactant should be developed in coordination with local experts.

6 Precautions to decrease the risk of neurologic injury

- Handle the baby gently.

- Avoid positioning the baby's legs higher than the head (Trendelenburg position).

- Avoid high airway pressures during PPV or CPAP.

- Use an oximeter and blood gases to monitor and adjust ventilation and oxygen concentration.

- Avoid rapid intravenous fluid infusions and hypertonic solutions.

7 After resuscitation and stabilization of a preterm baby,

- Monitor and control oxygen and ventilation.

- Monitor and control the baby's temperature.

- Monitor and control blood glucose.

- Monitor for apnea and bradycardia; intervene promptly if needed.

LESSON 9 REVIEW

1. You have turned on the radiant warmer in anticipation of the birth of a baby at 27 weeks' gestation. List 3 additional steps that will help maintain this baby's temperature.

   a. _____

   b. _____

   c. _____

2. A baby is delivered at 30 weeks' gestation. At 5 minutes of age, she is breathing, has a heart rate of 140 beats per minute, and is receiving CPAP with 30% oxygen. An oximeter on her right hand is reading 95% and is increasing. You should (decrease the oxygen concentration)/(begin positive-pressure ventilation).

3. A (self-inflating bag)/(T-piece resuscitator) can provide CPAP for a spontaneously breathing baby.

4. You may *decrease* the risk of neurologic injury in a premature newborn during and after resuscitation by (tilting the bed so the baby's legs are higher than the head)/(adjusting the bed so that the baby's legs are even or lower than the head).

5. A baby is born at 26 weeks' gestation. The initial steps of care, including gentle stimulation, have been completed and he is nearly 1-minute old. He is not breathing and his heart rate is 80 beats per minute. You should (start CPAP with a face mask)/ (start positive-pressure ventilation).

Answers

1. You can increase the room temperature, prepare a thermal mattress, prepare a polyethylene plastic bag or wrap, and pre-warm a transport incubator if the baby will be moved after birth.

2. You should decrease the oxygen concentration.

3. A T-piece resuscitator can provide CPAP for a spontaneously breathing baby.

4. Adjusting the bed so that the baby's legs are even or lower than the head may decrease the risk of neurologic injury.

5. You should start positive-pressure ventilation.

Additional Reading

American Academy of Pediatrics, American College of Obstetricians and Gynecologists. *Guidelines for Perinatal Care.* 7th ed. Elk Grove Village, IL: American Academy of Pediatrics, American College of Obstetricians and Gynecologists; 2012

Cummings J, Committee on Fetus and Newborn, American Academy of Pediatrics. Antenatal counseling regarding resuscitation and neonatal intensive care before 25 weeks of gestation. *Pediatrics.* 2015;136(3):588-595

Committee on Fetus and Newborn, American Academy of Pediatrcs. Respiratory support in preterm infants at birth. *Pediatrics.* 2014;133(1):171-174

Halamek LP. Prenatal consultation at the limits of viability. *NeoReviews.* 2003;4(6):e153-e156

Special Considerations

What you will learn

- When to suspect a pneumothorax or pleural effusion
- How to manage a life-threatening pneumothorax or pleural effusion
- How to manage a newborn with an airway obstruction
- How to manage congenital lung abnormalities that may complicate resuscitation
- How to manage the newborn with complications from maternal narcotic or anesthetic exposure
- How to apply this program's principles to babies who require resuscitation beyond the immediate newborn period or outside the hospital delivery room

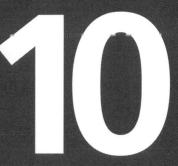

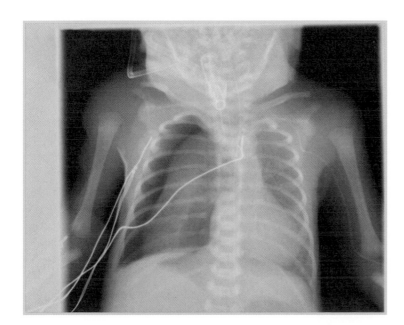

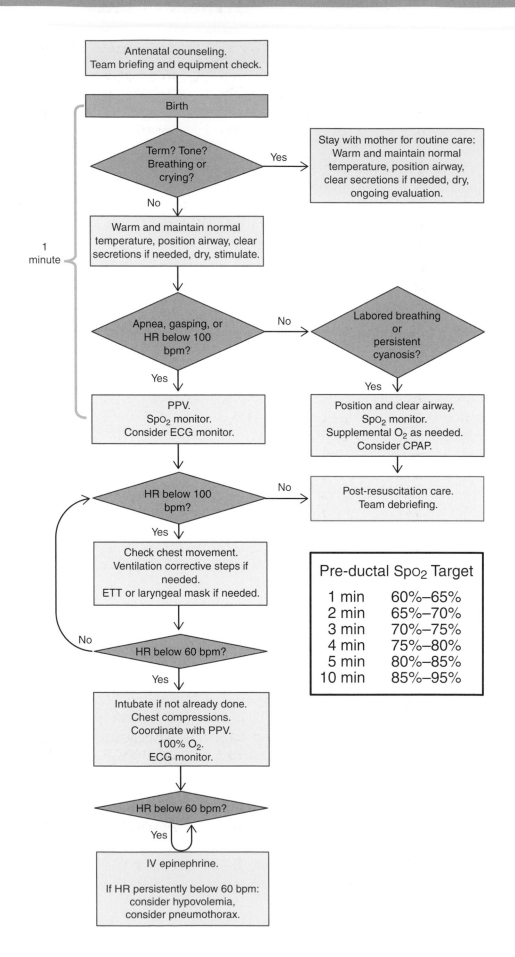

Antenatal counseling.
Team briefing and equipment check.

Birth

Term? Tone?
Breathing or
crying?

Yes → Stay with mother for routine care:
Warm and maintain normal
temperature, position airway,
clear secretions if needed, dry,
ongoing evaluation.

No

1 minute

Warm and maintain normal
temperature, position airway, clear
secretions if needed, dry, stimulate.

Apnea, gasping, or
HR below 100
bpm?

No → Labored breathing
or
persistent
cyanosis?

Yes

Yes

PPV.
SpO₂ monitor.
Consider ECG monitor.

Position and clear airway.
SpO₂ monitor.
Supplemental O₂ as needed.
Consider CPAP.

HR below 100
bpm?

No → Post-resuscitation care.
Team debriefing.

Yes

Check chest movement.
Ventilation corrective steps if
needed.
ETT or laryngeal mask if needed.

No

HR below 60 bpm?

Yes

Intubate if not already done.
Chest compressions.
Coordinate with PPV.
100% O₂.
ECG monitor.

HR below 60 bpm?

Yes

IV epinephrine.

If HR persistently below 60 bpm:
consider hypovolemia,
consider pneumothorax.

Pre-ductal SpO₂ Target

1 min	60%–65%
2 min	65%–70%
3 min	70%–75%
4 min	75%–80%
5 min	80%–85%
10 min	85%–95%

The following 2 cases are examples of less common circumstances that you may encounter during neonatal resuscitation. Because these scenarios do not occur frequently, it is important to be able to recognize them and be prepared to respond quickly and efficiently. As you read the cases, imagine yourself as part of the resuscitation team.

Case 1: A newborn with tension pneumothorax

A pregnant woman at 40 weeks' gestation is admitted in labor with a Category III fetal heart rate pattern. An emergency cesarean birth is planned. Your resuscitation team assembles in the operating room, completes a pre-resuscitation team briefing, and prepares equipment and supplies for a complex resuscitation. After birth, the umbilical cord is clamped and cut and a limp, apneic baby boy is handed to the team. One team member begins documenting the resuscitation events as they occur.

The initial steps are performed, but the baby remains limp without spontaneous respirations. You begin positive-pressure ventilation (PPV) with a face mask, but his heart rate does not improve. You perform the ventilation corrective steps and achieve chest movement after increasing the ventilating pressure; however, his heart rate remains 40 beats per minute (bpm). An endotracheal tube is rapidly placed for continued PPV, but there is no improvement in his heart rate or tone. Meanwhile, a team member has placed a pulse oximeter sensor on the baby's right hand, but the oximeter does not display a reliable signal. Electronic cardiac (ECG) monitor leads are placed on his chest and confirm the persistently low heart rate. Your team begins chest compressions while an umbilical venous catheter is prepared and inserted. The baby's heart rate does not improve after 60 seconds of coordinated compressions and ventilation with 100% oxygen. A dose of intravenous epinephrine is given through the umbilical catheter, followed by a normal saline flush, but the baby's condition still does not improve. The team reevaluates the placement of the endotracheal tube and the efficacy of ventilation and compressions while considering special circumstances that may complicate resuscitation. Listening to the chest, you recognize that breath sounds are absent on the right side. Your team suspects a life-threatening tension pneumothorax. Rapid transillumination of the chest confirms the suspicion and a team member quickly prepares a catheter-over-needle aspiration device. The catheter is inserted perpendicular to the chest wall just over the top of the rib in the fourth intercostal space at the anterior axillary line, connected to a 3-way stopcock, and 80 mL of air is aspirated from the chest. Upon decompression of the pneumothorax, the baby's heart rate rapidly improves and chest compressions are stopped. A small amount of air continues to flow through the catheter aspiration system and the baby is transferred to the nursery for a chest x-ray and additional treatment. Shortly afterward, you update the parents and conduct a debriefing to review your team's preparation, teamwork, and communication.

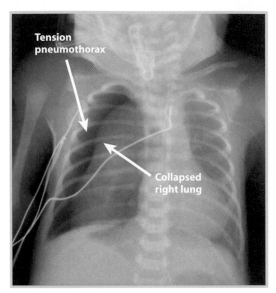

Figure 10.1. Pneumothorax causing collapse of the right lung

How do you identify a newborn with an air or fluid collection around the lung?

Abnormal air or fluid collections that prevent the newborn's lung from fully expanding within the chest can lead to severe respiratory distress and persistent bradycardia.

• **Pneumothorax**

It is not uncommon for small air leaks to develop as the newborn's lung fills with air. When air collects in the pleural space surrounding the lung, it is called a pneumothorax (Figure 10.1). Although a pneumothorax may occur spontaneously, the risk is increased by PPV, particularly in preterm babies, babies with meconium aspiration, and babies with other lung abnormalities.

A small pneumothorax may be asymptomatic or cause only mild respiratory distress. If the pneumothorax becomes larger, the pressure from the trapped air can cause the lung to collapse. If the pneumothorax becomes large enough, it can interfere with blood flow within the chest causing severe respiratory distress, oxygen desaturation, and bradycardia. This is called a tension pneumothorax. It is a life-threatening emergency and requires urgent treatment to evacuate the air.

You should consider the possibility of a pneumothorax if a baby fails to improve despite resuscitative measures or if a baby suddenly develops severe respiratory distress. Breath sounds may be diminished on the side of the pneumothorax, but breath sounds can be misleading because they are easily transmitted across the baby's chest and can sound normal even in the presence of a pneumothorax. If breath sounds are diminished, consider pneumothorax in addition to the other causes listed in Table 10-1. Transillumination of the chest is a rapid screening test that may be helpful. In a darkened room, hold a high-intensity fiber-optic light against the chest wall and compare the transmission of light on each side of the chest (Figure 10.2). During transillumination, light on the side with a pneumothorax will appear to spread further and glow brighter than the opposite side. In a life-threatening situation, a positive

Table 10-1. Causes of diminished breath sounds

- Inadequate ventilation technique
- Malpositioned endotracheal tube
- Pneumothorax
- Pleural effusion
- Tracheal obstruction
- Congenital diaphragmatic hernia
- Pulmonary hypoplasia or agenesis
- Enlarged heart
- Positive-pressure ventilation device leak or equipment failure

transillumination test can help to direct immediate treatment. Be careful when interpreting the results of transillumination in very premature babies because their thin skin may cause the chest to appear bright even in the absence of a pneumothorax. If a transilluminator is not immediately available and the baby is in severe distress, you may proceed with emergency treatment based on your clinical suspicion. If the baby is stable, the definitive diagnosis of a pneumothorax is made with a chest x-ray.

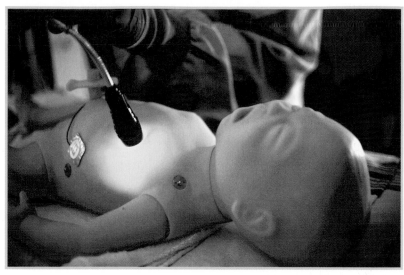

Figure 10.2. Positive transillumination of a left-sided pneumothorax. The light spreads and glows across a wide area.

A small pneumothorax usually will resolve spontaneously and often does not require treatment. The baby should be monitored for worsening distress. If the baby is maintaining normal oxygen saturation, supplemental oxygen is not indicated and does not result in earlier resolution of the pneumothorax. If a pneumothorax causes significant respiratory distress, bradycardia, or hypotension, it should be relieved urgently by placing a catheter into the pleural space and evacuating the air. If the baby has ongoing respiratory distress, placement of a thoracostomy tube attached to continuous suction may be required.

- **Pleural effusion**

Fluid that collects in the pleural space is called a pleural effusion (Figure 10.3). Similar to a pneumothorax, a large pleural effusion can prevent the lung from expanding. The fluid may be caused by edema, infection, or leakage from the baby's lymphatic system. Frequently, large pleural effusions are diagnosed before birth by ultrasound. There may be a history of severe fetal anemia, twin-to-twin transfusion, cardiac arrhythmia, congenital heart disease, congenital infection, or a genetic syndrome. You should suspect a pleural effusion if a newborn has respiratory distress and generalized body edema (hydrops fetalis). Excess fluid may also be present in the baby's abdomen (ascites) and around the baby's heart (pericardial effusion). Because the fluid collection interferes with lung expansion, breath sounds may be decreased on the affected side. The definitive diagnosis of a pleural effusion is made with a chest x-ray.

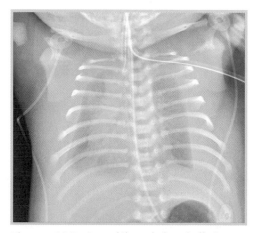

Figure 10.3. Large bilateral pleural effusions

A small pleural effusion may not require treatment. If respiratory distress is significant and does not resolve with intubation and PPV, you may need to insert a catheter into the pleural space to drain the fluid. If a large pleural effusion is identified before birth, emergency drainage may be required after birth. In this case, the baby should be born in a facility where emergency airway management and fluid drainage by an experienced team is immediately available in the delivery room.

How do you evacuate a pneumothorax or pleural effusion?

The air or fluid is aspirated by inserting a catheter into the pleural space on the affected side. This procedure is called *thoracentesis*. Ideally, thoracentesis should be performed using sterile technique with appropriate anesthetic for pain management; however, modifications may be required during emergency aspiration of a tension pneumothorax.

❶ Take a brief "time-out" and confirm the side that you plan to aspirate.

❷ Aspiration site and positioning

a. For a pneumothorax, the aspiration site is either the fourth intercostal space at the anterior axillary line or the second intercostal space at the mid-clavicular line (Figure 10.4). Using a small blanket roll, position the baby on his back (supine) with the affected side directed slightly upward to allow the air to rise to the upper (superior) portion of the chest.

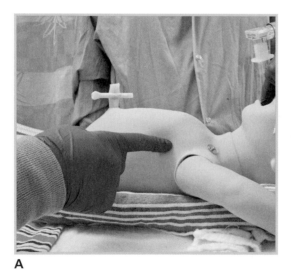
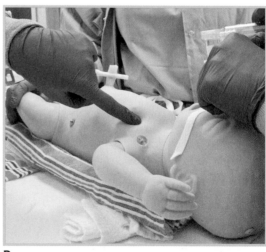

A   B

Figure 10.4. Locations for percutaneous aspiration of a pneumothorax. Fourth intercostal space at the anterior axillary line (A), second intercostal space at the mid-clavicular line (B).

b. For a pleural effusion, the aspiration site is the fifth or sixth intercostal space along the posterior axillary line. Place the baby on his back (supine) to allow the fluid to collect in the lower (posterior) portion of the chest (Figure 10.5).

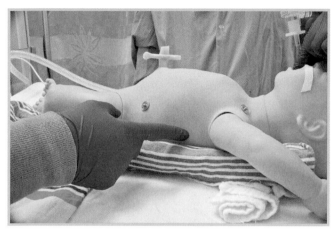

Figure 10.5. Location for aspiration of a pleural effusion

❸ Prepare the insertion site with topical antiseptic and sterile towels.

❹ Insert an 18- or 20-gauge percutaneous catheter-over-needle device perpendicular to the chest wall and just over the top of the rib. The needle is placed over the top of the rib, rather than below the rib, to avoid puncturing the blood vessels located under each rib.

a. For a pneumothorax, direct the catheter upward (Figure 10.6).

b. For a pleural effusion, direct catheter downward.

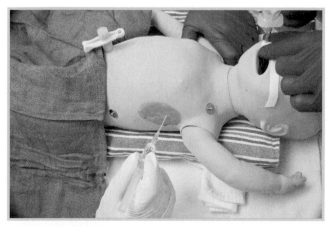

Figure 10.6. Aspiration of a pneumothorax. The needle is inserted over the rib and directed upward. *Note: The aspiration site is not covered with sterile towels for photographic purposes; however, modified sterile technique is acceptable for emergency aspiration.*

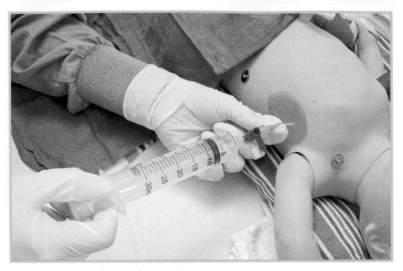

Figure 10.7. Syringe and stopcock assembly used to aspirate pneumothorax. The stopcock is opened between the catheter and syringe during aspiration. The stopcock is closed if the syringe becomes full and must be emptied. The same assembly is used to drain a pleural effusion.

⑤ Once the pleural space is entered, the needle is removed and a large syringe (20-60 mL) connected to a 3-way stopcock is attached to the catheter (Figure 10.7).

    a. When the stopcock is opened between the syringe and the catheter, the air or fluid can be evacuated.

    b. When the syringe is full, the stopcock may be closed to the chest while the syringe is emptied.

    c. After the syringe is emptied, the stopcock can be reopened to the chest and more fluid or air may be aspirated until the baby's condition has improved. To avoid accidental reinjection of air or fluid into the chest cavity, care must be taken when manipulating the stopcock.

    d. When evacuating a pleural effusion, maintain a sample of the fluid for diagnostic evaluation.

⑥ An x-ray should be obtained to document the presence or absence of residual pneumothorax or effusion.

If an appropriate catheter-over-needle device is not available, a small "butterfly" needle may be used. In this case, the syringe and stopcock will be connected to the tubing attached to the needle.

How do you manage a newborn with an airway obstruction?

Airway obstruction is a life-threatening emergency. The newborn's airway may be obstructed by thick secretions or a congenital anomaly that leads to an anatomic obstruction.

Thick secretions

Thick secretions, such as meconium, blood, mucus, or vernix, may cause complete tracheal obstruction. If you are attempting PPV, but the baby is not improving and the chest is not moving, perform each of the ventilation corrective steps (MR. SOPA), as described in Lesson 4, until you have successfully inflated the lungs. If you have correctly inserted an endotracheal tube for ventilation, but still cannot achieve chest movement, the trachea may be obstructed by thick secretions. As described in Lesson 5, you may attempt to remove secretions from the trachea using a suction catheter (5F-8F) inserted through the endotracheal tube. If the secretions are thick enough to completely obstruct the airway, you may not be able to clear them using a thin suction catheter. In this case, directly suction the trachea with a meconium aspirator attached to an endotracheal tube. Set the suction pressure to 80 to 100 mg Hg, connect suction tubing to the meconium aspirator, and attach the aspirator directly to the endotracheal tube connector. Some endotracheal tubes have an integrated aspiration device designed for suctioning the trachea. Occlude the aspirator's suction-control port with your finger. You may need to gradually withdraw the tube to remove secretions from the trachea and posterior pharynx before reinserting a new endotracheal tube for ventilation. Do not proceed to chest compressions until you have established an open airway and ventilation that inflates the lungs.

Anatomic obstructions

- **Robin sequence**

The Robin sequence describes a combination of facial anomalies that occur because the lower jaw (mandible) does not develop normally. The lower jaw is small and set back in relation to the upper jaw. The baby's tongue is positioned further back in the pharynx than normal and obstructs the airway (Figure 10.8). It is common for babies with the Robin sequence to also have a cleft palate. This combination of findings may be isolated or part of a genetic syndrome.

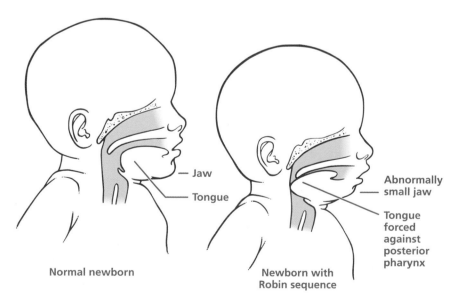

Jaw

Tongue

Normal newborn

Newborn with Robin sequence

Abnormally small jaw

Tongue forced against posterior pharynx

Figure 10.8. Newborn with normal anatomy (left) and newborn with Robin sequence (right)

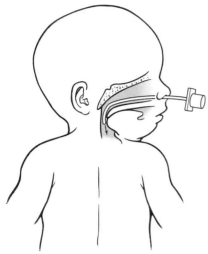

Figure 10.9. Endotracheal tube placed deep in posterior pharynx for relief of airway obstruction in a newborn with Robin sequence. The tube is in the nasopharynx, above the vocal cords, NOT in the trachea.

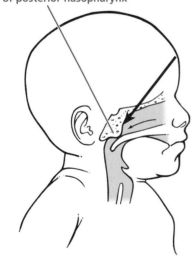

Congenital obstruction of posterior nasopharynx

Figure 10.10. Choanal atresia causing obstruction of the nasal airway

If a baby with Robin sequence has labored breathing, turn him onto his stomach (prone). In this position, the tongue may move forward and open the airway. If prone positioning is not successful, insert a small endotracheal tube (2.5 mm) through the nose with the tip placed deep in the posterior pharynx, past the base of the tongue, and above the vocal cords. It is not inserted into the trachea (Figure 10.9). A laryngoscope is not required to do this. This helps to relieve the airway obstruction.

If the baby has severe difficulty breathing and requires resuscitation, face-mask ventilation and endotracheal intubation may be very difficult. If none of the previous procedures results in adequate air movement, and attempts at face-mask ventilation and endotracheal intubation are unsuccessful, a **laryngeal mask** may provide a lifesaving rescue airway.

- **Choanal atresia**

Choanal atresia is a condition where the nasal airway is obstructed by bone or tissue (Figure 10.10). Because newborns normally breathe through their nose, babies with choanal atresia may have difficulty breathing unless they are crying and breathing through their mouth. In most cases, the obstruction occurs only on one side and does not cause significant symptoms in the newborn period. Babies with choanal atresia may present with cyclic episodes of obstruction, cyanosis, and oxygen desaturation that occur when they are sleeping or feeding and resolve when they are crying. If the obstruction is bilateral, the baby may have difficulty breathing immediately after birth; however, the presence of choanal atresia should not prevent you from achieving effective PPV with a face mask.

You can test for choanal atresia by passing a thin suction catheter into the posterior pharynx through the nares. If the catheter will not pass, choanal atresia may be present.

If the baby has bilateral choanal atresia and respiratory distress, you can keep the mouth and airway open by inserting one of the following into the baby's mouth—a feeding nipple or pacifier modified by cutting off the end (McGovern nipple) and secured with ties around the occiput (Figure 10.11), an oral endotracheal tube positioned with

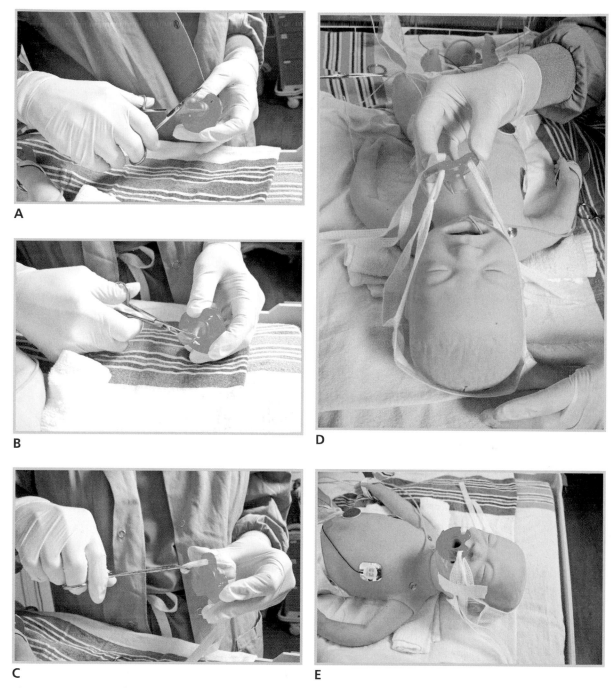

A

B

C

D

E

Figure 10.11. Modified pacifier (McGovern nipple) for temporary relief of airway obstruction in choanal atresia

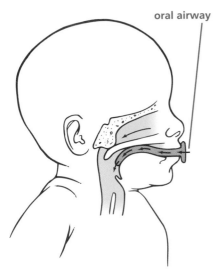

oral airway

Figure 10.12. Oral airway for temporary relief of airway obstruction in choanal atresia

the tip just beyond the tongue in the posterior pharynx, or a plastic oral (Guedel) airway (Figure 10.12). Each of these measures provides temporary stabilization until the baby can be evaluated by a specialist.

- **Other rare conditions**

Other conditions, such as oral, nasal, or neck masses, laryngeal and tracheal anomalies, and vascular rings that compress the trachea within the chest, have been reported as rare causes of airway compromise in the newborn. Some of these malformations will be evident by external examination. Depending on the location of the obstruction, it may be very difficult or impossible to achieve successful face-mask ventilation or to place an endotracheal tube. Special expertise and equipment may be required for successful intubation. If the obstruction is above the level of the vocal cords and you cannot ventilate or intubate the baby, placement of a **laryngeal mask** may provide a lifesaving rescue airway. If such problems are identified before birth, the baby should be born in a facility where emergency management of the airway by a trained multidisciplinary team is immediately available in the delivery room.

Review

① A newborn's heart rate is 50 beats per minute. He has not improved with ventilation through a face mask or a properly placed 3.5-mm endotracheal tube. His chest is not moving with positive-pressure ventilation. You should (suction the trachea using an 8F suction catheter or meconium aspirator)/(proceed immediately to chest compressions).

② A newborn has respiratory distress after birth. He has a small lower jaw and a cleft palate. The baby's respiratory distress may improve if you place a small endotracheal tube in the nose, advance it into the pharynx, and position him (supine [on his back])/(prone [on his stomach]).

③ You attended the birth of a baby that received positive-pressure ventilation during the first minutes of life. He improved and has been monitored in the nursery. A short time later, you are called because he has developed acute respiratory distress. You should suspect (a pneumothorax)/(a congenital heart defect) and should rapidly prepare (a needle aspiration device)/(epinephrine).

Answers

1 You should suction the trachea using an 8F suction catheter or meconium aspirator.

2 The baby's respiratory distress may improve if you place a small endotracheal tube in the nose, advance it into the pharynx, and position him prone (on his stomach).

3 You should suspect a pneumothorax and should rapidly prepare a needle aspiration device.

What abnormalities of fetal lung development can complicate resuscitation?

- **Congenital diaphragmatic hernia**

The diaphragm normally separates the abdominal and thoracic contents. When the diaphragm does not form correctly, the intestines, stomach, and liver can enter the chest and prevent the lungs from developing normally (Figure 10.13). This defect is called a congenital diaphragmatic hernia (CDH). The most common type of CDH occurs on the baby's left side. Frequently, the defect is identified by antenatal ultrasound, and the baby's birth can be planned at a high-risk center.

The baby may present with an unusually flat-appearing (scaphoid) abdomen, respiratory distress, and hypoxemia. If PPV is administered by face mask, gas enters the stomach and intestines. As these structures expand within the chest, lung inflation is increasingly inhibited and

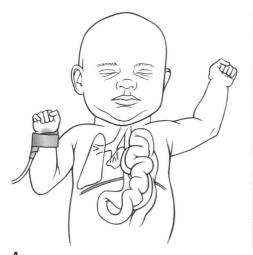

A

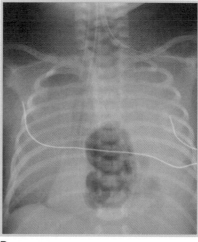

B

Figure 10.13. Congenital diaphragmatic hernia

breath sounds will be diminished on the side of the hernia. If the ventilating pressure is increased in an attempt to improve inflation, the baby may develop a pneumothorax. Pulmonary hypertension is commonly associated with a CDH and may contribute to severe hypoxemia.

> Babies with a known or suspected diaphragmatic hernia should not receive prolonged resuscitation with PPV by face mask.

Promptly intubate the trachea and place a large orogastric catheter (10F) to prevent gaseous distention (Figure 10.14). A double-lumen sump tube (Replogle tube) is most effective.

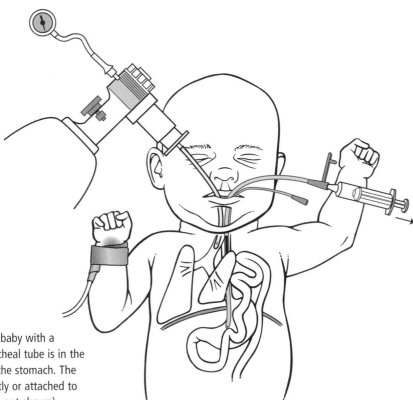

Figure 10.14. Stabilizing treatment for a baby with a congenital diaphragmatic hernia. An endotracheal tube is in the trachea and a double-lumen sump tube is in the stomach. The gastric drainage tube is aspirated intermittently or attached to vacuum suction. Both tubes are secured (tape not shown).

- **Pulmonary hypoplasia**

Normal lung development requires adequate space within the chest. Any condition that occupies space in the chest or causes a prolonged, severe decrease in amniotic fluid (oligohydramnios) may cause the lungs to be incompletely developed. This is called pulmonary hypoplasia. Examples of conditions causing pulmonary hypoplasia include congenital diaphragmatic hernia and obstruction or absence of both fetal kidneys. At the time of birth, the baby's chest may appear small and bell-shaped. If pulmonary hypoplasia was caused by oligohydramnios, the baby may have deformities of the hands, feet, nose, and ears caused by compression within the uterus. High inflating pressures are required to inflate the baby's lungs and this increases the risk of developing pneumothoraces. Severe pulmonary hypoplasia is incompatible with survival.

What do you do if a baby does not breathe or has decreased activity and the mother received a narcotic during labor?

Narcotics given to the laboring mother to relieve pain may cross the placenta and decrease the newborn's activity and respiratory drive. If a newborn has respiratory depression after maternal opiate exposure, manage the baby's airway and provide respiratory support with PPV as described in previous lessons. If the baby has prolonged apnea, insertion of an endotracheal tube or laryngeal mask may be required for ongoing respiratory support.

Although the narcotic antagonist naloxone has been used in this setting, there is insufficient evidence to evaluate the safety and efficacy of this practice. Very little is known about the pharmacology of naloxone in the newborn. Animal studies and case reports have raised concerns about complications from naloxone, including pulmonary edema, cardiac arrest, and seizures.

What do you do if a baby does not breathe or has decreased activity and the mother did not receive a narcotic during labor?

Other causes of neonatal depression should be considered. If PPV results in a normal heart rate and oxygen saturation, but the baby does not breathe spontaneously, the baby may have depressed respiratory drive or muscle activity due to hypoxia, severe acidosis, a structural brain abnormality, or a neuromuscular disorder. Medications given to the mother, such as magnesium sulfate and general anesthetics, can depress respirations in the newborn. There are no medications that reverse the effects of these drugs. Again, the focus is to provide airway support and effective ventilation until the medication's effect has resolved. Transport the baby to the nursery for further evaluation and management while administering PPV and monitoring the baby's heart rate and oxygen saturation.

Case 2: An emergency in the postpartum unit

A baby weighing 3,400 g was born in the hospital after an uncomplicated pregnancy and labor. The transitional period was uneventful and he remained with his mother to begin breastfeeding. At approximately 12 hours of age, his mother notices that he is not breathing and is unresponsive. She activates the bedside emergency alarm and a nurse responds immediately. The nurse turns on the room lights, opens the blankets to fully assess him, and finds that he is apneic and limp. She places him on a flat surface, opens his airway by placing his head in the "sniffing" position, clears his airway with a bulb syringe, and stimulates him by rubbing his back, but he does not improve. The nurse begins PPV with the neonatal self-inflating bag and mask supplied in the postpartum room.

The neonatal resuscitation team arrives in the room, receives information from the postpartum nurse, and quickly assesses the situation. One team member uses a stethoscope to listen to the baby's heart rate and breath sounds. Another team member brings an emergency cart with a pulse oximeter and ECG monitor. The pulse oximeter sensor is placed on the baby's right hand, and ECG monitor leads are attached to the baby's chest. The baby's heart rate is 80 bpm and rising, but the respiratory effort is still irregular and oxygen saturation is low. A blended oxygen source is attached to the resuscitation bag and the concentration is adjusted to achieve oxygen saturation >90%. The baby begins to have consistent respiratory effort and PPV is gradually weaned. He is given supplemental oxygen through the open tail reservoir of the self-inflating bag and transferred to the nursery in a pre-warmed incubator for additional evaluation and treatment. A team member stays with the baby's mother to obtain additional information, provide support, and answer questions. Shortly afterward, the care team conducts a debriefing to evaluate its readiness, teamwork, and communication.

Are resuscitation techniques different for babies born outside the hospital or beyond the immediate newborn period?

Throughout this program, you have learned about resuscitating babies who were born in the hospital and had difficulty making the transition to extrauterine life. Some babies may require resuscitation after being born outside the hospital and others will develop problems that require resuscitation after the immediate newborn period. Although scenarios encountered outside the delivery room present different challenges, the physiologic principles and basic steps remain the same throughout the neonatal period. *The initial priority for resuscitating babies during the neonatal period, regardless of location, should be to restore adequate ventilation.* Once adequate ventilation is ensured, obtain additional information about the baby's history to guide interventions.

Although this program is not designed to teach neonatal resuscitation in these other venues, some strategies for applying the principles that you have learned will be presented. More details are available through other American Academy of Pediatrics and American Heart Association programs, such as the Pediatric Education for Prehospital Professionals (PEPP), APLS: The Pediatric Emergency Medicine Resource, and Pediatric Advanced Life Support (PALS).

What are some of the different strategies needed to resuscitate babies outside the hospital or beyond the immediate newborn period?

- **Temperature management**

When babies are born outside the delivery room environment, maintaining body temperature may become a major challenge because you likely will not have a radiant warmer readily available. Some suggestions for minimizing heat loss are as follows:

- Turn up the heat source in the room or vehicle, if applicable.

- Dry the baby well with bath towels, a blanket, or clean clothing.

- Use the mother's body as a heat source. Consider placing the baby skin-to-skin on the mother's chest and covering both baby and mother with a clean sheet of food-grade plastic and a warm blanket.

- Emergency response teams should consider having polyethylene plastic wrap and portable thermal mattresses to help maintain temperature.

Maintaining normal body temperature is less difficult if the baby is not newly born because the baby's body is not wet. It is still important to prevent cooling during transport, especially during the winter months, by wrapping the baby in warm blankets and using a hat if available.

- **Clearing the airway**

If resuscitation is required outside a delivery room or nursery, vacuum suction may not be readily available. If secretions are obstructing the airway, use a bulb syringe or wipe the mouth and nose with a clean handkerchief or other cloth wrapped around your index finger.

- **Ventilation**

Most babies breathe spontaneously after birth. Drying the newborn and rubbing the back and extremities are acceptable methods of stimulation. Some babies born outside the hospital may require PPV to inflate their lungs. If a resuscitation bag-and-mask is not available, PPV can be administered by mouth-to-mouth-and-nose resuscitation. Place the baby in the "sniffing" position and form a tight seal with the resuscitator's mouth placed over the baby's mouth and nose. If the baby is large, it may be necessary to cover only the baby's mouth while the baby's nose is pinched to seal the airway. This technique poses a risk of transmitting infectious diseases.

- **Chest compressions**

Current PALS recommendations for infants call for a chest compression to ventilation ratio of 30:2 (single rescuer) or 15:2 (2 rescuers). This ratio was selected to decrease the educational complexity of resuscitation education for health care providers working with multiple age groups and for lay rescuers. During the first weeks following birth, respiratory failure is still the cause of nearly all cardiopulmonary arrests. In general, where differences exist between the Neonatal Resuscitation Program® (NRP®) and the recommendations presented in the PALS, APLS, and PEPP programs, you should apply the NRP recommendations during the immediate newborn period and during the time the baby is an inpatient following birth. If a newborn has cardiopulmonary arrest within the hospital during this period, the NRP recommends using a 3:1 compression to ventilation ratio unless there is a reason to suspect a primary cardiac etiology.

- **Vascular access**

Catheterization of the umbilical vessels generally is not an option outside the hospital or beyond the first several days after birth. In such cases, prompt insertion of an intraosseous needle into the tibia is an effective alternative.

If a baby is found unresponsive in a mother's room on the postpartum unit, should resuscitation be initiated in the mother's room or should the baby be carried to the nursery?

The decision to "scoop-and-run" to the nursery with a compromised newborn may seem like a reasonable approach, but this is not the best choice for several reasons. It is not safe to run down a hallway carrying a compromised newborn in your arms. This puts you and the newborn at risk for injury from a fall or a collision with another person, equipment, or passageway door. Every location where newborns receive care should have ready access to the equipment necessary to initiate resuscitation. Immediate access to a self-inflating resuscitation bag will allow a first responder to initiate PPV while the resuscitation team quickly assembles and brings additional equipment. As a team, determine when the baby is stable enough to be transported to the nursery area for further evaluation and management. Be prepared to support ventilation and monitor the baby's vital signs during transport. If there is a designated resuscitation space that is only steps away from every postpartum room, it may be appropriate to carefully move the compromised newborn directly to this location for immediate care. In all cases, the correct solution prioritizes a timely and efficient response and best serves the interests of the newborn's health and safety.

Each hospital should evaluate its readiness for resuscitating newborns in locations outside of the delivery rooms and nursery. Anticipate this potential scenario and develop a plan for how an emergency call will be initiated, how the appropriate team will be assembled, what equipment will be stored in the room, and what equipment will be stored in a nearby location (eg, code cart in the hallway). By simulating unusual or uncommon scenarios in different locations, you can make plans to address your system's weaknesses and improve your teamwork.

Focus on Teamwork

The special considerations described in this lesson highlight several opportunities for effective teams to use the NRP Key Behavioral skills.

Behavior	Example
Anticipate and plan. Use available information. Communicate effectively.	Through effective communication with the obstetric care provider, identify important antenatal risk factors, such as maternal narcotic exposure, abnormal amniotic fluid volume, and the results of prenatal ultrasound examinations.
	Share the information with your team so that you can anticipate high-risk deliveries and adequately prepare for resuscitation.
Use available resources.	Be aware of what resources are available to stabilize a newborn with a difficult airway. Where is the equipment stored?
	Develop a plan for delivery and resuscitation outside the delivery room area.
	If a baby suddenly deteriorates in the mother's postpartum room, plan how the mother and first responder will call for help.
	Consider how your resuscitation team will be notified about a neonatal emergency outside of your usual location. Who will respond and how will the necessary equipment arrive at the site of the emergency?
	Consider what you will do if there is no electrical power or compressed gas available at the site.

Key Points

1 Suspect a pneumothorax if a baby fails to improve despite resuscitative measures or suddenly develops severe respiratory distress. In an emergency, a pneumothorax may be detected by decreased breath sounds and increased transillumination on the affected side.

2 Suspect a pleural effusion if a newborn has respiratory distress and generalized edema (hydrops fetalis).

3 A pneumothorax or pleural effusion that causes cardiorespiratory compromise is treated by aspirating the air or fluid with a needle-catheter-stopcock assembly attached to a syringe and inserted into the chest.

4 If thick secretions obstruct the airway despite a correctly positioned endotracheal tube, attempt to remove the secretions using a suction catheter (5F-8F) inserted through the endotracheal tube. If the obstruction persists, directly suction the trachea with a meconium aspirator attached to the endotracheal tube. Do not proceed to chest compressions until the airway is clear and you have achieved ventilation that inflates and aerates the lungs.

5 Respiratory distress associated with the Robin sequence can be improved by placing the baby prone and inserting a small endotracheal tube (2.5 mm) into the nose so the tip is in the pharynx. If this does not result in adequate air movement, a laryngeal mask may provide a lifesaving airway. Endotracheal intubation is frequently difficult in this situation.

6 Respiratory distress associated with bilateral choanal atresia can be improved by inserting a modified feeding nipple or pacifier with the end cut off into the baby's mouth, an endotracheal tube into the mouth with the tip in the posterior pharynx, or an oral (Guedel) airway.

7 If a congenital diaphragmatic hernia (CDH) is suspected, avoid prolonged PPV with a face mask. Quickly intubate the trachea in the delivery room and insert an orogastric tube with suction to decompress the stomach and intestines.

8 If a mother received narcotics in labor and her baby is not breathing, provide airway support and assisted ventilation until the baby has adequate spontaneous respiratory effort.

9 Although resuscitation outside the delivery room presents different challenges, the physiologic principles and basic steps remain the same throughout the neonatal period. Restoring adequate ventilation is the priority when resuscitating newborns at birth in the delivery room, later in the nursery or the mother's room, or in other locations.

⑩ Additional strategies for resuscitating babies outside the delivery room include the following:

- Maintain temperature by drying the skin, placing the baby skin-to-skin with the mother, covering the baby with clean food-grade plastic and a warm blanket, using a thermal mattress, and raising the environmental temperature.

- Clear the airway, if necessary, using a bulb syringe or cloth on your finger.

- Use mouth-to-mouth-and-nose breathing for PPV if no mechanical device is available.

- Obtain emergency vascular access, if necessary, by placing an intraosseous needle in the tibia.

LESSON 10 REVIEW

1. A newborn's heart rate is 50 beats per minute. He has not improved with ventilation through a face mask or a properly placed 3.5-mm endotracheal tube. His chest is not moving with positive-pressure ventilation. You should (suction the trachea using an 8F suction catheter or meconium aspirator)/(proceed immediately to chest compressions).

2. A newborn has respiratory distress after birth. He has a small lower jaw and a cleft palate. The baby's respiratory distress may improve if you place a small endotracheal tube in the nose, advance it into the pharynx, and position him (supine [on his back])/(prone [on his stomach]).

3. You attended the birth of a baby that received positive-pressure ventilation during the first minutes of life. He improved and has been monitored in the nursery. A short time later, you are called because he has developed acute respiratory distress. You should suspect (a pneumothorax)/(a congenital heart defect) and should rapidly prepare (a needle aspiration device)/(epinephrine).

4. You attend the birth of a baby with antenatally diagnosed congenital diaphragmatic hernia. Promptly after birth, you should (begin face-mask ventilation and insert an orogastric tube in the stomach)/(intubate the trachea and insert an orogastric tube in the stomach).

5. A mother received a narcotic medication for pain relief 1 hour before delivery. After birth, the baby does not have spontaneous respirations and does not improve with stimulation. Your first priority is to (start positive-pressure ventilation)/(administer the narcotic antagonist naloxone).

6. A baby is found limp, blue, and cyanotic in his mother's room 12 hours after an uncomplicated vaginal birth. He does not improve after stimulation and suctioning his mouth/nose with a bulb syringe. Your first priority is to (restore adequate ventilation by beginning positive-pressure ventilation)/(restore adequate circulation by administering epinephrine).

Answers

1. You should suction the trachea using an 8F suction catheter or meconium aspirator.

2. The baby's respiratory distress may improve if you place a small endotracheal tube in the nose, advance it into the pharynx, and position him prone (on his stomach).

3. You should suspect a pneumothorax and should rapidly prepare a needle aspiration device.

4. Promptly after birth, you should intubate the trachea and insert an orogastric tube in the stomach.

5. Your first priority is to start positive-pressure ventilation.

6. Your first priority is to restore adequate ventilation by beginning positive-pressure ventilation.

Additional Reading

Abrams ME, Meredith KS, Kinnard P, Clark RH. Hydrops fetalis: a retrospective review of cases reported to a large national database and identification of risk factors associated with death *Pediatrics.* 2007;120(1):84-89

Benjamin JR, Bizzarro MJ, Cotton CM. Congenital diaphragmatic hernia: updates and outcomes. *NeoReviews.* 2011;12(8):e439-e452

Niwas R, Nadroo AM, Sutija VG, Guadvalli M, Narula P. Malposition of endotracheal tube: association with pneumothorax in ventilated neonates. *Arch Dis Child Fetal Neonatal Ed.* 2007;92(3):F233-234

Chinnadurai S, Goudy SL. Neonatal airway obstruction: overview of diagnosis and treatment. *NeoReviews.* 2013;14(3):e128-e137

Ethics and Care at the End of Life

What you will learn

- The ethical principles associated with neonatal resuscitation
- When it may be appropriate to withhold resuscitation
- What to do when the prognosis is uncertain
- What to do when a baby dies
- How to help parents and staff through the grieving process

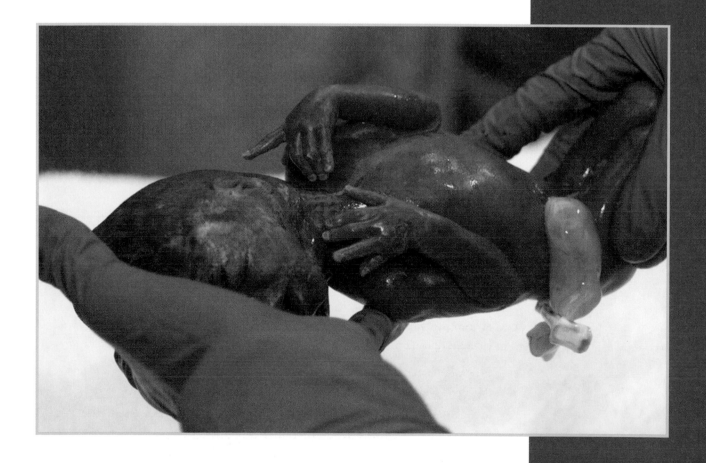

Although this lesson is directed at the resuscitation team member who guides medical decision making, all members of the team should understand the reasoning behind the decisions. As much as possible, there should be unified support of the parents during their very personal period of crisis. This lesson refers to "parents," although it is recognized that sometimes the mother or father is alone during the crisis and, other times, support will be available through extended family or significant others. This lesson is applicable to health care providers who participate in all aspects of care of pregnant women and newborns, including antenatal care providers, pediatricians doing preconception and prenatal consultations, inpatient perinatal care providers, and professionals providing care to families who have experienced a neonatal death.

It is important to recognize that the recommendations made in this lesson are determined, to an extent, by the cultural context and available resources and may require adaptation before being applied to other cultures and countries. These recommendations were based on mortality and morbidity data available at the time of publication. Decisions regarding initiation or non-initiation of resuscitation should be based on current local data and available therapies.

The following case is an example of the ethical considerations involved in neonatal resuscitation and how end-of-life care may be provided. As you read the case, imagine yourself as part of the care team.

Case: A baby who could not be resuscitated

A woman is admitted to the hospital at 23 weeks' gestation with contractions, fever, and ruptured membranes leaking purulent amniotic fluid. She has had consistent prenatal care and the gestational age was estimated by a first-trimester ultrasound. You meet with the obstetric care provider and discuss the pregnancy history. Together, you review current national and local data describing the anticipated short- and long-term outcomes at this extremely early gestation. Afterward, both of you meet with the parents to provide information, discuss goals, explain the treatment options, and develop a care plan. You explain that some parents might decide that resuscitation and intensive care are not in their baby's best interest in view of the high risk of mortality and morbidity and might, instead, choose palliative care focusing on the baby's comfort after birth. After considering the content of your discussion, the parents indicate that they "want everything done if there is any chance that our baby can live." You document your discussion in the medical chart and meet with your resuscitation team to review the care plan.

Your team performs a pre-resuscitation team briefing and prepares the equipment and supplies for a complex resuscitation. At the time of birth, the baby boy is limp and apneic, and has thin, gelatinous skin. He is carried to the radiant warmer and covered with plastic wrap. The initial steps are performed and positive-pressure ventilation (PPV) is administered. A team member places a pulse oximeter sensor and electronic cardiac (ECG) monitor leads. His heart rate is 40 beats per minute (bpm) and not improving. He is quickly intubated and PPV is continued; however, his heart rate does not increase and his oxygen saturation remains well below the target range. Although further resuscitation measures are provided, his heart rate gradually decreases. You explain the baby's condition to the parents and your assessment that resuscitation will not be successful. You agree to remove the endotracheal tube, wrap the baby in a clean blanket, and bring him to his parents to be held and comforted. The parents request a ceremonial blessing from the hospital clergy and this is quickly arranged. Staff members and additional family provide ongoing support. The baby is pronounced dead when no signs of life remain.

Later that day, you return to the parents' room, express condolences, answer their questions about the resuscitation attempt, and ask the parents about performing an autopsy. You offer to schedule a follow-up visit in several weeks to discuss the autopsy findings. The next day, a funeral home is identified. About 1 month later, you meet with the parents to discuss the results, answer questions, and talk about problems the parents and siblings may be having adjusting to their loss.

What ethical principles apply to neonatal resuscitation?

The ethical principles of neonatal resuscitation are the same as those followed in resuscitating an older child or adult. Common ethical principles that apply to all medical care include respecting an individual's rights to make choices that affect his or her life (autonomy), acting to benefit others (beneficence), avoiding harm (nonmaleficence), and treating people truthfully and fairly (justice). These principles underlie why we ask patients for informed consent before proceeding with treatment. Exceptions to this rule include life-threatening medical emergencies and situations where patients are not competent to make their own decisions. Neonatal resuscitation is a medical treatment often complicated by both of these exceptions.

What role should parents play in decisions about resuscitation?

Unlike adults, newborns cannot make decisions for themselves and cannot express their desires. A surrogate decision maker must be identified to assume the responsibility of guarding the newborn's best interests. Generally, parents are considered to be the best surrogate decision makers for their own babies and they should be involved in shared decision making whenever possible. For parents to fulfill this responsibility, they need relevant, accurate, and honest information about the risks and benefits of each treatment option. In addition, they must have adequate time to thoughtfully consider each option, ask questions, and seek other opinions. Unfortunately, the need for resuscitation is often an unexpected emergency with little opportunity to achieve fully informed consent before proceeding. Even when you have the opportunity to meet with parents, uncertainty about the extent of congenital anomalies, the actual gestational age, the likelihood of survival, and the potential for severe disabilities may make it difficult for parents to decide what is in their baby's best interest before the baby is born. Complete information may not be available until after birth and perhaps not for several hours or days. These uncertainties should be addressed with the parents when the initial treatment plan is developed and contingencies should be discussed. Parents and health care providers must be prepared to reevaluate their goals and plans based on the findings after birth and the baby's response to treatment. Discussions about the newborn's best interests may continue well beyond the delivery room.

What are the considerations involved in the decision whether to initiate resuscitation for an extremely premature baby?

Parents should be provided with accurate prognostic information using all relevant information affecting the prognosis. Antenatal outcome estimates for survival and disability among extremely premature babies have typically been based on gestational age and estimated weight. Unless the pregnancy was conceived by assisted reproductive technology where the date of fertilization or implantation can be defined, techniques used for obstetric dating are accurate to 3 to 5 days if applied in the first trimester, but only to ±1 to 2 weeks subsequently. Estimates of fetal weight are accurate only to ±15% to 20% and may be misleading if there is intrauterine growth restriction. Even small discrepancies of 1 or 2 weeks between estimated and actual gestational age, or 100 to 200 g difference in birth weight, may have implications for survival and long-term morbidity.

Gestational age and weight are not the only factors affecting prognosis. Maternal health, obstetric complications, and genetic factors also influence outcome. Scoring systems that include variables such as gender, use of antenatal steroids, and multiplicity have been developed in an effort to improve prognostic accuracy. Be cautious when interpreting results from different studies. Some investigators may describe the proportion of babies with each outcome based on the total number of live-born babies while others describe the same outcome based on the number of babies resuscitated, the number of babies admitted to the nursery, or the number surviving until discharge. By simply changing the inclusion criteria for the calculation, the likelihood of an adverse outcome will change. Remember that prognostic scores provide a range of plausible outcomes based on a sample of babies; however, they cannot definitively predict the outcome for any individual baby. Similarly, the baby's appearance at the time of birth is not an accurate predictor of survival or disability. Parents need to be informed that, despite your best efforts, the ability to give an accurate prognosis for a specific newborn either before or immediately after birth remains limited.

Are there situations in which it is ethical not to initiate resuscitation?

The birth of extremely premature babies and those with significant chromosomal abnormalities or congenital malformations frequently raises difficult questions about the initiation of resuscitation. Although general recommendations can guide practice, each situation is unique, and decision making should be individualized.

If the responsible physicians believe that there is no chance for survival, the initiation of resuscitation offers no benefit to the baby and should not be offered. Humane, compassionate, and culturally sensitive palliative care focused on ensuring the baby's comfort is the medically and ethically appropriate treatment. Examples may include birth at a confirmed gestational age of less than 22 weeks' gestation and some severe congenital malformations and chromosomal anomalies.

In conditions associated with a high risk of mortality or significant burden of morbidity for the baby, caregivers should discuss the risks and benefits of life-sustaining treatment with the parents and involve them in decision making about whether attempting resuscitation is in their baby's best interest. If there is agreement between the parents and the caregivers that intensive medical care will not improve the chances for the newborn's long-term survival or will pose an unacceptable burden on the child, it is ethical to provide compassionate palliative care and not initiate resuscitation. If the parents' preferences regarding resuscitation are either unknown or uncertain, resuscitation should be initiated pending further discussions. Examples may include birth between 22 and 24 weeks' gestation and some serious congenital and chromosomal anomalies.

The following statement from the American Medical Association (AMA) Code of Medical Ethics (AMA Opinion 2.215, 2010-2011) summarizes this approach to decision making and is endorsed by the Neonatal Resuscitation Program® (NRP®).

The primary consideration for decisions regarding life-sustaining treatment for seriously ill newborns should be what is best for the newborn.
Factors that should be weighed are as follows:
1. The chance that the therapy will succeed
2. The risks involved with treatment and nontreatment
3. The degree to which the therapy, if successful, will extend life
4. The pain and discomfort associated with the therapy
5. The anticipated quality of life for the newborn with and without treatment

What should you do if you are uncertain about the chances of survival or serious disability when you examine the baby after birth?

If parents are uncertain how to proceed, or your examination suggests that the prenatal assessment of disability was incorrect, initial resuscitation and stabilization allows you additional time to gather more complete clinical information and to review the situation with the parents and consultants.

Once you have resuscitated a baby, are you ethically obligated to continue life-sustaining therapies?

No, you are not ethically obligated to continue life-sustaining therapies. Withholding resuscitation and withdrawing life-sustaining treatment during or after resuscitation are ethically equivalent. If the responsible health care providers and parents determine that life-sustaining treatment is no longer in the baby's best interest, they may choose to redirect from curative to palliative care and focus on ensuring the baby's comfort.

What laws apply to neonatal resuscitation?

Medical ethics provide guidelines describing how health care providers should act within a society. Based on these guiding principles, governments create and enforce laws that describe how individuals must act. There is currently no federal law in the United States mandating delivery room resuscitation in all circumstances. There may be laws in the area where you practice that apply to the care of newborns in the delivery room. If you are uncertain about the laws in your area, you should consult your hospital ethics committee or attorney. In most circumstances, it is ethically and legally acceptable to withhold or withdraw resuscitation efforts if the parents and health care providers agree that further medical intervention would be futile, would merely prolong dying, or would not offer sufficient benefit to justify the burdens imposed on the baby.

Specific rights and responsibilities of minors, fathers, and unmarried partners may vary between states. You should meet with your hospital's legal counsel if you have questions about the regulations in the location where you practice.

How do you inform parents that their baby is dying?

Your role is to support the parents by being honest and speaking in an empathic and caring manner. Ask if they have chosen a name for their baby and, if they have, refer to the baby by name. Explain what treatment you have provided and your assessment of the baby's current condition. State clearly and without euphemism that, despite treatment, their baby is dying. Explain how you plan to care for their dying baby and what options are available.

Some parents may be interested in pursuing organ or tissue donation. Although many neonatal deaths will not meet eligibility criteria because of small size or the time interval between withdrawal of support and death, many potentially eligible donations have been lost because the neonatal team failed to make a timely referral to their organ procurement agency. When a neonatal death is anticipated, it is important to consult your regional organ procurement agency regarding eligibility criteria so that you can advise the parents about potential donation options.

How do you take care of a baby that is dying?

The most important goal is to minimize suffering by providing humane and compassionate care. Offer to bring the baby to the parent(s). Silence the alarms on monitors and medical equipment before removing them. Remove any unnecessary tubes, tape, monitors, or medical equipment, and gently clean the baby's mouth and face. If the cause of the baby's death is uncertain or the death will be investigated by the coroner or medical examiner, it may be important to leave all medical devices and tubes in place. Wrap the baby in a clean, warm blanket. Narcotics may be administered as needed, either orally, nasally or intravenously, to relieve the baby's discomfort. Prepare the parents for what they may see, feel, and hear when they hold their dying baby, including the possibility of gasping, agonal respirations, color changes, persistent heartbeat, and continuing movements. If the baby has obvious congenital anomalies, briefly explain to the parents what they will see. Help them look beyond any deformities by pointing out a good or memorable feature. Some units prepare a "memory box" for the parents with the baby's handprints or footprints, photographs, and other items.

Parents should be offered private time with the baby in a comfortable environment, but a health care provider should check at intervals to see if anything is needed. The baby's chest should be auscultated intermittently for at least 60 seconds, as a very slow heart rate may persist for hours. Disturbing noises such as phone calls, pagers, monitor alarms, and staff conversations should be minimized. When the parents are ready for you to take the baby, the baby should be taken to a designated, private location until ready to be transported to the morgue.

A member of the neonatal team should discuss the locally available options for performing a complete or limited autopsy. An autopsy can help determine the precise cause of death, confirm prenatal diagnoses, and reveal important new diagnoses. By further delineating the cause of death, an autopsy may reduce parental concerns and provide additional insight into the potential implications for future pregnancies.

It is very helpful to understand the cultural and religious expectations surrounding death in the community you serve. Some families grieve quietly while others are more demonstrative; however, all modes are acceptable and should be accommodated. Some parents may prefer to be alone, while others may want their other children, their extended family, friends, community members, and/or clergy to be with them. Families may request to take their baby to a hospital chapel or a more peaceful setting outside, or may ask for help with arrangements for blessings or rites for their dead or dying baby. You should be as flexible as you can in responding to their wishes.

It is helpful to anticipate this difficult situation in advance and develop a protocol. Plan which staff members will be responsible for providing palliative care and how other members of the team can provide support. Members of the neonatal team may play an important role even if the baby is born so prematurely that life-sustaining therapy is not indicated. They may offer the parents reassurance that the gestational age assessment is correct and use their expertise to help provide comfort care for the baby. Many nurseries develop a package of helpful information for staff members, including phone numbers for key support staff, instructions for completing the required administrative tasks, reminders about how to prepare the baby's body, and bereavement information for the family.

What follow-up arrangements should be planned for the parents?

Before the parents leave the hospital, make sure you have contact information for them, and provide them with details about how to contact the attending physician, bereavement professionals, and, if available, a perinatal loss support group. If your institution does not provide these services, it may be helpful to contact your regional perinatal referral center to obtain contact information for the parents. It is important to involve the family's primary care physician and/or obstetric provider so they can provide additional support. The attending physician may schedule a follow-up appointment to answer any unresolved questions, review results of the autopsy or other studies pending at the time of death, and assess the family's needs. Parents should be directed to the obstetric provider if they have questions regarding events and care before birth. Some hospitals sponsor parent-to-parent support groups and plan an annual memorial service, bringing together families who have suffered a perinatal loss. Recognize that some families may not want any additional contact from the hospital staff. This desire must be respected. Unexpected communications, such as a quality assurance survey from the hospital, or newsletters about baby care, may be an unwanted reminder of the family's loss.

How do you support the staff in the nursery after a perinatal death?

Staff members who participated in the care of the baby and family also need support. They will have feelings of sadness and may be feeling anger and guilt. Consider holding a debriefing session shortly after the baby's death so you can openly discuss questions and feelings in a professional, supportive, and nonjudgmental forum. However, speculation based on secondhand information should be avoided in such meetings, and questions and issues regarding care decisions and actions should be discussed only in a qualified peer review session and should follow hospital policy for such sessions.

Focus on Teamwork

The ethical considerations and end-of-life care described in this lesson highlight several opportunities for effective teams to use the NRP Key Behavioral skills.

Behavior	Example
Anticipate and plan.	Plan how you will provide antenatal counseling and manage difficult ethical decisions. Develop a protocol to use when caring for a dying baby and supporting the grieving family.
Communicate effectively.	When counseling parents, use clear language and terminology that they will understand. Visual aids and written materials may be helpful. Use an appropriately trained medical interpreter if the family is not proficient in English or has a hearing disability.
Use available information.	Review both national and local outcome data and understand their limitations. Use all available prognostic information.
Use available resources. Call for additional help when needed.	Become familiar with the resources in your hospital and community that can help to resolve conflicts, answer legal questions, and provide bereavement services. If necessary, consult with specialists at your regional referral center to obtain up-to-date outcome information.
Maintain professional behavior.	Ensure that all members of the health care team understand the treatment plan. Disagreements should be discussed in an appropriate forum. Consult the hospital ethics committee or legal counsel if necessary.
Know your environment.	Understand the cultural and religious expectations surrounding death in your community.

Key Points

1 The ethical principles of neonatal resuscitation are the same as those followed in resuscitating an older child or adult.

2 Parents are generally considered the best surrogate decision makers for their babies and should be involved in shared decision making whenever possible. For parents to fulfill this responsibility, they need relevant, accurate, and honest information about the risks and benefits of each treatment option.

3 Parents should be provided with accurate prognostic information using all relevant information affecting their baby's prognosis.

4 Parents need to be informed that, despite your best efforts, the ability to give an accurate prognosis for an extremely preterm baby remains limited either before or immediately after birth.

5 The primary consideration for decisions regarding life-sustaining treatment for seriously ill newborns should be what is best for the newborn.

6 If the responsible physicians believe that there is no chance for survival, initiation of resuscitation is not an ethical treatment option and should not be offered. Examples may include birth at a confirmed gestational age of less than 22 weeks' gestation and some severe congenital malformations and chromosomal anomalies.

7 In conditions associated with a high risk of mortality or significant burden of morbidity for the baby, parents should participate in the decision whether attempted resuscitation is in their baby's best interest. If there is agreement that intensive medical care will not improve the chances for the newborn's survival or will pose an unacceptable burden on the child, it is ethical to withhold resuscitation.

8 There may be laws in the area where you practice that apply to the care of newborns in the delivery room. If you are uncertain about the laws in your area, consult your hospital ethics committee or attorney.

9 Humane, compassionate, and culturally sensitive palliative care should be provided for all newborns for whom resuscitation is not initiated or is not successful.

Additional Reading

American Academy of Pediatrics and American College of Obstetricians and Gynecologists. *Guidelines for Perinatal Care.* 7th ed. Elk Grove Village, IL: American Academy of Pediatrics, American College of Obstetricians and Gynecologists; 2012

American Medical Association, Council on Ethical and Judicial Affairs. *Code of Medical Ethics: Current Opinions with Annotations,* 2010-2011 ed. Chicago, IL: American Medical Association (Opinion 2.215)

Cummings J, Committee on Fetus and Newborn, American Academy of Pediatrics. Antenatal counseling regarding resuscitation and intensive care before 25 weeks of gestation. *Pediatrics.* 2015;136(3):588-595

Carter BS, Jones PM. Evidence-based comfort care for neonates towards the end of life. *Semin Fetal and Neonatal Med.* 2013;18(2):88-92

Gold KJ. Navigating care after a baby dies: a systematic review of parent experiences with health providers. *J Perinatol.* 2007;27(4):230-237

Rysavy MA, Li L, Bell EF, et al. Between-hospital variation in treatment and outcomes in extremely preterm infants. *N Engl J Med.* 2015;372(19):1801-1811

Uthaya S, Mancini A, Beardsley C, Wood D, Ranmal R, Modi N. Managing palliation in the neonatal unit. *Arch Dis Child Fetal Neonatal Ed.* 2014;99(5):F349-F352

Younge N, Smith PB, Goldberg RN, et al. Impact of a palliative care program on end-of-life care in a neonatal intensive care unit. *J Perinatol.* 2015;35(3):218-222

Appendix

PEDIATRICS®

OFFICIAL JOURNAL OF THE AMERICAN ACADEMY OF PEDIATRICS

Part 13: Neonatal Resuscitation: 2015 American Heart Association Guidelines Update for Cardiopulmonary Resuscitation and Emergency Cardiovascular Care (Reprint)

Myra H. Wyckoff, Khalid Aziz, Marilyn B. Escobedo, Vishal S. Kapadia, John Kattwinkel, Jeffrey M. Perlman, Wendy M. Simon, Gary M. Weiner and Jeanette G. Zaichkin

Pediatrics 2015;136;S196; originally published online October 14, 2015;
DOI: 10.1542/peds.2015-3373G

The online version of this article, along with updated information and services, is located on the World Wide Web at:
/content/136/Supplement_2/S196.full.html

PEDIATRICS is the official journal of the American Academy of Pediatrics. A monthly publication, it has been published continuously since 1948. PEDIATRICS is owned, published, and trademarked by the American Academy of Pediatrics, 141 Northwest Point Boulevard, Elk Grove Village, Illinois, 60007. Copyright © 2015 by the American Academy of Pediatrics. All rights reserved. Print ISSN: 0031-4005. Online ISSN: 1098-4275.

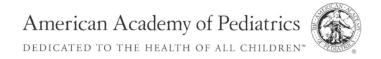

American Academy of Pediatrics
DEDICATED TO THE HEALTH OF ALL CHILDREN™

Part 13: Neonatal Resuscitation
2015 American Heart Association Guidelines Update for Cardiopulmonary Resuscitation and Emergency Cardiovascular Care (Reprint)

Reprint: The American Heart Association requests that this document be cited as follows: Wyckoff MH, Aziz K, Escobedo MB, Kapadia VS, Kattwinkel J, Perlman JM, Simon WM, Weiner GM, Zaichkin, JG. Part 13: neonatal resuscitation: 2015 American Heart Association Guidelines Update for Cardiopulmonary Resuscitation and Emergency Cardiovascular Care. *Circulation*. 2015;132(suppl 2):S543–S560.

Reprinted with permission of the American Heart Association, Inc. This article has been co-published in *Circulation*.

AUTHORS: Myra H. Wyckoff, Chair; Khalid Aziz; Marilyn B. Escobedo; Vishal S. Kapadia; John Kattwinkel; Jeffrey M. Perlman; Wendy M. Simon; Gary M. Weiner; Jeanette G. Zaichkin

KEY WORD

cardiopulmonary resuscitation

www.pediatrics.org/cgi/doi/10.1542/peds.2015-3373G

doi:10.1542/peds.2015-3373G

PEDIATRICS (ISSN Numbers: Print, 0031-4005; Online, 1098-4275).

(*Circulation*. 2015;132[suppl 2]:S543–S560. DOI: 10.1161/CIR. 0000000000000267.)

INTRODUCTION

The following guidelines are a summary of the evidence presented in the *2015 International Consensus on Cardiopulmonary Resuscitation and Emergency Cardiovascular Care Science With Treatment Recommendations* (CoSTR).[1,2] Throughout the online version of this publication, live links are provided so the reader can connect directly to systematic reviews on the International Liaison Committee on Resuscitation (ILCOR) Scientific Evidence Evaluation and Review System (SEERS) website. These links are indicated by a combination of letters and numbers (eg, NRP 787). We encourage readers to use the links and review the evidence and appendices.

These guidelines apply primarily to newly born infants transitioning from intrauterine to extrauterine life. The recommendations are also applicable to neonates who have completed newborn transition and require resuscitation during the first weeks after birth.[3] Practitioners who resuscitate infants at birth or at any time during the initial hospitalization should consider following these guidelines. For purposes of these guidelines, the terms *newborn* and *neonate* apply to any infant during the initial hospitalization. The term *newly born* applies specifically to an infant at the time of birth.[3]

Immediately after birth, infants who are breathing and crying may undergo delayed cord clamping (see Umbilical Cord Management section). However, until more evidence is available, infants who are not breathing or crying should have the cord clamped (unless part of a delayed cord clamping research protocol), so that resuscitation measures can commence promptly.

Approximately 10% of newborns require some assistance to begin breathing at birth. Less than 1% require extensive resuscitation measures,[4] such as cardiac compressions and medications. Although most newly born infants successfully transition from intrauterine to extrauterine life without special help, because of the large total number of births, a significant number will require some degree of resuscitation.[2]

Newly born infants who do not require resuscitation can be generally identified upon delivery by rapidly assessing the answers to the following 3 questions:

- Term gestation?
- Good tone?
- Breathing or crying?

If the answer to all 3 questions is "yes," the newly born infant may stay with the mother for routine care. Routine care means the infant is dried, placed skin to skin with the mother, and covered with dry linen to maintain a normal temperature. Observation of breathing, activity, and color must be ongoing.

If the answer to any of these assessment questions is "no," the infant should be moved to a radiant warmer to receive 1 or more of the following 4 actions in sequence:

A. Initial steps in stabilization (warm and maintain normal temperature, position, clear secretions only if copious and/or obstructing the airway, dry, stimulate)

B. Ventilate and oxygenate

C. Initiate chest compressions

D. Administer epinephrine and/or volume

Approximately 60 seconds ("the Golden Minute") are allotted for completing the initial steps, reevaluating, and beginning ventilation if required (Figure 1). Although the 60-second mark is not precisely defined by science, it is important to avoid unnecessary delay in initiation of ventilation, because this is *the* most important step for successful resuscitation of the newly born who has not responded to the initial steps. The decision to progress beyond the initial steps is determined by simultaneous assessment of 2 vital characteristics: respirations (apnea, gasping, or labored or unlabored breathing) and heart rate (less than 100/min). Methods to accurately assess the heart rate will

be discussed in detail in the section on Assessment of Heart Rate. Once positive-pressure ventilation (PPV) or supplementary oxygen administration is started, assessment should consist of simultaneous evaluation of 3 vital characteristics: heart rate, respirations, and oxygen saturation, as determined by pulse oximetry and discussed under Assessment of Oxygen Need and Administration of Oxygen. The most sensitive indicator of a successful response to each step is an increase in heart rate.[3]

Neonatal Resuscitation Algorithm—2015 Update

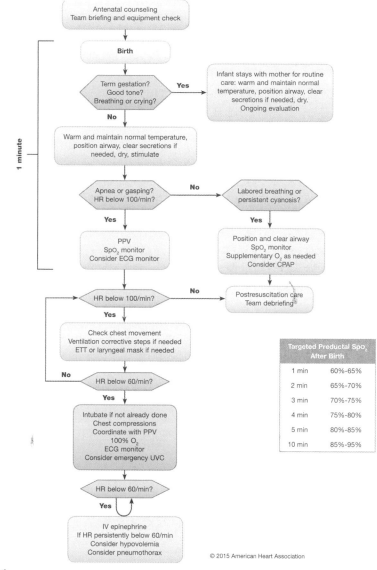

© 2015 American Heart Association

Figure 1
Neonatal Resuscitation Algorithm—2015 Update.

ANTICIPATION OF RESUSCITATION NEED

Readiness for neonatal resuscitation requires assessment of perinatal risk, a system to assemble the appropriate personnel based on that risk, an organized method for ensuring immediate access to supplies and equipment, and standardization of behavioral skills that help assure effective teamwork and communication.

Every birth should be attended by at least 1 person who can perform the initial steps of newborn resuscitation and PPV, and whose only responsibility is care of the newborn. In the presence of significant perinatal risk factors that increase the likelihood of the need for resuscitation,[5,6] additional personnel with resuscitation skills, including chest compressions, endotracheal intubation, and umbilical vein catheter insertion, should be immediately available. Furthermore, because a newborn without apparent risk factors may unexpectedly require resuscitation, each institution should have a procedure in place for rapidly mobilizing a team with complete newborn resuscitation skills for any birth.

The neonatal resuscitation provider and/or team is at a major disadvantage if supplies are missing or equipment is not functioning. A standardized checklist to ensure that all necessary supplies and equipment are present and functioning may be helpful. A known perinatal risk factor, such as preterm birth, requires preparation of supplies specific to thermoregulation and respiratory support for this vulnerable population.

When perinatal risk factors are identified, a team should be mobilized and a team leader identified. As time permits, the leader should conduct a presuscitation briefing, identify interventions that may be required, and assign roles and responsibilities to the team members.[7,8] During resuscitation, it is vital that the team demonstrates effective communication and teamwork skills to help ensure quality and patient safety.

UMBILICAL CORD MANAGEMENT[NRP 787, NRP 849]

Until recent years, a common practice has been to clamp the umbilical cord soon after birth to quickly transfer the infant to the neonatal team for stabilization. This immediate clamping was deemed particularly important for infants at high risk for difficulty with transition and those most likely to require resuscitation, such as infants born preterm. During the 2010 CoSTR review, evidence began to emerge suggesting that delayed cord clamping (DCC) might be beneficial for infants who did not need immediate resuscitation at birth.[7]

The 2015 ILCOR systematic review[NRP 787] confirms that DCC is associated with less intraventricular hemorrhage (IVH) of any grade, higher blood pressure and blood volume, less need for transfusion after birth, and less necrotizing enterocolitis. There was no evidence of decreased mortality or decreased incidence of severe IVH.[1,2] The studies were judged to be very low quality (downgraded for imprecision and very high risk of bias). The only negative consequence appears to be a slightly increased level of bilirubin, associated with more need for phototherapy. These findings have led to national recommendations that DCC be practiced when possible.[9,10] A major problem with essentially all of these studies has been that infants who were thought to require resuscitation were either withdrawn from the randomized controlled trials or electively were not enrolled. Therefore, there is no evidence regarding safety or utility of DCC for infants requiring resuscitation and some concern that the delay in establishing ventilation may be harmful. Some studies have suggested that cord "milking" might accomplish goals similar to DCC,[11–13] but there is insufficient evidence of either its safety or utility to suggest its routine use in the newly born, particularly in extremely preterm infants.

In summary, from the evidence reviewed in the 2010 CoSTR[7] and subsequent review of DCC and cord milking in preterm newborns in the 2015 ILCOR systematic review,[1,2] DCC for longer than 30 seconds is reasonable for both term and preterm infants who do not require resuscitation at birth (Class IIa, Level of Evidence [LOE] C-LD). There is insufficient evidence to recommend an approach to cord clamping for infants who require resuscitation at birth, and more randomized trials involving such infants are encouraged. In light of the limited information regarding the safety of rapid changes in blood volume for extremely preterm infants, we suggest against the routine use of cord milking for infants born at less than 29 weeks of gestation outside of a research setting. Further study is warranted because cord milking may improve initial mean blood pressure and hematologic indices and reduce intracranial hemorrhage, but thus far there is no evidence for improvement in long-term outcomes (Class IIb, LOE C-LD).

INITIAL STEPS

The initial steps of newborn resuscitation are to maintain normal temperature of the infant, position the infant in a "sniffing" position to open the airway, clear secretions if needed with a bulb syringe or suction catheter, dry the infant (unless preterm and covered in plastic wrap), and stimulate the infant to breathe. Current examination of the evidence for these practices is summarized below.

Importance of Maintaining Normal Temperature in the Delivery Room[NRP 589]

It has long been recognized (since Budin's 1907 publication of *The Nursling*)[14] that the admission temperature of newly born nonasphyxiated infants is a strong predictor of mortality at all gestational ages.[15–49] Preterm infants are especially vulnerable. Hypothermia is also associated with serious morbidities, such as increased risk of IVH,[19,26,39,50–54] respiratory issues,[15,19,21,50,55–60] hypoglycemia,[15,44,60–64] and late-onset sepsis.[33,65]

Because of this, admission temperature should be recorded as a predictor of outcomes as well as a quality indicator (Class I, LOE B-NR.) It is recommended that the temperature of newly born nonasphyxiated infants be maintained between 36.5°C and 37.5°C after birth through admission and stabilization (Class I, LOE C-LD).

Interventions to Maintain Newborn Temperature in the Delivery Room[NRP 599]

The use of radiant warmers and plastic wrap with a cap has improved but not eliminated the risk of hypothermia in preterm infants in the delivery room. Other strategies have been introduced, which include increased room temperature, thermal mattresses, and the use of warmed humidified resuscitation gases. Various combinations of these strategies may be reasonable to prevent hypothermia in infants born at less than 32 weeks of gestation (Class IIb, LOE B-R, B-NR, C-LD). Compared with plastic wrap and radiant warmer, the addition of a thermal mattress,[66–70] warmed humidified gases,[71,72] and increased room temperature plus cap plus thermal mattress[55,57,59,73] were all effective in reducing hypothermia. For all the studies, hyperthermia was a concern, but harm was not shown. Hyperthermia (greater than 38.0°C) should be avoided due to the potential associated risks (Class III: Harm, LOE C-EO).

Warming Hypothermic Newborns to Restore Normal Temperature[NRP 858]

The traditional recommendation for the method of rewarming neonates who are hypothermic after resuscitation has been that slower is preferable to faster rewarming to avoid complications such as apnea and arrhythmias. However, there is insufficient current evidence to recommend a preference for either rapid (0.5°C/h or greater) or slow rewarming (less than 0.5°C/h) of

unintentionally hypothermic newborns (temperature less than 36°C) at hospital admission. Either approach to rewarming may be reasonable (Class IIb, LOE C-LD).

Effect of Maternal Hypothermia and Hyperthermia on the Neonate[NRP 804]

Maternal hyperthermia in labor is associated with adverse neonatal effects. These include increased mortality,[74,75] neonatal seizures,[74–80] and adverse neurologic states like encephalopathy.[81–84] Maternal hypothermia in labor has not been shown to be associated with clinically significant adverse neonatal outcomes at the time of birth.[85–89] Although maternal hyperthermia is associated with adverse neonatal outcomes, there is insufficient evidence to make a recommendation on the management of maternal hyperthermia.

Maintaining Normothermia in Resource-Limited Settings[NRP 793]

The ability to maintain temperature in resource-limited settings after birth is a significant problem,[40] with a dose-dependent increase in mortality for temperatures below 36.5°C. Premature newborns are at much higher risk than those born at term. Simple interventions to prevent hypothermia during transition (birth until 1 to 2 hours of life) reduce mortality. During transition, the use of plastic wraps[90–92] and the use of skin-to-skin contact[93–100] reduce hypothermia.

In resource-limited settings, to maintain body temperature or prevent hypothermia during transition (birth until 1 to 2 hours of life) in well newborn infants, it may be reasonable to put them in a clean food-grade plastic bag up to the level of the neck and swaddle them after drying (Class IIb, LOE C-LD). Another option that may be reasonable is to nurse such newborns with skin-to-skin contact or kangaroo mother care (Class IIb, LOE C-LD). There are no data

examining the use of plastic wraps or skin-to-skin contact during resuscitation/stabilization in resource-limited settings.

Clearing the Airway

When Amniotic Fluid Is Clear

This topic was last reviewed in 2010.[3] Suctioning immediately after birth, whether with a bulb syringe or suction catheter, may be considered only if the airway appears obstructed or if PPV is required. Avoiding unnecessary suctioning helps prevent the risk of induced bradycardia due to suctioning of the nasopharynx.[101,102] Deterioration of pulmonary compliance, oxygenation, and cerebral blood flow velocity shown to accompany tracheal suction in intubated infants in the neonatal intensive care unit also suggests the need for caution in the use of suction immediately after birth.[103–105] This recommendation remains unchanged. Please refer to the 2010 CoSTR for the latest science review.[7,8]

When Meconium Is Present[NRP 865]

Since the mid-1970s, interventions to decrease the mortality and morbidity of meconium aspiration syndrome in infants who are born through meconium-stained amniotic fluid have been recommended. The practice of universal oropharyngeal suctioning of the fetus on the perineum followed by routine intubation and suctioning of the trachea at birth was generally practiced for many years. This practice was abandoned over a decade ago after a large multicenter, multinational randomized clinical trial provided evidence that newborns born through meconium-stained amniotic fluid who were vigorous at birth did not benefit from intervention and could avoid the risk of intubation.[106]

Because the presence of meconium-stained amniotic fluid may indicate fetal distress and increases the risk that the infant will require resuscitation after birth, a team that includes an individual skilled in tracheal intubation should be present at the time of birth. If the infant is vigorous with good respiratory effort and muscle tone, the infant may stay with the mother to receive the initial steps of newborn care. Gentle clearing of meconium from the mouth and nose with a bulb syringe may be done if necessary.

However, if the infant born through meconium-stained amniotic fluid presents with poor muscle tone and inadequate breathing efforts, the initial steps of resuscitation should be completed under the radiant warmer. PPV should be initiated if the infant is not breathing or the heart rate is less than 100/min after the initial steps are completed.

Routine intubation for tracheal suction in this setting is not suggested, because there is insufficient evidence to continue recommending this practice (Class IIb, LOE C-LD). In making this suggested change, greater value has been placed on harm avoidance (ie, delays in providing bag-mask ventilation, potential harm of the procedure) over the unknown benefit of the intervention of routine tracheal intubation and suctioning. Therefore, emphasis should be made on initiating ventilation within the first minute of life in nonbreathing or ineffectively breathing infants.

Although a definitive randomized clinical trial is still needed, current published human evidence does not support a recommendation for routine intervention of intubation and suction for the nonvigorous newborn with meconium-stained amniotic fluid.[107–116] Appropriate intervention to support ventilation and oxygenation should be initiated as indicated for each individual infant. This may include intubation and suction if the airway is obstructed.

Assessment of Heart Rate[NRP 898]

Immediately after birth, assessment of the newborn's heart rate is used to evaluate the effectiveness of spontaneous respiratory effort and determine the need for subsequent interventions. During resuscitation, an increase in the newborn's heart rate is considered the most sensitive indicator of a successful response to each intervention. Therefore, identifying a rapid, reliable, and accurate method to measure the newborn's heart rate is critically important. In previous treatment guidelines, auscultation of the precordium was recommended as the preferred physical examination method, and pulse oximetry was recommended as an adjunct to provide a noninvasive, rapid, and continuous assessment of heart rate during resuscitation.[3]

The 2015 ILCOR systematic review evaluated 1 study comparing clinical assessment with electrocardiography (ECG) in the delivery room[117] and 5 studies comparing simultaneous pulse oximetry and ECG.[118–122] Clinical assessment was found to be both unreliable and inaccurate. Among healthy newborns, providers frequently could not palpate the umbilical pulse and underestimated the newborn's heart rate by auscultation or palpation.[117] Four studies found that 3-lead ECG displayed a reliable heart rate faster than pulse oximetry.[118,120–122] In 2 studies, ECG was more likely to detect the newborn's heart rate during the first minute of life.[120,121] Although the mean differences between the series of heart rates measured by ECG and pulse oximetry were small, pulse oximetry tended to underestimate the newborn's heart rate and would have led to potentially unnecessary interventions.[118,119,122] During the first 2 minutes of life, pulse oximetry frequently displayed the newborn's heart rate below either 60/min or 100/min, while a simultaneous ECG showed the heart rate greater than 100/min.[122]

Many of the newborns included in the studies did not require resuscitation, and very few required chest compressions.

The majority of the studies did not report any difficulties with applying the leads.[118–120]

During resuscitation of term and preterm newborns, the use of 3-lead ECG for the rapid and accurate measurement of the newborn's heart rate may be reasonable (Class IIb, LOE C-LD). The use of ECG does not replace the need for pulse oximetry to evaluate the newborn's oxygenation.

Assessment of Oxygen Need and Administration of Oxygen

Use of Pulse Oximetry

This topic was last reviewed in 2010.[3] It is recommended that oximetry be used when resuscitation can be anticipated, when PPV is administered, when central cyanosis persists beyond the first 5 to 10 minutes of life, or when supplementary oxygen is administered.

Administration of Oxygen

Term Infants

This topic was last reviewed in 2010.[3] It is reasonable to initiate resuscitation with air (21% oxygen at sea level). Supplementary oxygen may be administered and titrated to achieve a preductal oxygen saturation approximating the interquartile range measured in healthy term infants after vaginal birth at sea level.[7,8,123]

Preterm[NRP 864]

Meta-analysis of 7 randomized trials that compared initiating resuscitation of preterm newborns (less than 35 weeks of gestation) with high oxygen (65% or greater) and low oxygen (21% to 30%) showed no improvement in survival to hospital discharge with the use of high oxygen.[124–130] Similarly, in the subset of studies that evaluated these outcomes, no benefit was seen for the prevention of bronchopulmonary dysplasia,[125,127–130] IVH,[125,128–130] or retinopathy of prematurity.[125,128,129]

When oxygen targeting was used as a cointervention, the oxygen concentration of resuscitation gas and the preductal oxygen saturation were similar between the high-oxygen and low-oxygen groups within the first 10 minutes of life.[125,128–130]

In all studies, irrespective of whether air or high oxygen (including 100%) was used to initiate resuscitation, most infants were in approximately 30% oxygen by the time of stabilization. Resuscitation of preterm newborns of less than 35 weeks of gestation should be initiated with low oxygen (21% to 30%), and the oxygen concentration should be titrated to achieve preductal oxygen saturation approximating the interquartile range measured in healthy term infants after vaginal birth at sea level[123] (Class I, LOE B-R). Initiating resuscitation of preterm newborns with high oxygen (65% or greater) is not recommended (Class III: No Benefit, LOE B-R). This recommendation reflects a preference for not exposing preterm newborns to additional oxygen without data demonstrating a proven benefit for important outcomes.

POSITIVE PRESSURE VENTILATION

Initial Breaths[NRP 809]

Several recent animal studies have suggested that a longer sustained inflation may be beneficial for establishing functional residual capacity during transition from fluid-filled to air-filled lungs after birth.[131,132] Some clinicians have suggested applying this technique for transition of human newborns. Review of the literature in 2015 identified 3 randomized controlled trials[133–135] and 2 cohort studies[136,137] that demonstrated a benefit of sustained inflation for reducing need for mechanical ventilation (very low quality of evidence, downgraded for variability of interventions). However, no benefit was found for reduction of mortality, bronchopulmonary dysplasia, or air leak.

One cohort study[156] suggested that the need for intubation was less after sustained inflation.

There are insufficient data regarding short and long-term safety and the most appropriate duration and pressure of inflation to support routine application of sustained inflation of greater than 5 seconds' duration to the transitioning newborn (Class IIb, LOE B-R). Further studies using carefully designed protocols are needed.

End-Expiratory Pressure[NRP 897]

Administration of PPV is the standard recommended treatment for both preterm and term infants who are apneic. A flow-inflating or self-inflating resuscitation bag or T-piece resuscitator are appropriate devices to use for PPV. In the 2010 Guidelines[3] and based on experience with delivering PPV in the neonatal intensive care unit, the use of positive end-expiratory pressure (PEEP) was speculated to be beneficial when PPV is administered to the newly born, but no published evidence was available to support this recommendation. PEEP was evaluated again in 2015, and 2 randomized controlled trials[138,139] suggested that addition of PEEP during delivery room resuscitation of preterm newborns resulted in no improvement in mortality, no less need for cardiac drugs or chest compressions, no more rapid improvement in heart rate, no less need for intubation, no change in pulmonary air leaks, no less chronic lung disease, and no effect on Apgar scores, although the studies were underpowered to have sufficient confidence in a no-difference conclusion. However, 1 of the trials[139] provided low-quality evidence that the maximum amount of supplementary oxygen required to achieve target oxygen saturation may be slightly less when using PEEP. In 2015, the Neonatal Resuscitation ILCOR and Guidelines Task Forces repeated their 2010 recommendation that, when

PPV is administered to preterm newborns, use of approximately 5 cm H_2O PEEP is suggested (Class IIb, LOE B-R). This will require the addition of a PEEP valve for self-inflating bags.

Assisted-Ventilation Devices and Advanced Airways[NRP 870, NRP 806]

PPV can be delivered effectively with a flow-inflating bag, self-inflating bag, or T-piece resuscitator[138,139] (Class IIa, LOE B-R). The most appropriate choice may be guided by available resources, local expertise, and preferences. The self-inflating bag remains the only device that can be used when a compressed gas source is not available. Unlike flow-inflating bags or T-piece resuscitators, self-inflating bags cannot deliver continuous positive airway pressure (CPAP) and may not be able to achieve PEEP reliably during PPV, even with a PEEP valve.[140–143] However, it may take more practice to use a flow-inflating bag effectively. In addition to ease of use, T-piece resuscitators can consistently provide target inflation pressures and longer inspiratory times in mechanical models,[144–146] but there is insufficient evidence to suggest that these qualities result in improved clinical outcomes.[138,139]

Use of respiratory mechanics monitors have been reported to prevent excessive pressures and tidal volumes[147] and exhaled CO_2 monitors may help assess that actual gas exchange is occurring during face-mask PPV attempts.[148] Although use of such devices is feasible, thus far their effectiveness, particularly in changing important outcomes, has not been established (Class IIb, LOE C-LD).

Laryngeal Mask[NRP 618]

Laryngeal masks, which fit over the laryngeal inlet, can facilitate effective ventilation in term and preterm newborns at 34 weeks or more of gestation. Data are limited for their use in preterm infants delivered at less than 34 weeks of gestation or who weigh less than 2000 g. A laryngeal mask may be considered as an alternative to tracheal intubation if face-mask ventilation is unsuccessful in achieving effective ventilation[149] (Class IIb, LOE B-R). A laryngeal mask is recommended during resuscitation of term and preterm newborns at 34 weeks or more of gestation when tracheal intubation is unsuccessful or is not feasible (Class I, LOE C-EO). Use of the laryngeal mask has not been evaluated during chest compressions or for administration of emergency medications.

Endotracheal Tube Placement

During neonatal resuscitation, endotracheal intubation may be indicated when bag-mask ventilation is ineffective or prolonged, when chest compressions are performed, or for special circumstances such as congenital diaphragmatic hernia. When PPV is provided through an endotracheal tube, the best indicator of successful endotracheal intubation with successful inflation and aeration of the lungs is a prompt increase in heart rate. Although last reviewed in 2010,[3] exhaled CO_2 detection remains the most reliable method of confirmation of endotracheal tube placement.[7,8] Failure to detect exhaled CO_2 in neonates with adequate cardiac output strongly suggests esophageal intubation. Poor or absent pulmonary blood flow (eg, during cardiac arrest) may result in failure to detect exhaled CO_2 despite correct tube placement in the trachea and may result in unnecessary extubation and reintubation in these critically ill newborns.[3] Clinical assessment such as chest movement, presence of equal breath sounds bilaterally, and condensation in the endotracheal tube are additional indicators of correct endotracheal tube placement.

Continuous Positive Airway Pressure[NRP 590]

Three randomized controlled trials enrolling 2358 preterm infants born at less than 30 weeks of gestation demonstrated that starting newborns on CPAP may be beneficial when compared with endotracheal intubation and PPV.[150–152] Starting CPAP resulted in decreased rate of intubation in the delivery room, decreased duration of mechanical ventilation with potential benefit of reduction of death and/or bronchopulmonary dysplasia, and no significant increase in air leak or severe IVH. Based on this evidence, spontaneously breathing preterm infants with respiratory distress may be supported with CPAP initially rather than routine intubation for administering PPV (Class IIb, LOE B-R).

CHEST COMPRESSIONS[NRP 605, NRP 895, NRP 738, NRP 862]

If the heart rate is less than 60/min despite adequate ventilation (via endotracheal tube if possible), chest compressions are indicated. Because ventilation is the most effective action in neonatal resuscitation and because chest compressions are likely to compete with effective ventilation, rescuers should ensure that assisted ventilation is being delivered optimally before starting chest compressions.[3]

Compressions are delivered on the lower third of the sternum[153–156] to a depth of approximately one third of the anterior-posterior diameter of the chest (Class IIb, LOE C-LD).[157] Two techniques have been described: compression with 2 thumbs with the fingers encircling the chest and supporting the back (the 2-thumb technique) or compression with 2 fingers with a second hand supporting the back (the 2-finger technique). Because the 2-thumb technique generates higher blood pressure and coronary perfusion pressure with less rescuer fatigue, the 2 thumb–encircling

hands technique is suggested as the preferred method[158–172] (Class IIb, LOE C-LD). Because the 2-thumb technique can be continued from the head of the bed while the umbilicus is accessed for insertion of an umbilical catheter, the 2-finger technique is no longer needed.

It is still suggested that compressions and ventilations be coordinated to avoid simultaneous delivery. The chest should be allowed to re-expand fully during relaxation, but the rescuer's thumbs should not leave the chest. The Neonatal Resuscitation ILCOR and Guidelines Task Forces continue to support use of a 3:1 ratio of compressions to ventilation, with 90 compressions and 30 breaths to achieve approximately 120 events per minute to maximize ventilation at an achievable rate[173–178] (Class IIa, LOE C-LD). Thus, each event will be allotted approximately a half of a second, with exhalation occurring during the first compression after each ventilation. A 3:1 compression-to-ventilation ratio is used for neonatal resuscitation where compromise of gas exchange is nearly always the primary cause of cardiovascular collapse, but rescuers may consider using higher ratios (eg, 15:2) if the arrest is believed to be of cardiac origin (Class IIb, LOE C-EO).

The Neonatal Guidelines Writing Group endorses increasing the oxygen concentration to 100% whenever chest compressions are provided (Class IIa, LOE C-EO). There are no available clinical studies regarding oxygen use during neonatal CPR. Animal evidence shows no advantage to 100% oxygen during CPR.[179–186] However, by the time resuscitation of a newborn infant has reached the stage of chest compressions, efforts to achieve return of spontaneous circulation using effective ventilation with low-concentration oxygen should have been attempted. Thus, it would appear sensible to try increasing the supplementary oxygen concentration. To reduce the risks of complications associated with hyperoxia, the supplementary oxygen concentration should be weaned as soon as the heart rate recovers (Class I, LOE C-LD).

The current measure for determining successful progress in neonatal resuscitation is to assess the heart rate response. Other devices, such as end-tidal CO_2 monitoring and pulse oximetry, may be useful techniques to determine when return of spontaneous circulation occurs.[187–191] However, in asystolic/bradycardic neonates, we suggest against the routine use of any single feedback device such as $ETCO_2$ monitors or pulse oximeters for detection of return of spontaneous circulation, as their usefulness for this purpose in neonates has not been well established (Class IIb, LOE C-LD).

MEDICATIONS

Drugs are rarely indicated in resuscitation of the newly born infant. Bradycardia in the newborn infant is usually the result of inadequate lung inflation or profound hypoxemia, and establishing adequate ventilation is the most important step to correct it. However, if the heart rate remains less than 60/min despite adequate ventilation with 100% oxygen (preferably through an endotracheal tube) and chest compressions, administration of epinephrine or volume, or both, is indicated.[3]

Epinephrine

This topic was last reviewed in 2010.[3] Dosing recommendations remain unchanged from 2010.[7,8] Intravenous administration of epinephrine may be considered at a dose of 0.01 to 0.03 mg/kg of 1:10 000 epinephrine. If endotracheal administration is attempted while intravenous access is being established, higher dosing at 0.05 to 0.1 mg/kg may be reasonable. Given the lack of supportive data for endotracheal epinephrine, it is reasonable to provide drugs by the intravenous route as soon as venous access is established.

VOLUME EXPANSION

This topic was last reviewed in 2010.[3] Dosing recommendations remain unchanged from 2010.[7,8] Volume expansion may be considered when blood loss is known or suspected (pale skin, poor perfusion, weak pulse) and the infant's heart rate has not responded adequately to other resuscitative measures. An isotonic crystalloid solution or blood may be considered for volume expansion in the delivery room. The recommended dose is 10 mL/kg, which may need to be repeated. When resuscitating premature infants, it is reasonable to avoid giving volume expanders rapidly, because rapid infusions of large volumes have been associated with IVH.[3]

POSTRESUSCITATION CARE

Infants who require resuscitation are at risk of deterioration after their vital signs have returned to normal. Once effective ventilation and/or the circulation has been established, the infant should be maintained in or transferred to an environment where close monitoring and anticipatory care can be provided.

Glucose

In the 2010 Guidelines, the potential role of glucose in modulating neurologic outcome after hypoxia-ischemia was identified. Lower glucose levels were associated with an increased risk for brain injury, while increased glucose levels may be protective. However, it was not possible to recommend a specific protective target glucose concentration range. There are no new data to change this recommendation.[7,8]

Induced Therapeutic Hypothermia

Resource-Abundant Areas

Induced therapeutic hypothermia was last reviewed in 2010; at that time it was recommended that infants born at more than 36 weeks of gestation with evolving moderate-to-severe hypoxic-ischemic encephalopathy should be offered therapeutic hypothermia under clearly defined protocols similar to those used in published clinical trials and in facilities with the capabilities for multidisciplinary care and longitudinal follow-up (Class IIa, LOE A).[7,8] This recommendation remains unchanged.

Resource-Limited Areas[NRP 734]

Evidence suggests that use of therapeutic hypothermia in resource-limited settings (ie, lack of qualified staff, inadequate equipment, etc) may be considered and offered under clearly defined protocols similar to those used in published clinical trials and in facilities with the capabilities for multidisciplinary care and longitudinal follow-up[192–195] (Class IIb, LOE B-R).

GUIDELINES FOR WITHHOLDING AND DISCONTINUING

Data reviewed for the 2010 Guidelines regarding management of neonates born at the margins of viability or those with conditions that predict a high risk of mortality or morbidity document wide variation in attitudes and practice by region and availability of resources. Additionally, parents desire a larger role in decisions related to initiation of resuscitation and continuation of support of severely compromised newborns. Noninitiation of resuscitation and discontinuation of life-sustaining treatment during or after resuscitation are considered ethically equivalent. The 2010 Guidelines provide suggestions for when resuscitation is not indicated, when it is nearly always indicated, and that under circumstances when outcome remains unclear, that the desires of the parents should be supported. No new data have been published that would justify a change to these guidelines as published in 2010.[7,8]

Antenatal assignment of prognosis for survival and/or disability of the neonate born extremely preterm has generally been made on the basis of gestational age alone. Scoring systems for including additional variables such as gender, use of maternal antenatal steroids, and multiplicity have been developed in an effort to improve prognostic accuracy. Indeed, it was suggested in the 2010 Guidelines that decisions regarding morbidity and risks of morbidity may be augmented by the use of published tools based on data from specific populations.

Withholding Resuscitation[NRP 805]

There is no evidence to support the prospective use of any particular delivery room prognostic score presently available over gestational age assessment alone, in preterm infants at less than 25 weeks of gestation. Importantly, no score has been shown to improve the clinician's ability to estimate likelihood of survival through the first 18 to 22 months after birth. However, in individual cases, when counseling a family and constructing a prognosis for survival at gestations below 25 weeks, it is reasonable to consider variables such as perceived accuracy of gestational age assignment, the presence or absence of chorioamnionitis, and the level of care available for location of delivery. Decisions about appropriateness of resuscitation below 25 weeks

of gestation will be influenced by region-specific guidelines. In making this statement, a higher value was placed on the lack of evidence for a generalized prospective approach to changing important outcomes over improved retrospective accuracy and locally validated counseling policies. The most useful data for antenatal counseling provides outcome figures for infants alive at the onset of labor, not only for those born alive or admitted to a neonatal intensive care unit[196–200] (Class IIb, LOE C-LD).

Discontinuing Resuscitative Efforts[NRP 896]

An Apgar score of 0 at 10 minutes is a strong predictor of mortality and morbidity in late preterm and term infants. We suggest that, in infants with an Apgar score of 0 after 10 minutes of resuscitation, if the heart rate remains undetectable, it may be reasonable to stop assisted ventilation; however, the decision to continue or discontinue resuscitative efforts must be individualized. Variables to be considered may include whether the resuscitation was considered optimal; availability of advanced neonatal care, such as therapeutic hypothermia; specific circumstances before delivery (eg, known timing of the insult); and wishes expressed by the family[201–206] (Class IIb, LOE C-LD).

BRIEFING/DEBRIEFING

This topic was last reviewed in 2010.[3] It is still suggested that briefing and debriefing techniques be used whenever possible for neonatal resuscitation.

STRUCTURE OF EDUCATIONAL PROGRAMS TO TEACH NEONATAL RESUSCITATION

Instructors[NRP 867]

In studies that looked at the preparation of instructors for the training of healthcare providers, there was no association between the preparation provided and instructor or learner performance.[207–214] Until more research is available to clarify the optimal instructor training methodology, it is suggested that neonatal resuscitation instructors be trained using timely, objective, structured, and individually targeted verbal and/or written feedback (Class IIb, LOE C-EO).

Resuscitation Providers[NRP 859]

The 2010 Guidelines suggested that simulation should become a standard component in neonatal resuscitation training.[3,6,215] Studies that explored how frequently healthcare providers or healthcare students should train showed no differences in patient outcomes (LOE C-EO) but were able to show some advantages in psychomotor performance (LOE B-R) and knowledge and confidence (LOE C-LD) when focused training occurred every 6 months or more frequently.[216–231] It is therefore suggested that neonatal resuscitation task training occur more frequently than the current 2-year interval (Class IIb, LOE B-R).

REFERENCES

1. Perlman JM, Wyllie J, Kattwinkel J, Wyckoff MH, Aziz K, Guinsburg R, Kim HS, Liley HG, Mildenhall L, Simon WM, Szyld E, Tamura M, Velaphi S; on behalf of the Neonatal Resuscitation Chapter Collaborators. Part 7: neonatal resuscitation: 2015 International Consensus on Cardiopulmonary Resuscitation and Emergency Cardiovascular Care Science With Treatment Recommendations. *Circulation.* 2015;132(suppl 1):S204–S241. doi: 10.1161/CIR.0000000000000276.

2. Wyllie J, Perlman JM, Kattwinkel J, Wyckoff MH, Aziz K, Guinsburg R, Kim HS, Liley HG, Mildenhall L, Simon WM, Szyld E, Tamura M, Velaphi S; on behalf of the Neonatal Resuscitation Chapter Collaborators. Part 7: neonatal resuscitation: 2015 International Consensus on Cardiopulmonary Resuscitation and Emergency Cardiovascular Care Science With Treatment Recommendations. *Resuscitation.* 2015. In press.

3. Kattwinkel J, Perlman JM, Aziz K, Colby C, Fairchild K, Gallagher J, Hazinski MF, Halamek LP, Kumar P, Little G, McGowan

JL, Nightengale R, Ramirez MM, Ringer S, Simon WM, Weiner GM, Wyckoff M, Zaichkin J. Part 15: neonatal resuscitation: 2010 American Heart Association Guidelines for Cardiopulmonary Resuscitation and Emergency Cardiovascular Care. *Circulation.* 2010;122(suppl 3):S909–S919. doi: 10.1161/CIRCULATIONAHA.110.971119.

4. Barber CA, Wyckoff MH. Use and efficacy of endotracheal versus intravenous epinephrine during neonatal cardiopulmonary resuscitation in the delivery room. *Pediatrics.* 2006;118:1028–1034. doi: 10.1542/peds.2006-0416.

5. Aziz K, Chadwick M, Baker M, Andrews W. Ante- and intra-partum factors that predict increased need for neonatal resuscitation. *Resuscitation.* 2008;79:444–452. doi: 10.1016/j.resuscitation.2008.08.004.

6. Zaichkin J, ed. *Instructor Manual for Neonatal Resuscitation.* Chicago, IL: American Academy of Pediatrics;2011.

7. Perlman JM, Wyllie J, Kattwinkel J, Atkins DL, Chameides L, Goldsmith JP, Guinsburg R, Hazinski MF, Morley C, Richmond S, Simon WM, Singhal N, Szyld E, Tamura M, Velaphi S; Neonatal Resuscitation Chapter Collaborators. Part 11: neonatal resuscitation: 2010 International Consensus on Cardiopulmonary Resuscitation and Emergency Cardiovascular Care Science With Treatment Recommendations. *Circulation.* 2010;122(suppl 2): S516–S538. doi: 10.1161/CIRCULATIONAHA.110.971127.

8. Wyllie J, Perlman JM, Kattwinkel J, Atkins DL, Chameides L, Goldsmith JP, Guinsburg R, Hazinski MF, Morley C, Richmond S, Simon WM, Singhal N, Szyld E, Tamura M, Velaphi S; Neonatal Resuscitation Chapter Collaborators. Part 11: neonatal resuscitation: 2010 International Consensus on Cardiopulmonary Resuscitation and Emergency Cardiovascular Care Science With Treatment Recommendations. *Resuscitation.* 2010;81 suppl 1:e260–e287. doi: 10.1016/j.resuscitation.2010.08.029.

9. Committee Opinion No.543: Timing of umbilical cord clamping after birth. *Obstet Gynecol.* 2012;120:1522–1526.

10. American Academy of Pediatrics. Statement of endorsement: timing of umbilical cord clamping after birth. *Pediatrics.* 2013;131:e1323.

11. Hosono S, Mugishima H, Fujita H, Hosono A, Minato M, Okada T, Takahashi S, Harada K. Umbilical cord milking reduces the need for red cell transfusions and improves neonatal adaptation in infants born at less than 29 weeks' gestation: a randomised controlled trial. *Arch Dis Child Fetal Neonatal Ed.* 2008;93:F14–F19. doi: 10.1136/adc.2006.108902.

12. Katheria AC, Leone TA, Woelkers D, Garey DM, Rich W, Finer NN. The effects of umbilical cord milking on hemodynamics and neonatal outcomes in premature neonates. *J Pediatr.* 2014;164:1045–1050. e1. doi: 10.1016/j.jpeds.2014.01.024.

13. March MI, Hacker MR, Parson AW, Modest AM, de Veciana M. The effects of umbilical cord milking in extremely preterm infants: a randomized controlled trial. *J Perinatol.* 2013;33:763–767. doi: 10.1038/jp.2013.70.

14. Budin P. *The Nursling. The Feeding and Hygiene of Premature and Full-term Infants. Translation by WJ Maloney.* London: The Caxton Publishing Co;1907.

15. A Abd-El Hamid S, Badr-El Din MM, Dabous NI, Saad KM. Effect of the use of a polyethylene wrap on the morbidity and mortality of very low birth weight infants in Alexandria University Children's Hospital. *J Egypt Public Health Assoc.* 2012;87:104–108.

16. Acolet D, Elbourne D, McIntosh N, Weindling M, Korkodilos M, Haviland J, Modder J, Macintosh M; Confidential Enquiry Into Maternal and Child Health. Project 27/28: inquiry into quality of neonatal care and its effect on the survival of infants who were born at 27 and 28 weeks in England, Wales, and Northern Ireland. *Pediatrics.* 2005;116:1457–1465. doi: 10.1542/peds.2004-2691.

17. Bateman DA, O'Bryan L, Nicholas SW, Heagarty MC. Outcome of unattended out-of-hospital births in Harlem. *Arch Pediatr Adolesc Med.* 1994;148:147–152.

18. Bhoopalam PS, Watkinson M. Babies born before arrival at hospital. *Br J Obstet Gynaecol.* 1991;98:57–64.

19. Boo NY, Guat-Sim Cheah I; Malaysian National Neonatal Registry. Admission hypothermia among VLBW infants in Malaysian NICUs. *J Trop Pediatr.* 2013;59:447–452. doi: 10.1093/tropej/fmt051.

20. Buetow KC, Kelein SW. Effects of maintenenance of "normal" skin temperature on survival of infants of low birth weight. *Pediatr.* 1964;33:163–169.

21. Costeloe K, Hennessy E, Gibson AT, Marlow N, Wilkinson AR. The EPICure study: outcomes to discharge from hospital for infants born at the threshold of viability. *Pediatrics.* 2000;106:659–671.

22. Costeloe KL, Hennessy EM, Haider S, Stacey F, Marlow N, Draper ES. Short term outcomes after extreme preterm birth in England: comparison of two birth cohorts in 1995 and 2006 (the EPICure studies). *BMJ.* 2012;345:e7976.

23. da Mota Silveira SM, Gonçalves de Mello MJ, de Arruda Vidal S, de Frias PG, Cattaneo A. Hypothermia on admission: a risk factor for death in newborns referred to the Pernambuco Institute of Mother and Child Health. *J Trop Pediatr.* 2003;49:115–120.

24. Daga AS, Daga SR, Patole SK. Determinants of death among admissions to intensive care unit for newborns. *J Trop Pediatr.* 1991;37:53–56.

25. de Almeida MF, Guinsburg R, Sancho GA, Rosa IR, Lamy ZC, Martinez FE, da Silva RP, Ferrari LS, de Souza Rugolo LM, Abdallah VO, Silveira Rde C; Brazilian Network on Neonatal Research. Hypothermia and early neonatal mortality in preterm infants. *J Pediatr.* 2014;164:271–5.e1. doi: 10.1016/j.jpeds.2013.09.049.

26. García-Muñoz Rodrigo F, Rivero Rodríguez S, Siles Quesada C. [Hypothermia risk factors in the very low weight newborn and associated morbidity and mortality in a neonatal care unit]. *An Pediatr (Barc).* 2014,00:144 150. doi: 10.1016/j.anpedi.2013.06.029.

27. Harms K, Osmers R, Kron M, Schill M, Kuhn W, Speer CP, Schröter W. [Mortality of premature infants 1980-1990: analysis of data from the Göttingen perinatal center]. *Z Geburtshilfe Perinatol.* 1994; 198:126–133.

28. Hazan J, Maag U, Chessex P. Association between hypothermia and mortality rate of premature infants–revisited. *Am J Obstet Gynecol.* 1991;164(1 pt 1):111–112.

29. Jones P, Alberti C, Julé L, Chabernaud JL, Lodé N, Sieurin A, Dauger S. Mortality in out-of-hospital premature births. *Acta Paediatr.* 2011;100:181–187. doi: 10.1111/j.1651-2227.2010.02003.x.

30. Kalimba E, Ballot D. Survival of extremely low-birth-weight infants. *South African Journal of Child Health.* 2013;7:13–16.

31. Kambarami R, Chidede O. Neonatal hypothermia levels and risk factors for mortality in a tropical country. *Cent Afr J Med.* 2003;49:103–106.

32. Kent AL, Williams J. Increasing ambient operating theatre temperature and wrapping in polyethylene improves admission temperature in premature infants. *J Paediatr Child Health.* 2008; 44:325–331. doi: 10.1111/j.1440-1754.2007.01264.x.

33. Laptook AR, Salhab W, Bhaskar B; Neonatal Research Network. Admission temperature of low birth weight infants: predictors and associated morbidities. *Pediatrics.* 2007;119:e643–e649. doi: 10.1542/peds.2006-0943.

34. Lee HC, Ho QT, Rhine WD. A quality improvement project to improve admission temperatures in very low birth weight infants. *J Perinatol.* 2008;28:754–758. doi: 10.1038/jp.2008.92.

35. Levi S, Taylor W, Robinson LE, Levy LI. Analysis of morbidity and outcome of infants weighing less than 800 grams at birth. *South Med J.* 1984;77:975–978.

36. Manani M, Jegatheesan P, DeSandre G, Song D, Showalter L, Govindaswami B. Elimination of admission hypothermia in preterm very-low-birth-weight infants by standardization of delivery room management. *Perm J.* 2013;17:8–13. doi: 10.7812/TPP/12-130.

37. Manji KP, Kisenge R. Neonatal hypothermia on admission to a special care unit in Dar-es-Salaam, Tanzania: a cause for concern. *Cent Afr J Med.* 2003;49:23–27.

38. Mathur NB, Krishnamurthy S, Mishra TK. Evaluation of WHO classification of hypothermia in sick extramural neonates as predictor of fatality. *J Trop Pediatr.* 2005; 51:341–345. doi: 10.1093/tropej/fmi049.

39. Miller SS, Lee HC, Gould JB. Hypothermia in very low birth weight infants: distribution, risk factors and outcomes. *J Perinatol.* 2011;31 suppl 1:S49–S56. doi: 10.1038/jp.2010.177.

40. Mullany LC, Katz J, Khatry SK, LeClerq SC, Darmstadt GL, Tielsch JM. Risk of mortality associated with neonatal hypothermia in southern Nepal. *Arch Pediatr Adolesc Med.* 2010;164:650–656. doi: 10.1001/archpediatrics.2010.103.

41. Nayeri F, Nili F. Hypothermia at birth and its associated complications in newborn infants: a follow-up study. *Iran J Public Health.* 2006;35:48–52.

42. Obladen M, Heemann U, Hennecke KH, Hanssler L. [Causes of neonatal mortality 1981-1983: a regional analysis]. *Z Geburtshilfe Perinatol.* 1985;189:181–187.

43. Ogunlesi TA, Ogunfowora OB, Adekanmbi FA, Fetuga BM, Olanrewaju DM. Point-of-admission hypothermia among high-risk Nigerian newborns. *BMC Pediatr.* 2008;8:40. doi: 10.1186/1471-2431-8-40.

44. Pal DK, Manandhar DS, Rajbhandari S, Land JM, Patel N, de L Costello AM. Neonatal hypoglycaemia in Nepal 1. Prevalence and risk factors. *Arch Dis Child Fetal Neonatal Ed.* 2000;82:F46–F51.

45. Shah S, Zemichael O, Meng HD. Factors associated with mortality and length of stay in hospitalised neonates in Eritrea, Africa: a cross-sectional study. *BMJ Open.* 2012;2. doi: 10.1136/bmjopen-2011-000792.

46. Singh A, Yadav A, Singh A. Utilization of postnatal care for newborns and its association with neonatal mortality in India: an analytical appraisal. *BMC Pregnancy Childbirth.* 2012;12:33. doi: 10.1186/1471-2393-12-33.

47. Sodemann M, Nielsen J, Veirum J, Jakobsen MS, Biai S, Aaby P. Hypothermia of newborns is associated with excess mortality in the first 2 months of life in Guinea-Bissau, West Africa. *Trop Med Int Health.* 2008;13:980–986. doi: 10.1111/j.1365-3156.2008.02113.x.

48. Stanley FJ, Alberman EV. Infants of very low birthweight. I: Perinatal factors affecting survival. *Dev Med Child Neurol.* 1978;20:300–312.

49. Wyckoff MH, Perlman JM. Effective ventilation and temperature control are vital to outborn resuscitation. *Prehosp Emerg Care.* 2004;8:191–195.

50. Bartels DB, Kreienbrock L, Dammann O, Wenzlaff P, Poets CF. Population based study on the outcome of small for gestational age newborns. *Arch Dis Child Fetal Neonatal Ed.* 2005;90:F53–F59. doi: 10.1136/adc.2004.053892.

51. Carroll PD, Nankervis CA, Giannone PJ, Cordero L. Use of polyethylene bags in extremely low birth weight infant resuscitation for the prevention of hypothermia. *J Reprod Med.* 2010;55:9–13.

52. Gleissner M, Jorch G, Avenarius S. Risk factors for intraventricular hemorrhage in a birth cohort of 3721 premature infants. *J Perinat Med.* 2000;28:104–110. doi: 10.1515/JPM.2000.013.

53. Herting E, Speer CP, Harms K, Robertson B, Curstedt T, Halliday HL, Compagnone D, Gefeller O, McClure G, Reid M. Factors influencing morbidity and mortality in infants with severe respiratory distress syndrome treated with single or multiple doses of a natural porcine surfactant. *Biol Neonate.* 1992;61 suppl 1:26–30.

54. Van de Bor M, Van Bel F, Lineman R, Ruys JH. Perinatal factors and periventricular-intraventricular hemorrhage in preterm infants. *Am J Dis Child.* 1986;140:1125–1130.

55. DeMauro SB, Douglas E, Karp K, Schmidt B, Patel J, Kronberger A, Scarboro R, Posencheg M. Improving delivery room management for very preterm infants. *Pediatrics.* 2013;132:e1018–e1025. doi: 10.1542/peds.2013-0686.

56. Harms K, Herting E, Kron M, Schill M, Schiffmann H. [Importance of pre- and perinatal risk factors in respiratory distress syndrome of premature infants. A logical regression analysis of 1100 cases]. *Z Geburtshilfe Neonatol.* 1997; 201:258–262.

57. Lee HC, Powers RJ, Bennett MV, Finer NN, Halamek LP, Nisbet C, Crockett M, Chance K, Blackney D, von Köhler C, Kurtin P, Sharek PJ. Implementation methods for delivery room management: a quality improvement comparison study. *Pediatrics.* 2014;134:e1378–e1386. doi: 10.1542/peds.2014-0863.

58. Reilly MC, Vohra S, Rac VE, Dunn M, Ferrelli K, Kiss A, Vincer M, Wimmer J, Zayack D, Soll RF; Vermont Oxford Network Heat Loss Prevention (HeLP) Trial Study Group. Randomized trial of occlusive wrap for heat loss prevention in preterm infants. *J Pediatr.* 2015;166:262–8.e2. doi: 10.1016/j.jpeds.2014.09.068.

59. Russo A, McCready M, Torres L, Theuriere C, Venturini S, Spaight M, Hemway RJ, Handrinos S, Perlmutter D, Huynh T, Grunebaum A, Perlman J. Reducing hypothermia in preterm infants following delivery. *Pediatrics.* 2014;133:e1055–e1062. doi: 10.1542/peds.2013-2544.

60. Zayeri F, Kazemnejad A, Ganjali M, Babaei G, Khanafshar N, Nayeri F. Hypothermia in Iranian newborns. Incidence, risk factors and related complications. *Saudi Med J.* 2005;26:1367–1371.

61. Anderson S, Shakya KN, Shrestha LN, Costello AM. Hypoglycaemia: a common problem among uncomplicated newborn infants in Nepal. *J Trop Pediatr.* 1993;39: 273–277.

62. Lazić-Mitrović T, Djukić M, Cutura N, Andjelić S, Curković A, Soldo V, Radlović N. [Transitory hypothermia as early prognostic factor in term newborns with intrauterine growth retardation]. *Srp Arh Celok Lek.* 2010;138:604–608.

63. Lenclen R, Mazraani M, Jugie M, Couderc S, Hoenn E, Carbajal R, Blanc P, Paupe A. [Use of a polyethylene bag: a way to improve the thermal environment of the premature newborn at the delivery room]. *Arch Pediatr.* 2002;9:238–244.

64. Sasidharan CK, Gokul E, Sabitha S. Incidence and risk factors for neonatal hypoglycaemia in Kerala, India. *Ceylon Med J.* 2004;49:110–113.

65. Mullany LC. Neonatal hypothermia in low-resource settings. *Semin Perinatol.* 2010; 34:426–433. doi: 10.1053/j.semperi.2010.09.007.

66. McCarthy LK, Molloy EJ, Twomey AR, Murphy JF, O'Donnell CP. A randomized trial of exothermic mattresses for preterm newborns in polyethylene bags. *Pediatrics.* 2013;132:e135–e141. doi: 10.1542/peds.2013-0279.

67. Billimoria Z, Chawla S, Bajaj M, Natarajan G. Improving admission temperature in

extremely low birth weight infants: a hospital-based multi-intervention quality improvement project. *J Perinat Med.* 2013; 41:455–460. doi: 10.1515/jpm-2012-0259.

68. Chawla S, Amaram A, Gopal SP, Natarajan G. Safety and efficacy of Trans-warmer mattress for preterm neonates: results of a randomized controlled trial. *J Perinatol.* 2011;31:780–784. doi: 10.1038/jp.2011.33.

69. Ibrahim CP, Yoxall CW. Use of self-heating gel mattresses eliminates admission hypothermia in infants born below 28 weeks gestation. *Eur J Pediatr.* 2010;169:795–799. doi: 10.1007/s00431-009-1113-y.

70. Singh A, Duckett J, Newton T, Watkinson M. Improving neonatal unit admission temperatures in preterm babies: exothermic mattresses, polythene bags or a traditional approach? *J Perinatol.* 2010;30:45–49. doi: 10.1038/jp.2009.94.

71. Meyer MP, Payton MJ, Salmon A, Hutchinson C, de Klerk A. A clinical comparison of radiant warmer and incubator care for preterm infants from birth to 1800 grams. *Pediatrics.* 2001;108:395–401.

72. te Pas AB, Lopriore E, Dito I, Morley CJ, Walther FJ. Humidified and heated air during stabilization at birth improves temperature in preterm infants. *Pediatrics.* 2010;125:e1427–e1432. doi: 10.1542/peds.2009-2656.

73. Pinheiro JM, Furdon SA, Boynton S, Dugan R, Reu-Donlon C, Jensen S. Decreasing hypothermia during delivery room stabilization of preterm neonates. *Pediatrics.* 2014;133:e218–e226. doi: 10.1542/peds.2013-1293.

74. Petrova A, Demissie K, Rhoads GG, Smulian JC, Marcella S, Ananth CV. Association of maternal fever during labor with neonatal and infant morbidity and mortality. *Obstet Gynecol.* 2001;98:20–27.

75. Alexander JM, McIntire DM, Leveno KJ. Chorioamnionitis and the prognosis for term infants. *Obstet Gynecol.* 1999;94:274–278.

76. Greenwell EA, Wyshak G, Ringer SA, Johnson LC, Rivkin MJ, Lieberman E. Intrapartum temperature elevation, epidural use, and adverse outcome in term infants. *Pediatrics.* 2012;129:e447–e454. doi: 10.1542/peds.2010-2301.

77. Goetzl L, Manevich Y, Roedner C, Praktish A, Hebbar I, Townsend DM. Maternal and fetal oxidative stress and intrapartum term fever. *Am J Obstet Gynecol.* 2010;202: 363.e1–363.e5. doi: 10.1016/j.ajog.2010.01.034.

78. Glass HC, Pham TN, Danielsen B, Towner D, Glidden D, Wu YW. Antenatal and intrapartum risk factors for seizures in term newborns: a population-based study, California 1998-2002. *J Pediatr.* 2009;154:24–28.e1. doi: 10.1016/j.jpeds.2008.07.008.

79. Lieberman E, Lang J, Richardson DK, Frigoletto FD, Heffner LJ, Cohen A. Intrapartum maternal fever and neonatal outcome. *Pediatrics.* 2000;105(1 pt 1):8–13.

80. Lieberman E, Eichenwald E, Mathur G, Richardson D, Heffner L, Cohen A. Intrapartum fever and unexplained seizures in term infants. *Pediatrics.* 2000;106:983–988.

81. Badawi N, Kurinczuk JJ, Keogh JM, Alessandri LM, O'Sullivan F, Burton PR, Pemberton PJ, Stanley FJ. Intrapartum risk factors for newborn encephalopathy: the Western Australian case-control study. *BMJ.* 1998;317:1554–1558.

82. Impey L, Greenwood C, MacQuillan K, Reynolds M, Sheil O. Fever in labour and neonatal encephalopathy: a prospective cohort study. *BJOG.* 2001;108:594–597.

83. Impey LW, Greenwood CE, Black RS, Yeh PS, Sheil O, Doyle P. The relationship between intrapartum maternal fever and neonatal acidosis as risk factors for neonatal encephalopathy. *Am J Obstet Gynecol.* 2008; 198:49.e1–49.e6. doi: 10.1016/j.ajog.2007.06.011.

84. Linder N, Fridman E, Makhoul A, Lubin D, Klinger G, Laron-Kenet T, Yogev Y, Melamed N. Management of term newborns following maternal intrapartum fever. *J Matern Fetal Neonatal Med.* 2013;26:207–210. doi: 10.3109/14767058.2012.722727.

85. Butwick AJ, Lipman SS, Carvalho B. Intraoperative forced air-warming during cesarean delivery under spinal anesthesia does not prevent maternal hypothermia. *Anesth Analg.* 2007;105:1413–1419, table of contents. doi: 10.1213/01.ane.0000286167.96410.27.

86. Fallis WM, Hamelin K, Symonds J, Wang X. Maternal and newborn outcomes related to maternal warming during cesarean delivery. *J Obstet Gynecol Neonatal Nurs.* 2006;35:324–331. doi: 10.1111/j.1552-6909.2006.00052.x.

87. Horn EP, Schroeder F, Gottschalk A, Sessler DI, Hiltmeyer N, Standl T, Schulte am Esch J. Active warming during cesarean delivery. *Anesth Analg.* 2002;94:409–414, table of contents.

88. Woolnough M, Allam J, Hemingway C, Cox M, Yentis SM. Intra-operative fluid warming in elective caesarean section: a blinded randomised controlled trial. *Int J Obstet Anesth.* 2009;18:346–351. doi: 10.1016/j.ijoa.2009.02.009.

89. Yokoyama K, Suzuki M, Shimada Y, Matsushima T, Bito H, Sakamoto A. Effect of administration of pre-warmed intravenous fluids on the frequency of hypothermia following spinal anesthesia for Cesarean delivery. *J Clin Anesth.* 2009;21: 242–248. doi: 10.1016/j.jclinane.2008.12.010.

90. Belsches TC, Tilly AE, Miller TR, Kambeyanda RH, Leadford A, Manasyan A, Chomba E, Ramani M, Ambalavanan N, Carlo WA. Randomized trial of plastic bags to prevent term neonatal hypothermia in a resource-poor setting. *Pediatrics.* 2013; 132:e656–e661. doi: 10.1542/peds.2013-0172.

91. Leadford AE, Warren JB, Manasyan A, Chomba E, Salas AA, Schelonka R, Carlo WA. Plastic bags for prevention of hypothermia in preterm and low birth weight infants. *Pediatrics.* 2013;132:e128–e134. doi: 10.1542/peds.2012-2030.

92. Raman S, Shahla A. Temperature drop in normal term newborn infants born at the University Hospital, Kuala Lumpur. *Aust N Z J Obstet Gynaecol.* 1992;32:117–119.

93. Bergman NJ, Linley LL, Fawcus SR. Randomized controlled trial of skin-to-skin contact from birth versus conventional incubator for physiological stabilization in 1200- to 2199-gram newborns. *Acta Paediatr.* 2004;93:779–785.

94. Fardig JA. A comparison of skin-to-skin contact and radiant heaters in promoting neonatal thermoregulation. *J Nurse Midwifery.* 1980;25:19–28.

95. Christensson K, Siles C, Moreno L, Belaustequi A, De La Fuente P, Lagercrantz H, Puyol P, Winberg J. Temperature, metabolic adaptation and crying in healthy full-term newborns cared for skin-to-skin or in a cot. *Acta Paediatr.* 1992;81:488–493.

96. Christensson K. Fathers can effectively achieve heat conservation in healthy newborn infants. *Acta Paediatr.* 1996;85: 1354–1360.

97. Bystrova K, Widström AM, Matthiesen AS, Ransjö-Arvidson AB, Welles-Nyström B, Wassberg C, Vorontsov I, Uvnäs-Moberg K. Skin-to-skin contact may reduce negative consequences of "the stress of being born": a study on temperature in newborn infants, subjected to different ward routines in St. Petersburg. *Acta Paediatr.* 2003;92:320–326.

98. Gouchon S, Gregori D, Picotto A, Patrucco G, Nangeroni M, Di Giulio P. Skin-to-skin contact after cesarean delivery: an experimental study. *Nurs Res.* 2010;59:78–84. doi: 10.1097/NNR.0b013e3181d1a8bc.

99. Marín Gabriel MA, Llana Martín I, López Escobar A, Fernández Villalba E, Romero

291

Blanco I, Touza Pol P. Randomized controlled trial of early skin-to-skin contact: effects on the mother and the newborn. *Acta Paediatr.* 2010;99:1630–1634. doi: 10.1111/j.1651-2227.2009.01597.x.

100. Nimbalkar SM, Patel VK, Patel DV, Nimbalkar AS, Sethi A, Phatak A. Effect of early skin-to-skin contact following normal delivery on incidence of hypothermia in neonates more than 1800 g: randomized control trial. *J Perinatol.* 2014;34:364–368. doi: 10.1038/jp.2014.15.

101. Gungor S, Kurt E, Teksoz E, Goktolga U, Ceyhan T, Baser I. Oronasopharyngeal suction versus no suction in normal and term infants delivered by elective cesarean section: a prospective randomized controlled trial. *Gynecol Obstet Invest.* 2006;61:9–14. doi: 10.1159/000087604.

102. Waltman PA, Brewer JM, Rogers BP, May WL. Building evidence for practice: a pilot study of newborn bulb suctioning at birth. *J Midwifery Womens Health.* 2004;49:32–38. doi: 10.1016/j.jmwh.2003.10.003.

103. Carrasco M, Martell M, Estol PC. Oronasopharyngeal suction at birth: effects on arterial oxygen saturation. *J Pediatr.* 1997; 130:832–834.

104. Perlman JM, Volpe JJ. Suctioning in the preterm infant: effects on cerebral blood flow velocity, intracranial pressure, and arterial blood pressure. *Pediatrics.* 1983;72:329–334.

105. Simbruner G, Coradello H, Fodor M, Havelec L, Lubec G, Pollak A. Effect of tracheal suction on oxygenation, circulation, and lung mechanics in newborn infants. *Arch Dis Child.* 1981;56:326–330.

106. Vain NE, Szyld EG, Prudent LM, Wiswell TE, Aguilar AM, Vivas NI. Oropharyngeal and nasopharyngeal suctioning of meconium-stained neonates before delivery of their shoulders: multicentre, randomised controlled trial. *Lancet.* 2004;364:597–602. doi: 10.1016/S0140-6736(04)16852-9.

107. Al Takroni AM, Parvathi CK, Mendis KB, Hassan S, Reddy I, Kudair HA. Selective tracheal suctioning to prevent meconium aspiration syndrome. *Int J Gynaecol Obstet.* 1998;63:259–263.

108. Chettri S, Adhisivam B, Bhat BV. Endotracheal suction for nonvigorous neonates born through meconium stained amniotic fluid: a randomized controlled trial. *J Pediatr.* 2015;166:1208–1213.e1. doi: 10.1016/j.jpeds.2014.12.076.

109. Davis RO, Philips JB 3rd, Harris BA Jr, Wilson ER, Huddleston JF. Fatal meconium aspiration syndrome occurring despite airway management considered appropriate. *Am J Obstet Gynecol.* 1985;151:731–736.

110. Dooley SL, Pesavento DJ, Depp R, Socol ML, Tamura RK, Wiringa KS. Meconium below the vocal cords at delivery: correlation with intrapartum events. *Am J Obstet Gynecol.* 1985;153:767–770.

111. Hageman JR, Conley M, Francis K, Stenske J, Wolf I, Santi V, Farrell EE. Delivery room management of meconium staining of the amniotic fluid and the development of meconium aspiration syndrome. *J Perinatol.* 1988;8:127–131.

112. Manganaro R, Mamì C, Palmara A, Paolata A, Gemelli M. Incidence of meconium aspiration syndrome in term meconium-stained babies managed at birth with selective tracheal intubation. *J Perinat Med.* 2001;29:465–468. doi: 10.1515/JPM.2001.065.

113. Peng TC, Gutcher GR, Van Dorsten JP. A selective aggressive approach to the neonate exposed to meconium-stained amniotic fluid. *Am J Obstet Gynecol.* 1996;175:296–301; discussion 301.

114. Rossi EM, Philipson EH, Williams TG, Kalhan SC. Meconium aspiration syndrome: intrapartum and neonatal attributes. *Am J Obstet Gynecol.* 1989;161:1106–1110.

115. Suresh GK, Sarkar S. Delivery room management of infants born through thin meconium stained liquor. *Indian Pediatr.* 1994;31:1177–1181.

116. Yoder BA. Meconium-stained amniotic fluid and respiratory complications: impact of selective tracheal suction. *Obstet Gynecol.* 1994;83:77–84.

117. Kamlin CO, O'Donnell CP, Everest NJ, Davis PG, Morley CJ. Accuracy of clinical assessment of infant heart rate in the delivery room. *Resuscitation.* 2006;71:319–321. doi: 10.1016/j.resuscitation.2006.04.015.

118. Dawson JA, Saraswat A, Simionato L, Thio M, Kamlin CO, Owen LS, Schmölzer GM, Davis PG. Comparison of heart rate and oxygen saturation measurements from Masimo and Nellcor pulse oximeters in newly born term infants. *Acta Paediatr.* 2013;102:955–960. doi: 10.1111/apa.12329.

119. Kamlin CO, Dawson JA, O'Donnell CP, Morley CJ, Donath SM, Sekhon J, Davis PG. Accuracy of pulse oximetry measurement of heart rate of newborn infants in the delivery room. *J Pediatr.* 2008;152:756–760. doi: 10.1016/j.jpeds.2008.01.002.

120. Katheria A, Rich W, Finer N. Electrocardiogram provides a continuous heart rate faster than oximetry during neonatal resuscitation. *Pediatrics.* 2012;130:e1177–e1181. doi: 10.1542/peds.2012-0784.

121. Mizumoto H, Tomotaki S, Shibata H, Ueda K, Akashi R, Uchio H, Hata D. Electrocardiogram shows reliable heart rates much earlier than pulse oximetry during neonatal resuscitation. *Pediatr Int.* 2012;54:205–207. doi: 10.1111/j.1442-200X.2011.03506.x.

122. van Vonderen JJ, Hooper SB, Kroese JK, Roest AA, Narayen IC, van Zwet EW, te Pas AB. Pulse oximetry measures a lower heart rate at birth compared with electrocardiography. *J Pediatr.* 2015;166:49–53. doi: 10.1016/j.jpeds.2014.09.015.

123. Mariani G, Dik PB, Ezquer A, Aguirre A, Esteban ML, Perez C, Fernandez Jonusas S, Fustiñana C. Pre-ductal and post-ductal O2 saturation in healthy term neonates after birth. *J Pediatr.* 2007;150:418–421. doi: 10.1016/j.jpeds.2006.12.015.

124. Armanian AM, Badiee Z. Resuscitation of preterm newborns with low concentration oxygen versus high concentration oxygen. *J Res Pharm Pract.* 2012;1:25–29. doi: 10.4103/2279-042X.99674.

125. Kapadia VS, Chalak LF, Sparks JE, Allen JR, Savani RC, Wyckoff MH. Resuscitation of preterm neonates with limited versus high oxygen strategy. *Pediatrics.* 2013;132:e1488–e1496. doi: 10.1542/peds.2013-0978.

126. Lundstrøm KE, Pryds O, Greisen G. Oxygen at birth and prolonged cerebral vasoconstriction in preterm infants. *Arch Dis Child Fetal Neonatal Ed.* 1995;73:F81–F86.

127. Rabi Y, Singhal N, Nettel-Aguirre A. Room-air versus oxygen administration for resuscitation of preterm infants: the ROAR study. *Pediatrics.* 2011;128:e374–e381. doi: 10.1542/peds.2010-3130.

128. Rook D, Schierbeek H, Vento M, Vlaardingerbroek H, van der Eijk AC, Longini M, Buonocore G, Escobar J, van Goudoever JB, Vermeulen MJ. Resuscitation of preterm infants with different inspired oxygen fractions. *J Pediatr.* 2014;164:1322–6.e3. doi: 10.1016/j.jpeds.2014.02.019.

129. Vento M, Moro M, Escrig R, Arruza L, Villar G, Izquierdo I, Roberts LJ 2nd, Arduini A, Escobar JJ, Sastre J, Asensi MA. Preterm resuscitation with low oxygen causes less oxidative stress, inflammation, and chronic lung disease. *Pediatrics.* 2009;124:e439–e449. doi: 10.1542/peds.2009-0434.

130. Wang CL, Anderson C, Leone TA, Rich W, Govindaswami B, Finer NN. Resuscitation of preterm neonates by using room air or 100% oxygen. *Pediatrics.* 2008;121:1083–1089. doi: 10.1542/peds.2007-1460.

131. Klingenberg C, Sobotka KS, Ong T, Allison BJ, Schmölzer GM, Moss TJ, Polglase GR, Dawson JA, Davis PG, Hooper SB. Effect of sustained inflation duration; resuscitation of near-term asphyxiated lambs. *Arch Dis Child Fetal Neonatal Ed.* 2013;98:

F222–F227. doi: 10.1136/archdischild 2012 301787.

132. te Pas AB, Siew M, Wallace MJ, Kitchen MJ, Fouras A, Lewis RA, Yagi N, Uesugi K, Donath S, Davis PG, Morley CJ, Hooper SB. Effect of sustained inflation length on establishing functional residual capacity at birth in ventilated premature rabbits. *Pediatr Res.* 2009;66:295–300. doi: 10.1203/ PDR.0b013e3181b1bca4.

133. Harling AE, Beresford MW, Vince GS, Bates M, Yoxall CW. Does sustained lung inflation at resuscitation reduce lung injury in the preterm infant? *Arch Dis Child Fetal Neonatal Ed.* 2005;90:F406–F410. doi: 10.1136/ adc.2004.059303.

134. Lindner W, Högel J, Pohlandt F. Sustained pressure-controlled inflation or intermittent mandatory ventilation in preterm infants in the delivery room? A randomized, controlled trial on initial respiratory support via nasopharyngeal tube. *Acta Paediatr.* 2005;94:303–309.

135. Lista G, Boni L, Scopesi F, Mosca F, Trevisanuto D, Messner H, Vento G, Magaldi R, Del Vecchio A, Agosti M, Gizzi C, Sandri F, Biban P, Bellettato M, Gazzolo D, Boldrini A, Dani C; SLI Trial Investigators. Sustained lung inflation at birth for preterm infants: a randomized clinical trial. *Pediatrics.* 2015;135: e457–e464. doi: 10.1542/peds.2014-1692.

136. Lindner W, Vossbeck S, Hummler H, Pohlandt F. Delivery room management of extremely low birth weight infants: spontaneous breathing or intubation? *Pediatrics.* 1999;103(5 pt 1):961–967.

137. Lista G, Fontana P, Castoldi F, Cavigioli F, Dani C. Does sustained lung inflation at birth improve outcome of preterm infants at risk for respiratory distress syndrome? *Neonatology.* 2011;99:45–50. doi: 10.1159/ 000298312.

138. Dawson JA, Schmölzer GM, Kamlin CO, Te Pas AB, O'Donnell CP, Donath SM, Davis PG, Morley CJ. Oxygenation with T-piece versus self-inflating bag for ventilation of extremely preterm infants at birth: a randomized controlled trial. *J Pediatr.* 2011; 158:912–918.e1. doi: 10.1016/j.jpeds.2010. 12.003.

139. Szyld E, Aguilar A, Musante GA, Vain N, Prudent L, Fabres J, Carlo WA; Delivery Room Ventilation Devices Trial Group. Comparison of devices for newborn ventilation in the delivery room. *J Pediatr.* 2014;165: 234–239.e3. doi: 10.1016/j.jpeds. 2014.02.035.

140. Dawson JA, Gerber A, Kamlin CO, Davis PG, Morley CJ. Providing PEEP during neonatal resuscitation: which device is best? *J*

Paediatr Child Health. 2011:47:698–703. doi: 10.1111/j.1440-1754.2011.02036.x.

141. Morley CJ, Dawson JA, Stewart MJ, Hussain F, Davis PG. The effect of a PEEP valve on a Laerdal neonatal self-inflating resuscitation bag. *J Paediatr Child Health.* 2010;46:51–56. doi: 10.1111/j.1440-1754.2009. 01617.x.

142. Bennett S, Finer NN, Rich W, Vaucher Y. A comparison of three neonatal resuscitation devices. *Resuscitation.* 2005;67: 113–118. doi: 10.1016/j.resuscitation.2005. 02.016.

143. Kelm M, Proquitté H, Schmalisch G, Roehr CC. Reliability of two common PEEP-generating devices used in neonatal resuscitation. *Klin Padiatr.* 2009;221:415– 418. doi: 10.1055/s-0029-1233493.

144. Oddie S, Wyllie J, Scally A. Use of self-inflating bags for neonatal resuscitation. *Resuscitation.* 2005;67:109–112. doi: 10.1016/ j.resuscitation.2005.05.004.

145. Hussey SG, Ryan CA, Murphy BP. Comparison of three manual ventilation devices using an intubated mannequin. *Arch Dis Child Fetal Neonatal Ed.* 2004;89:F490– F493. doi: 10.1136/adc.2003.047712.

146. Finer NN, Rich W, Craft A, Henderson C. Comparison of methods of bag and mask ventilation for neonatal resuscitation. *Resuscitation.* 2001;49:299–305.

147. Schmölzer GM, Morley CJ, Wong C, Dawson JA, Kamlin CO, Donath SM, Hooper SB, Davis PG. Respiratory function monitor guidance of mask ventilation in the delivery room: a feasibility study. *J Pediatr.* 2012;160:377–381.e2. doi: 10.1016/j.jpeds. 2011.09.017.

148. Kong JY, Rich W, Finer NN, Leone TA. Quantitative end-tidal carbon dioxide monitoring in the delivery room: a randomized controlled trial. *J Pediatr.* 2013; 163:104–8.e1. doi: 10.1016/j.jpeds.2012. 12.016.

149. Esmail N, Saleh M, et al. Laryngeal mask airway versus endotracheal intubation for Apgar score improvement in neonatal resuscitation. *Egypt J Anesth.* 2002;18: 115–121.

150. Morley CJ, Davis PG, Doyle LW, Brion LP, Hascoet JM, Carlin JB; COIN Trial Investigators. Nasal CPAP or intubation at birth for very preterm infants. *N Engl J Med.* 2008;358:700–708. doi: 10.1056/ NEJMoa072788.

151. SUPPORT Study Group of the Eunice Kennedy Shriver NICHD Neonatal Research Network, Finer NN, Carlo WA, Walsh MC, Rich W, Gantz MG, Laptook AR, Yoder BA, Faix RG, Das A, Poole WK, Donovan EF, Newman NS, Ambalavanan N, Frantz ID

3rd, Buchter S, Sanchez PJ, Kennedy KA, Laroia N, Poindexter BB, Cotten CM, Van Meurs KP, Duara S, Narendran V, Sood BG, O'Shea TM, Bell EF, Bhandari V, Watterberg KL, Higgins RD. Early CPAP versus surfactant in extremely preterm infants. *N Engl J Med.* 2010;362:1970–1979.

152. Dunn MS, Kaempf J, de Klerk A, de Klerk R, Reilly M, Howard D, Ferrelli K, O'Conor J, Soll RF; Vermont Oxford Network DRM Study Group. Randomized trial comparing 3 approaches to the initial respiratory management of preterm neonates. *Pediatrics.* 2011;128:e1069–e1076. doi: 10.1542/ peds.2010-3848.

153. Orlowski JP. Optimum position for external cardiac compression in infants and young children. *Ann Emerg Med.* 1986;15: 667–673.

154. Phillips GW, Zideman DA. Relation of infant heart to sternum: its significance in cardiopulmonary resuscitation. *Lancet.* 1986; 1:1024–1025.

155. Saini SS, Gupta N, Kumar P, Bhalla AK, Kaur H. A comparison of two-fingers technique and two-thumbs encircling hands technique of chest compression in neonates. *J Perinatol.* 2012;32:690–694. doi: 10.1038/jp.2011.167.

156. You Y. Optimum location for chest compressions during two-rescuer infant cardiopulmonary resuscitation. *Resuscitation.* 2009;80:1378–1381. doi: 10.1016/j.resuscitation. 2009.08.013.

157. Meyer A, Nadkarni V, Pollock A, Babbs C, Nishisaki A, Braga M, Berg RA, Ades A. Evaluation of the Neonatal Resuscitation Program's recommended chest compression depth using computerized tomography imaging. *Resuscitation.* 2010;81: 544–548. doi: 10.1016/j.resuscitation.2010.01. 032.

158. Christman C, Hemway RJ, Wyckoff MH, Perlman JM. The two-thumb is superior to the two-finger method for administering chest compressions in a manikin model of neonatal resuscitation. *Arch Dis Child Fetal Neonatal Ed.* 2011;96:F99–F101. doi: 10. 1136/adc.2009.180406.

159. David R. Closed chest cardiac massage in the newborn infant. *Pediatrics.* 1988;81: 552–554.

160. Dellimore K, Heunis S, Gohier F, Archer E, de Villiers A, Smith J, Scheffer C. Development of a diagnostic glove for unobtrusive measurement of chest compression force and depth during neonatal CPR. *Conf Proc IEEE Eng Med Biol Soc.* 2013;2013:350–353. doi: 10.1109/EMBC.2013.6609509.

161. Dorfsman ML, Menegazzi JJ, Wadas RJ, Auble TE. Two-thumb vs. two-finger chest

compression in an infant model of prolonged cardiopulmonary resuscitation. *Acad Emerg Med.* 2000;7:1077–1082.

162. Houri PK, Frank LR, Menegazzi JJ, Taylor R. A randomized, controlled trial of two-thumb vs two-finger chest compression in a swine infant model of cardiac arrest [see comment]. *Prehosp Emerg Care.* 1997;1:65–67.

163. Martin PS, Kemp AM, Theobald PS, Maguire SA, Jones MD. Do chest compressions during simulated infant CPR comply with international recommendations? *Arch Dis Child.* 2013;98:576–581. doi: 10.1136/archdischild-2012-302583.

164. Martin PS, Kemp AM, Theobald PS, Maguire SA, Jones MD. Does a more "physiological" infant manikin design effect chest compression quality and create a potential for thoracic over-compression during simulated infant CPR? *Resuscitation.* 2013;84:666–671. doi: 10.1016/j.resuscitation.2012.10.005.

165. Martin P, Theobald P, Kemp A, Maguire S, Maconochie I, Jones M. Real-time feedback can improve infant manikin cardiopulmonary resuscitation by up to 79%–a randomised controlled trial. *Resuscitation.* 2013;84:1125–1130. doi: 10.1016/j.resuscitation.2013.03.029.

166. Menegazzi JJ, Auble TE, Nicklas KA, Hosack GM, Rack L, Goode JS. Two-thumb versus two-finger chest compression during CRP in a swine infant model of cardiac arrest. *Ann Emerg Med.* 1993;22:240–243.

167. MOYA F, JAMES LS, BURNARD ED, HANKS EC. Cardiac massage in the newborn infant through the intact chest. *Am J Obstet Gynecol.* 1962;84:798–803.

168. Park J, Yoon C, Lee JC, Jung JY, Kim do K, Kwak YH, Kim HC. Manikin-integrated digital measuring system for assessment of infant cardiopulmonary resuscitation techniques. *IEEE J Biomed Health Inform.* 2014;18:1659–1667. doi: 10.1109/JBHI.2013.2288641.

169. Thaler MM, Stobie GH. An improved technic of external cardiac compression in infants and young children. *N Engl J Med.* 1963;269: 606–610. doi: 10.1056/NEJM196309192691204.

170. Todres ID, Rogers MC. Methods of external cardiac massage in the newborn infant. *J Pediatr.* 1975;86:781–782.

171. Udassi S, Udassi JP, Lamb MA, Theriaque DW, Shuster JJ, Zaritsky AL, Haque IU. Two-thumb technique is superior to two-finger technique during lone rescuer infant manikin CPR. *Resuscitation.* 2010;81:712–717. doi: 10.1016/j.resuscitation.2009.12.029.

172. Whitelaw CC, Slywka B, Goldsmith LJ. Comparison of a two-finger versus two-thumb method for chest compressions by healthcare providers in an infant mechanical model. *Resuscitation.* 2000;43:213–216.

173. Dannevig I, Solevåg AL, Saugstad OD, Nakstad B. Lung injury in asphyxiated newborn pigs resuscitated from cardiac arrest—the impact of supplementary oxygen, longer ventilation intervals and chest compressions at different compression-to-ventilation ratios. *Open Respir Med J.* 2012;6:89–96. doi: 10.2174/1874306401206010089.

174. Dannevig I, Solevåg AL, Sonerud T, Saugstad OD, Nakstad B. Brain inflammation induced by severe asphyxia in newborn pigs and the impact of alternative resuscitation strategies on the newborn central nervous system. *Pediatr Res.* 2013;73:163–170. doi: 10.1038/pr.2012.167.

175. Hemway RJ, Christman C, Perlman J. The 3:1 is superior to a 15:2 ratio in a newborn manikin model in terms of quality of chest compressions and number of ventilations. *Arch Dis Child Fetal Neonatal Ed.* 2013;98:F42–F45. doi: 10.1136/archdischild-2011-301334.

176. Solevåg AL, Dannevig I, Wyckoff M, Saugstad OD, Nakstad B. Extended series of cardiac compressions during CPR in a swine model of perinatal asphyxia. *Resuscitation.* 2010; 81:1571–1576. doi: 10.1016/j.resuscitation.2010.06.007.

177. Solevåg AL, Dannevig I, Wyckoff M, Saugstad OD, Nakstad B. Return of spontaneous circulation with a compression: ventilation ratio of 15:2 versus 3:1 in newborn pigs with cardiac arrest due to asphyxia. *Arch Dis Child Fetal Neonatal Ed.* 2011;96:F417–F421. doi: 10.1136/adc.2010.200386.

178. Solevåg AL, Madland JM, Gjærum E, Nakstad B. Minute ventilation at different compression to ventilation ratios, different ventilation rates, and continuous chest compressions with asynchronous ventilation in a newborn manikin. *Scand J Trauma Resusc Emerg Med.* 2012;20:73. doi: 10.1186/1757-7241-20-73.

179. Lakshminrusimha S, Steinhorn RH, Wedgwood S, Savorgnan F, Nair J, Mathew B, Gugino SF, Russell JA, Swartz DD. Pulmonary hemodynamics and vascular reactivity in asphyxiated term lambs resuscitated with 21 and 100% oxygen. *J Appl Physiol (1985).* 2011;111:1441–1447. doi: 10.1152/japplphysiol.00711.2011.

180. Linner R, Werner O, Perez-de-Sa V, Cunha-Goncalves D. Circulatory recovery is as fast with air ventilation as with 100% oxygen after asphyxia-induced cardiac arrest in piglets. *Pediatr Res.* 2009;66:391–394. doi: 10.1203/PDR.0b013e3181b3b110.

181. Lipinski CA, Hicks SD, Callaway CW. Normoxic ventilation during resuscitation and outcome from asphyxial cardiac arrest in rats. *Resuscitation.* 1999;42:221–229.

182. Perez-de-Sa V, Cunha-Goncalves D, Nordh A, Hansson S, Larsson A, Ley D, Fellman V, Werner O. High brain tissue oxygen tension during ventilation with 100% oxygen after fetal asphyxia in newborn sheep. *Pediatr Res.* 2009;65:57–61.

183. Solevåg AL, Dannevig I, Nakstad B, Saugstad OD. Resuscitation of severely asphyctic newborn pigs with cardiac arrest by using 21% or 100% oxygen. *Neonatology.* 2010;98:64–72. doi: 10.1159/000275560.

184. Temesvári P, Karg E, Bódi I, Németh I, Pintér S, Lazics K, Domoki F, Bari F. Impaired early neurologic outcome in newborn piglets reoxygenated with 100% oxygen compared with room air after pneumothorax-induced asphyxia. *Pediatr Res.* 2001;49:812–819. doi: 10.1203/00006450-200106000-00017.

185. Walson KH, Tang M, Glumac A, Alexander H, Manole MD, Ma L, Hsia CJ, Clark RS, Kochanek PM, Kagan VE, Bayr H. Normoxic versus hyperoxic resuscitation in pediatric asphyxial cardiac arrest: effects on oxidative stress. *Crit Care Med.* 2011;39: 335–343. doi: 10.1097/CCM.0b013e3181ffda0e.

186. Yeh ST, Cawley RJ, Aune SE, Angelos MG. Oxygen requirement during cardiopulmonary resuscitation (CPR) to effect return of spontaneous circulation. *Resuscitation.* 2009; 80:951–955. doi: 10.1016/j.resuscitation.2009.05.001.

187. Berg RA, Henry C, Otto CW, Sanders AB, Kern KB, Hilwig RW, Ewy GA. Initial end-tidal CO2 is markedly elevated during cardiopulmonary resuscitation after asphyxial cardiac arrest. *Pediatr Emerg Care.* 1996;12: 245–248.

188. Bhende MS, Karasic DG, Menegazzi JJ. Evaluation of an end-tidal CO2 detector during cardiopulmonary resuscitation in a canine model for pediatric cardiac arrest. *Pediatr Emerg Care.* 1995;11:365–368.

189. Bhende MS, Thompson AE. Evaluation of an end-tidal CO2 detector during pediatric cardiopulmonary resuscitation. *Pediatrics.* 1995;95:395–399.

190. Bhende MS, Karasic DG, Karasic RB. End-tidal carbon dioxide changes during cardiopulmonary resuscitation after experimental

asphyxial cardiac arrest. *Am J Emerg Med.* 1996;14:349–350. doi: 10.1016/S0735-6757(96)90046-7.

191. Chalak LF, Barber CA, Hynan L, Garcia D, Christie L, Wyckoff MH. End-tidal CO$_2$ detection of an audible heart rate during neonatal cardiopulmonary resuscitation after asystole in asphyxiated piglets. *Pediatr Res.* 2011;69(5 pt 1):401–405. doi: 10.1203/PDR.0b013e3182125f7f.

192. Jacobs SE, Morley CJ, Inder TE, Stewart MJ, Smith KR, McNamara PJ, Wright IM, Kirpalani HM, Darlow BA, Doyle LW; Infant Cooling Evaluation Collaboration. Whole-body hypothermia for term and near-term newborns with hypoxic-ischemic encephalopathy: a randomized controlled trial. *Arch Pediatr Adolesc Med.* 2011;165:692–700. doi: 10.1001/archpediatrics.2011.43.

193. Bharadwaj SK, Bhat BV. Therapeutic hypothermia using gel packs for term neonates with hypoxic ischaemic encephalopathy in resource-limited settings: a randomized controlled trial. *J Trop Pediatr.* 2012;58:382–388. doi: 10.1093/tropej/fms005.

194. Robertson NJ, Hagmann CF, Acolet D, Allen E, Nyombi N, Elbourne D, Costello A, Jacobs I, Nakakeeto M, Cowan F. Pilot randomized trial of therapeutic hypothermia with serial cranial ultrasound and 18-22 month follow-up for neonatal encephalopathy in a low resource hospital setting in Uganda: study protocol. *Trials.* 2011;12:138. doi: 10.1186/1745-6215-12-138.

195. Thayyil S, Shankaran S, Wade A, Cowan FM, Ayer M, Sathccsan K, Srccjith C, Eylcs H, Taylor AM, Bainbridge A, Cady EB, Robertson NJ, Price D, Balraj G. Whole-body cooling in neonatal encephalopathy using phase changing material. *Arch Dis Child Fetal Neonatal Ed.* 2013;98:F280–F281. doi: 10.1136/archdischild-2013-303840.

196. Bottoms SF, Paul RH, Mercer BM, MacPherson CA, Caritis SN, Moawad AH, Van Dorsten JP, Hauth JC, Thurnau GR, Miodovnik M, Meis PM, Roberts JM, McNellis D, Iams JD. Obstetric determinants of neonatal survival: antenatal predictors of neonatal survival and morbidity in extremely low birth weight infants. *Am J Obstet Gynecol.* 1999;180 (3 pt 1):665–669.

197. Ambalavanan N, Carlo WA, Bobashev G, Mathias E, Liu B, Poole K, Fanaroff AA, Stoll BJ, Ehrenkranz R, Wright LL; National Institute of Child Health and Human Development Neonatal Research Network. Prediction of death for extremely low birth weight neonates. *Pediatrics.* 2005;116:1367–1373. doi: 10.1542/peds.2004-2099.

198. Manktelow BN, Seaton SE, Field DJ, Draper ES. Population-based estimates of in-unit survival for very preterm infants. *Pediatrics.* 2013;131:e425–e432. doi: 10.1542/peds.2012-2189.

199. Medlock S, Ravelli AC, Tamminga P, Mol BW, Abu-Hanna A. Prediction of mortality in very premature infants: a systematic review of prediction models. *PLoS One.* 2011;6:e23441. doi: 10.1371/journal.pone.0023441.

200. Tyson JE, Parikh NA, Langer J, Green C, Higgins RD; National Institute of Child Health and Human Development Neonatal Research Network. Intensive care for extreme prematurity—moving beyond gestational age. *N Engl J Med.* 2008;358:1672–1681. doi: 10.1056/NEJMoa073059.

201. Casalaz DM, Marlow N, Speidel BD. Outcome of resuscitation following unexpected apparent stillbirth. *Arch Dis Child Fetal Neonatal Ed.* 1998;78:F112–F115.

202. Harrington DJ, Redman CW, Moulden M, Greenwood CE. The long-term outcome in surviving infants with Apgar zero at 10 minutes: a systematic review of the literature and hospital-based cohort. *Am J Obstet Gynecol.* 2007;196:463.e1–463.e5. doi: 10.1016/j.ajog.2006.10.877.

203. Kasdorf E, Laptook A, Azzopardi D, Jacobs S, Perlman JM. Improving infant outcome with a 10 min Apgar of 0. *Arch Dis Child Fetal Neonatal Ed.* 2015;100:F102–F105. doi: 10.1136/archdischild-2014-306687.

204. Laptook AR, Shankaran S, Ambalavanan N, Carlo WA, McDonald SA, Higgins RD, Das A; Hypothermia Subcommittee of the NICHD Neonatal Research Network. Outcome of term infants using apgar scores at 10 minutes following hypoxic-ischemic encephalopathy. *Pediatrics.* 2009;124:1619–1626. doi: 10.1542/peds.2009-0934.

205. Patel H, Beeby PJ. Resuscitation beyond 10 minutes of term babies born without signs of life. *J Paediatr Child Health.* 2004;40:136–138.

206. Sarkar S, Bhagat I, Dechert RE, Barks JD. Predicting death despite therapeutic hypothermia in infants with hypoxic-ischaemic encephalopathy. *Arch Dis Child Fetal Neonatal Ed.* 2010;95:F423–F428. doi: 10.1136/adc.2010.182725.

207. Breckwoldt J, Svensson J, Lingemann C, Gruber H. Does clinical teacher training always improve teaching effectiveness as opposed to no teacher training? A randomized controlled study. *BMC Med Educ.* 2014;14:6. doi: 10.1186/1472-6920-14-6.

208. Boerboom TB, Jaarsma D, Dolmans DH, Scherpbier AJ, Mastenbroek NJ, Van Beukelen P. Peer group reflection helps clinical teachers to critically reflect on their teaching. *Med Teach.* 2011;33:e615–e623. doi: 10.3109/0142159X.2011.610840.

209. Litzelman DK, Stratos GA, Marriott DJ, Lazaridis EN, Skeff KM. Beneficial and harmful effects of augmented feedback on physicians' clinical-teaching performances. *Acad Med.* 1998;73:324–332.

210. Naji SA, Maguire GP, Fairbairn SA, Goldberg DP, Faragher EB. Training clinical teachers in psychiatry to teach interviewing skills to medical students. *Med Educ.* 1986;20:140–147.

211. Schum TR, Yindra KJ. Relationship between systematic feedback to faculty and ratings of clinical teaching. *Acad Med.* 1996;71:1100–1102.

212. Skeff KM, Stratos G, Campbell M, Cooke M, Jones HW III. Evaluation of the seminar method to improve clinical teaching. *J Gen Intern Med.* 1986;1:315–322.

213. Lye P, Heidenreich C, Wang-Cheng R, Bragg D, Simpson D; Advanced Faculty Development Group. Experienced clinical educators improve their clinical teaching effectiveness. *Ambul Pediatr.* 2003;3:93–97.

214. Regan-Smith M, Hirschmann K, Iobst W. Direct observation of faculty with feedback: an effective means of improving patient-centered and learner-centered teaching skills. *Teach Learn Med.* 2007;19:278–286. doi: 10.1080/10401330701366739.

215. American Academy of Pediatrics, American Heart Association. *Textbook of Neonatal Resuscitation (NRP).* Chicago, IL: American Academy of Pediatrics;2011.

216. Berden HJ, Willems FF, Hendrick JM, Pijls NH, Knape JT. How frequently should basic cardiopulmonary resuscitation training be repeated to maintain adequate skills? *BMJ.* 1993;306:1576–1577.

217. Ernst KD, Cline WL, Dannaway DC, Davis EM, Anderson MP, Atchley CB, Thompson BM. Weekly and consecutive day neonatal intubation training: comparable on a pediatrics clerkship. *Acad Med.* 2014;89:505–510. doi: 10.1097/ACM.0000000000000150.

218. Kaczorowski J, Levitt C, Hammond M, Outerbridge E, Grad R, Rothman A, Graves L. Retention of neonatal resuscitation skills and knowledge: a randomized controlled trial. *Fam Med.* 1998;30:705–711.

219. Kovacs G, Bullock G, Ackroyd-Stolarz S, Cain E, Petrie D. A randomized controlled trial on the effect of educational interventions in promoting airway management skill maintenance. *Ann Emerg Med.* 2000;36:301–309. doi: 10.1067/mem.2000.109339.

220. Montgomery C, Kardong-Edgren SE, Oermann MH, Odom-Maryon T. Student satisfaction and self report of CPR competency:

295

HeartCode BLS courses, instructor-led CPR courses, and monthly voice advisory manikin practice for CPR skill maintenance. *Int J Nurs Educ Scholarsh.* 2012;9. doi: 10.1515/1548-923X.2361.

221. Oermann MH, Kardong-Edgren SE, Odom-Maryon T. Effects of monthly practice on nursing students' CPR psychomotor skill performance. *Resuscitation.* 2011;82:447–453. doi: 10.1016/j.resuscitation. 2010.11.022.

222. Stross JK. Maintaining competency in advanced cardiac life support skills. *JAMA.* 1983;249:3339–3341.

223. Su E, Schmidt TA, Mann NC, Zechnich AD. A randomized controlled trial to assess decay in acquired knowledge among paramedics completing a pediatric resuscitation course. *Acad Emerg Med.* 2000;7:779–786.

224. Sutton RM, Niles D, Meaney PA, Aplenc R, French B, Abella BS, Lengetti EL, Berg RA, Helfaer MA, Nadkarni V. "Booster" training: evaluation of instructor-led bedside cardiopulmonary resuscitation skill training and automated corrective feedback to improve cardiopulmonary resuscitation compliance of Pediatric Basic Life Support providers during simulated cardiac arrest. *Pediatr Crit Care Med.* 2011;12:e116–e121. doi: 10.1097/PCC.0b013e3181e91271.

225. Turner NM, Scheffer R, Custers E, Cate OT. Use of unannounced spaced telephone testing to improve retention of knowledge after life-support courses. *Med Teach.* 2011;33: 731–737. doi: 10.3109/0142159X.2010.542521.

226. Lubin J, Carter R. The feasibility of daily mannequin practice to improve intubation success. *Air Med J.* 2009;28:195–197. doi: 10.1016/j.amj.2009.03.006.

227. Mosley CM, Shaw BN. A longitudinal cohort study to investigate the retention of knowledge and skills following attendance on the Newborn Life support course. *Arch Dis Child.* 2013;98:582–586. doi: 10.1136/archdischild-2012-303263.

228. Nadel FM, Lavelle JM, Fein JA, Giardino AP, Decker JM, Durbin DR. Teaching resuscitation to pediatric residents: the effects of an intervention. *Arch Pediatr Adolesc Med.* 2000; 154:1049–1054.

229. Niles D, Sutton RM, Donoghue A, Kalsi MS, Roberts K, Boyle L, Nishisaki A, Arbogast KB, Helfaer M, Nadkarni V. "Rolling Refreshers": a novel approach to maintain CPR psychomotor skill competence. *Resuscitation.* 2009;80: 909–912. doi: 10.1016/j.resuscitation.2009.04.021.

230. Nishisaki A, Donoghue AJ, Colborn S, Watson C, Meyer A, Brown CA 3rd, Helfaer MA, Walls RM, Nadkarni VM. Effect of just-in-time simulation training on tracheal intubation procedure safety in the pediatric intensive care unit. *Anesthesiology.* 2010;113:214–223. doi: 10.1097/ALN.0b013e3181e19bf2.

231. O'Donnell CM, Skinner AC. An evaluation of a short course in resuscitation training in a district general hospital. *Resuscitation.* 1993;26:193–201.

DISCLOSURES

Part 13: Neonatal Resuscitation: 2015 Guidelines Update Writing Group Disclosures

Writing Group Member	Employment	Research Grant	Other Research Support	Speakers' Bureau/ Honoraria	Expert Witness	Ownership Interest	Consultant/ Advisory Board	Other
Myra H. Wyckoff	UT Southwestern Medical School	None	None	None	None	None	None	None
Khalid Aziz	Royal Alexandra Hospital	None	None	None	None	None	None	None
Marilyn B. Escobedo	University of Oklahoma Medical School	None	None	None	None	None	None	None
Vishal S. Kapadia	UT Southwestern	None	Neonatal Resuscitation Program*; NIH/NCATS KL2TR001103†	None	None	None	None	None
John Kattwinkel	University of Virginia Health System	None	None	None	None	None	None	None
Jeffrey M. Perlman	Weill Cornell Medical College	None	Laerdal Foundation for Global Health*	None	None	None	None	None
Wendy M. Simon	American Academy of Pediatrics	None	None	None	None	None	None	None
Gary M. Weiner	University of Michigan	None	None	None	None	None	American Academy of Pediatrics†	None
Jeannette G. Zaichkin	Self-employed	None	None	None	None	None	American Academy of Pediatrics†	None

This table represents the relationships of writing group members that may be perceived as actual or reasonably perceived conflicts of interest as reported on the Disclosure Questionnaire, which all members of the writing group are required to complete and submit. A relationship is considered to be "significant" if (a) the person receives $10 000 or more during any 12-month period, or 5% or more of the person's gross income; or (b) the person owns 5% or more of the voting stock or share of the entity, or owns $10 000 or more of the fair market value of the entity. A relationship is considered to be "modest" if it is less than "significant" under the preceding definition.

* Modest.
† Significant.

2015 Guidelines Update: Part 13 Recommendations

Year Last Reviewed	Topic	Recommendation	Comments
2015	Umbilical Cord Management	In summary, from the evidence reviewed in the 2010 CoSTR and subsequent review of DCC and cord milking in preterm newborns in the 2015 ILCOR systematic review, DCC for longer than 30 seconds is reasonable for both term and preterm infants who do not require resuscitation at birth (Class IIa, LOE C-LD).	new for 2015
2015	Umbilical Cord Management	There is insufficient evidence to recommend an approach to cord clamping for infants who require resuscitation at birth and more randomized trials involving such infants are encouraged. In light of the limited information regarding the safety of rapid changes in blood volume for extremely preterm infants, we suggest against the routine use of cord milking for infants born at less than 29 weeks of gestation outside of a research setting. Further study is warranted because cord milking may improve initial mean blood pressure, hematologic indices, and reduce intracranial hemorrhage, but thus far there is no evidence for improvement in long-term outcomes (Class IIb, LOE C-LD).	new for 2015
2015	Importance of Maintaining Normal Temperature in the Delivery Room	Preterm infants are especially vulnerable. Hypothermia is also associated with serious morbidities, such as increased respiratory issues, hypoglycemia, and late-onset sepsis. Because of this, admission temperature should be recorded as a predictor of outcomes as well as a quality indicator (Class I, LOE B-NR).	new for 2015
2015	Importance of Maintaining Normal Temperature in the Delivery Room	It is recommended that the temperature of newly born nonasphyxiated infants be maintained between 36.5°C and 37.5°C after birth through admission and stabilization (Class I, LOE C-LD).	new for 2015
2015	Interventions to Maintain Newborn Temperature in the Delivery Room	The use of radiant warmers and plastic wrap with a cap has improved but not eliminated the risk of hypothermia in preterms in the delivery room. Other strategies have been introduced, which include increased room temperature, thermal mattresses, and the use of warmed humidified resuscitation gases. Various combinations of these strategies may be reasonable to prevent hypothermia in infants born at less than 32 weeks of gestation (Class IIb, LOE B-R, B-NR, C-LD).	updated for 2015
2015	Interventions to Maintain Newborn Temperature in the Delivery Room	Compared with plastic wrap and radiant warmer, the addition of a thermal mattress, warmed humidified gases and increased room temperature plus cap plus thermal mattress were all effective in reducing hypothermia. For all the studies, hyperthermia was a concern, but harm was not shown. Hyperthermia (greater than 38.0°C) should be avoided due to the potential associated risks (Class III: Harm, LOE C-EO).	updated for 2015
2015	Warming Hypothermic Newborns to Restore Normal Temperature	The traditional recommendation for the method of rewarming neonates who are hypothermic after resuscitation has been that slower is preferable to faster rewarming to avoid complications such as apnea and arrhythmias. However, there is insufficient current evidence to recommend a preference for either rapid (0.5°C/h or greater) or slow rewarming (less than 0.5°C/h) of unintentionally hypothermic newborns (temperature less than 36°C) at hospital admission. Either approach to rewarming may be reasonable (Class IIb, LOE C-LD).	new for 2015
2015	Maintaining Normothermia in Resource-Limited Settings	In resource-limited settings, to maintain body temperature or prevent hypothermia during transition (birth until 1 to 2 hours of life) in well newborn infants, it may be reasonable to put them in a clean food-grade plastic bag up to the level of the neck and swaddle them after drying (Class IIb, LOE C-LD).	new for 2015
2015	Maintaining Normothermia in Resource-Limited Settings	Another option that may be reasonable is to nurse such newborns with skin-to-skin contact or kangaroo mother care (Class IIb, LOE C-LD).	new for 2015

Appendix Continued

Year Last Reviewed	Topic	Recommendation	Comments
2015	Clearing the Airway When Meconium Is Present	However, if the infant born through meconium-stained amniotic fluid presents with poor muscle tone and inadequate breathing efforts, the initial steps of resuscitation should be completed under the radiant warmer. PPV should be initiated if the infant is not breathing or the heart rate is less than 100/min after the initial steps are completed. Routine intubation for tracheal suction in this setting is not suggested, because there is insufficient evidence to continue recommending this practice (Class IIb, LOE C-LD).	updated for 2015
2015	Assessment of Heart Rate	During resuscitation of term and preterm newborns, the use of 3-lead ECG for the rapid and accurate measurement of the newborn's heart rate may be reasonable (Class IIb, LOE C-LD).	new for 2015
2015	Administration of Oxygen in Preterm Infants	In all studies, irrespective of whether air or high oxygen (including 100%) was used to initiate resuscitation, most infants were in approximately 30% oxygen by the time of stabilization. Resuscitation of preterm newborns of less than 35 weeks of gestation should be initiated with low oxygen (21% to 30%), and the oxygen concentration should be titrated to achieve preductal oxygen saturation approximating the interquartile range measured in healthy term infants after vaginal birth at sea level (Class I, LOE B-R).	new for 2015
2015	Administration of Oxygen	Initiating resuscitation of preterm newborns with high oxygen (65% or greater) is not recommended (Class III: No Benefit, LOE B-R).	new for 2015
2015	Positive Pressure Ventilation (PPV)	There is insufficient data regarding short and long-term safety and the most appropriate duration and pressure of inflation to support routine application of sustained inflation of greater than 5 seconds' duration to the transitioning newborn (Class IIb, LOE B-R).	new for 2015
2015	Positive Pressure Ventilation (PPV)	In 2015, the Neonatal Resuscitation ILCOR and Guidelines Task Forces repeated their 2010 recommendation that, when PPV is administered to preterm newborns, approximately 5 cm H_2O PEEP is suggested (Class IIb, LOE B-R).	updated for 2015
2015	Positive Pressure Ventilation (PPV)	PPV can be delivered effectively with a flow-inflating bag, self-inflating bag, or T-piece resuscitator (Class IIa, LOE B-R).	updated for 2015
2015	Positive Pressure Ventilation (PPV)	Use of respiratory mechanics monitors have been reported to prevent excessive pressures and tidal volumes and exhaled CO_2 monitors may help assess that actual gas exchange is occurring during face-mask PPV attempts. Although use of such devices is feasible, thus far their effectiveness, particularly in changing important outcomes, has not been established (Class IIb, LOE C-LD).	new for 2015
2015	Positive Pressure Ventilation (PPV)	Laryngeal masks, which fit over the laryngeal inlet, can achieve effective ventilation in term and preterm newborns at 34 weeks or more of gestation. Data are limited for their use in preterm infants delivered at less than 34 weeks of gestation or who weigh less than 2000 g. A laryngeal mask may be considered as an alternative to tracheal intubation if face-mask ventilation is unsuccessful in achieving effective ventilation (Class IIb, LOE B-R).	updated for 2015
2015	Positive Pressure Ventilation (PPV)	A laryngeal mask is recommended during resuscitation of term and preterm newborns at 34 weeks or more of gestation when tracheal intubation is unsuccessful or is not feasible (Class I, LOE C-EO).	updated for 2015
2015	CPAP	Based on this evidence, spontaneously breathing preterm infants with respiratory distress may be supported with CPAP initially rather than routine intubation for administering PPV (Class IIb, LOE B-R).	updated for 2015
2015	Chest Compressions	Compressions are delivered on the lower third of the sternum to a depth of approximately one third of the anterior-posterior diameter of the chest (Class IIb, LOE C-LD).	updated for 2015

Appendix Continued

Year Last Reviewed	Topic	Recommendation	Comments
2015	Chest Compressions	Because the 2-thumb technique generates higher blood pressures and coronary perfusion pressure with less rescuer fatigue, the 2 thumb–encircling hands technique is suggested as the preferred method (Class IIb, LOE C-LD).	updated for 2015
2015	Chest Compressions	It is still suggested that compressions and ventilations be coordinated to avoid simultaneous delivery. The chest should be allowed to re-expand fully during relaxation, but the rescuer's thumbs should not leave the chest. The Neonatal Resuscitation ILCOR and Guidelines Task Forces continue to support use of a 3:1 ratio of compressions to ventilation, with 90 compressions and 30 breaths to achieve approximately 120 events per minute to maximize ventilation at an achievable rate (Class IIa, LOE C-LD).	updated for 2015
2015	Chest Compressions	A 3:1 compression-to-ventilation ratio is used for neonatal resuscitation where compromise of gas exchange is nearly always the primary cause of cardiovascular collapse, but rescuers may consider using higher ratios (eg, 15:2) if the arrest is believed to be of cardiac origin (Class IIb, LOE C-EO).	updated for 2015
2015	Chest Compressions	The Neonatal Guidelines Writing Group endorses increasing the oxygen concentration to 100% whenever chest compressions are provided (Class IIa, LOE C-EO).	new for 2015
2015	Chest Compressions	To reduce the risks of complications associated with hyperoxia the supplementary oxygen concentration should be weaned as soon as the heart rate recovers (Class I, LOE C-LD).	new for 2015
2015	Chest Compressions	The current measure for determining successful progress in neonatal resuscitation is to assess the heart rate response. Other devices, such as end-tidal CO_2 monitoring and pulse oximetry, may be useful techniques to determine when return of spontaneous circulation occurs. However, in asystolic/bradycardic neonates, we suggest against the routine use of any single feedback device such as $ETCO_2$ monitors or pulse oximeters for detection of return of spontaneous circulation, as their usefulness for this purpose in neonates has not been well established (Class IIb, LOE C-LD).	new for 2015
2015	Induced Therapeutic Hypothermia Resource-Limited Areas	Evidence suggests that use of therapeutic hypothermia in resource-limited settings (ie, lack of qualified staff, inadequate equipment, etc) may be considered and offered under clearly defined protocols similar to those used in published clinical trials and in facilities with the capabilities for multidisciplinary care and longitudinal follow-up (Class IIb, LOE-B-R).	new for 2015
2015	Guidelines for Withholding and Discontinuing	However, in individual cases, when counseling a family and constructing a prognosis for survival at gestations below 25 weeks, it is reasonable to consider variables such as perceived accuracy of gestational age assignment, the presence or absence of chorioamnionitis, and the level of care available for location of delivery. It is also recognized that decisions about appropriateness of resuscitation below 25 weeks of gestation will be influenced by region-specific guidelines. In making this statement, a higher value was placed on the lack of evidence for a generalized prospective approach to changing important outcomes over improved retrospective accuracy and locally validated counseling policies. The most useful data for antenatal counseling provides outcome figures for infants alive at the onset of labor, not only for those born alive or admitted to a neonatal intensive care unit (Class IIb, LOE C-LD).	new for 2015
2015	Guidelines for Withholding and Discontinuing	We suggest that, in infants with an Apgar score of 0 after 10 minutes of resuscitation, if the heart rate remain undetectable, it may be reasonable to stop assisted ventilations; however, the decision to continue or discontinue resuscitative efforts must be individualized. Variables to be considered may include whether the resuscitation was considered optimal; availability of advanced neonatal care, such as therapeutic hypothermia; specific circumstances before delivery (eg, known timing of the insult); and wishes expressed by the family (Class IIb, LOE C-LD).	updated for 2015

Appendix Continued

Year Last Reviewed	Topic	Recommendation	Comments
2015	Structure of Educational Programs to Teach Neonatal Resuscitation: Instructors	Until more research is available to clarify the optimal instructor training methodology, it is suggested that neonatal resuscitation instructors be trained using timely, objective, structured, and individually targeted verbal and/or written feedback (Class IIb, LOE C-EO).	new for 2015
2015	Structure of Educational Programs to Teach Neonatal Resuscitation: Providers	Studies that explored how frequently healthcare providers or healthcare students should train showed no differences in patient outcomes (LOE C-EO) but were able to show some advantages in psychomotor performance (LOE B-R) and knowledge and confidence (LOE C-LD) when focused training occurred every 6 months or more frequently. It is therefore suggested that neonatal resuscitation task training occur more frequently than the current 2-year interval (Class IIb, LOE B-R, LOE C-EO, LOE C-LD).	new for 2015

The following recommendations were not reviewed in 2015. For more information, see the *2010 AHA Guidelines for CPR and ECC*, "Part 15: Neonatal Resuscitation."

Year Last Reviewed	Topic	Recommendation	Comments
2010	Temperature Control	All resuscitation procedures, including endotracheal intubation, chest compression, and insertion of intravenous lines, can be performed with these temperature-controlling interventions in place (Class IIb, LOE C).	not reviewed in 2015
2010	Clearing the Airway When Amniotic Fluid Is Clear	Suctioning immediately after birth, whether with a bulb syringe or suction catheter, may be considered only if the airway appears obstructed or if PPV is required (Class IIb, LOE C).	not reviewed in 2015
2010	Assessment of Oxygen Need and Administration of Oxygen	It is recommended that oximetry be used when resuscitation can be anticipated, when PPV is administered, when central cyanosis persists beyond the first 5 to 10 minutes of life, or when supplementary oxygen is administered (Class I, LOE B).	not reviewed in 2015
2010	Administration of Oxygen in Term Infants	It is reasonable to initiate resuscitation with air (21% oxygen at sea level; Class IIb, LOE C).	not reviewed in 2015
2010	Administration of Oxygen in Term Infants	Supplementary oxygen may be administered and titrated to achieve a preductal oxygen saturation approximating the interquartile range measured in healthy term infants after vaginal birth at sea level (Class IIb, LOE B).	not reviewed in 2015
2010	Initial Breaths and Assisted Ventilation	Inflation pressure should be monitored; an initial inflation pressure of 20 cm H_2O may be effective, but $\geq$30 to 40 cm H_2O may be required in some term babies without spontaneous ventilation (Class IIb, LOE C).	not reviewed in 2015
2010	Initial Breaths and Assisted Ventilation	In summary, assisted ventilation should be delivered at a rate of 40 to 60 breaths per minute to promptly achieve or maintain a heart rate of 100 per minute (Class IIb, LOE C).	not reviewed in 2015
2010	Assisted-Ventilation Devices	Target inflation pressures and long inspiratory times are more consistently achieved in mechanical models when T-piece devices are used rather than bags, although the clinical implications of these findings are not clear (Class IIb, LOE C).	not reviewed in 2015
2010	Assisted-Ventilation Devices	Resuscitators are insensitive to changes in lung compliance, regardless of the device being used (Class IIb, LOE C).	not reviewed in 2015
2010	Endotracheal Tube Placement	Although last reviewed in 2010, exhaled CO_2 detection remains the most reliable method of confirmation of endotracheal tube placement (Class IIa, LOE B).	not reviewed in 2015
2010	Chest Compressions	Respirations, heart rate, and oxygenation should be reassessed periodically, and coordinated chest compressions and ventilations should continue until the spontaneous heart rate is <60 per minute (Class IIb, LOE C).	not reviewed in 2015
2010	Epinephrine	Dosing recommendations remain unchanged from 2010. Intravenous administration of epinephrine may be considered at a dose of 0.01 to 0.03 mg/kg of 1:10 000 epinephrine. If an endotracheal administration route is attempted while intravenous access is being established, higher dosing will be needed at 0.05 to 0.1 mg/kg (Class IIb, LOE C).	not reviewed in 2015
2010	Epinephrine	Given the lack of supportive data for endotracheal epinephrine, it is reasonable to provide drugs by the intravenous route as soon as venous access is established (Class IIb, LOE C).	not reviewed in 2015
2010	Volume Expansion	Volume expansion may be considered when blood loss is known or suspected (pale skin, poor perfusion, weak pulse) and the infant's heart rate has not responded adequately to other resuscitative measures (Class IIb, LOE C).	not reviewed in 2015

301

Appendix Continued

Year Last Reviewed	Topic	Recommendation	Comments
2010	Volume Expansion	An isotonic crystalloid solution or blood may be useful for volume expansion in the delivery room (Class IIb, LOE C).	not reviewed in 2015
2010	Volume Expansion	The recommended dose is 10 mL/kg, which may need to be repeated. When resuscitating premature infants, care should be taken to avoid giving volume expanders rapidly, because rapid infusions of large volumes have been associated with IVH (Class IIb, LOE C).	not reviewed in 2015
2010	Induced Therapeutic Hypothermia Resource-Abundant Areas	Induced therapeutic hypothermia was last reviewed in 2010; at that time it was recommended that infants born at more than 36 weeks of gestation with evolving moderate-to-severe hypoxic-ischemic encephalopathy should be offered therapeutic hypothermia under clearly defined protocols similar to those used in published clinical trials and in facilities with the capabilities for multidisciplinary care and longitudinal follow-up (Class IIa, LOE A).	not reviewed in 2015
2010	Guidelines for Withholding and Discontinuing	The 2010 Guidelines provide suggestions for when resuscitation is not indicated, when it is nearly always indicated, and that under circumstances when outcome remains unclear, that the desires of the parents should be supported (Class IIb, LOE C).	not reviewed in 2015
2010	Briefing/Debriefing	It is still suggested that briefing and debriefing techniques be used whenever possible for neonatal resuscitation (Class IIb, LOE C).	not reviewed in 2015

302

Part 13: Neonatal Resuscitation: 2015 American Heart Association Guidelines Update for Cardiopulmonary Resuscitation and Emergency Cardiovascular Care (Reprint)

Myra H. Wyckoff, Khalid Aziz, Marilyn B. Escobedo, Vishal S. Kapadia, John Kattwinkel, Jeffrey M. Perlman, Wendy M. Simon, Gary M. Weiner and Jeanette G. Zaichkin

Pediatrics 2015;136;S196; originally published online October 14, 2015;
DOI: 10.1542/peds.2015-3373G

Updated Information & Services	including high resolution figures, can be found at: /content/136/Supplement_2/S196.full.html
References	This article cites 223 articles, 62 of which can be accessed free at: /content/136/Supplement_2/S196.full.html#ref-list-1
Permissions & Licensing	Information about reproducing this article in parts (figures, tables) or in its entirety can be found online at: /site/misc/Permissions.xhtml
Reprints	Information about ordering reprints can be found online: /site/misc/reprints.xhtml

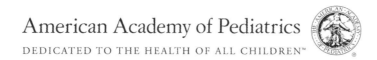

American Academy of Pediatrics
DEDICATED TO THE HEALTH OF ALL CHILDREN™

Index

congenital neuromuscular disorder, 257
continuous positive airway pressure
     (CPAP), 8, 50, 67, 68,
     226–227.
   administered after initial
     stabilization period, 88
   administered during initial
     stabilization period, 87–88
   avoiding excessive pressure during,
     234
   distinction from PEEP, 86–87
   indication for, 72
   orogastric tube for, 89–90
   in post-resuscitation care, 215
   in preterm babies, 229, 232
   in response to labored breathing or
     persistently low oxygen
     saturation, 50
   spontaneous breathing and, 86–87
CPAP. See continuous positive airway
     pressure (CPAP)
cricoid cartilage, 117, 119, 127, 148
crying, initial, 38
crystalloid fluid, 190
cyanosis, 36, 46–47, 60

D

death, newborn, 266–267
   follow-up arrangements for parents
     after, 273–274
   how to care for baby until, 272–273
   informing parents about impending,
     271
   organ donation after, 271
   palliative care and, 266, 269,
     270–271, 273
   and situations in which it is ethical
     not to initiate resuscitation,
     269–270
   support for nursery staff after, 274
delayed umbilical cord clamping
     (DCC), 36–37
delivery. See also birth
   high risk, 20
   personnel present at, 19–20
   supplies and equipment available at,
     21
   uncomplicated, 19, 35, 51, 258
devices, resuscitation, 48, 50, 68–72
dextrose, intravenous, 218
diaphragm, 255–257
dobutamine, 218
documentation, accurate, 12
dopamine, 218
double-lumen sump tube for congenital
     diaphragmatic hernia,
     256–257

drying of newborns, 42
ductus arteriosus, 4, 6, 7

E

ECG. See electrocardiogram (ECG)
ECMO. See extracorporeal membrane
     oxygenation (ECMO)
electrocardiogram (ECG), 47, 165
   checking heart rate during
     compressions, 172
   for monitoring baby's response to
     positive-pressure ventilation,
     81
   for preterm babies, 229
   tension pneumothorax and, 245
electrolyte disturbances, 219
end of life, ethics and care at, 266–274
endotracheal intubation, 53, 83,
     117–118, 226
   assisting with, 138–139
   bilateral breath sounds confirming
     placement of, 85, 86, 159, 160,
     172, 176
   carbon dioxide detector, 132–133,
     174
   epinephrine administration via, 187,
     188
   equipment for, 119–122
   how to confirm placement in the
     trachea, 132
   how to perform, 125
   insertion of tube, 129–130
     depth, 134–135
   performance checklist, 156–161
   positioning for, 123–124
     improper, 133–134
   preparation of laryngoscope for,
     123
   prior to starting chest compressions,
     149
   to remove thick secretions,
     250–251
   resuscitation with PPV using, 117
   for Robin sequence, 252
   securing tube in, 130–131,
     136–138
   sedative premedication before, 149
   for suction, 139
   time allowed for attempting, 131
   ventilating through, 131
   when to consider using, 118
   worsening condition after, 140
epiglottis, 119
epinephrine, 4
   administration, 188
   concentration, 187
   dose, 188, 202

function of, 186
   indication, 187
   preparation, 187
   route of administration, 187–188,
     202
   summary, 189
   what to do if baby not responding
     after giving, 191–192
   what to expect after giving,
     188–189
equipment, neonatal resuscitation, 21,
     25–27
esophagus, 119
ethics, 14, 266–267
   critical care interventions, 221
   with dying baby, 202
   of initiating resuscitation for
     extremely preterm babies,
     268–269
   and laws related to neonatal
     resuscitation, 271
   obligation to continue
     life-sustaining therapies,
     270–271
   principles applied to neonatal
     resuscitation, 267
   in resuscitating a newborn at
     threshold of viability, 238
   and role parents should play in
     decisions about resuscitation,
     268
   situations in which it is ethical not
     to initiate resuscitation,
     269–270
   what to do if uncertain about
     chances of survival or serious
     disability, 270
   when uncertain about chances of
     survival or serious disability
     of preterm babies, 238
extracorporeal membrane oxygenation
     (ECMO), 217
extremely preterm babies, 227–228
   counseling parents before birth of,
     237–238
   decisions regarding initiating
     resuscitation for, 268–269
   and situations in which it is ethical
     not to initiate resuscitation,
     269–270

F

face masks. See masks
feeding problems, 218
fetal heart rate, 28
fetal lungs, 4, 255–256
fetal monitoring, 3